Studying the Organisation and Delivery of Health Services

A Reader

How should health services be funded? How should they be organised? Who should receive health services? Who should deliver services?

Research into the delivery and organisation of health care is a vital component in responding to such questions and in the improvement of health services. The most appropriate method for such research is often not a quantitative approach or the randomised control trial, although these have their place; rather, a broad range of methods needs to be deployed, drawing on the expertise of different disciplines.

Studying the Organisation and Delivery of Health Services brings together thirty examples of high-quality research into service delivery and organisation using a range of methods and from a wide range of disciplines, including organisational studies, epidemiology, sociology, history, health economics, anthropology and policy studies. Expert editorial commentary highlights different themes and methodological issues.

This unique Reader covers six main areas of research:

- Organising services around the user
- User involvement in health care
- Workforce
- Evaluating models of service delivery
- Quality management and the management of change
- Studying health care organisations

This Reader is a companion volume to *Studying the Organisation and Delivery of Health Services: Research Methods* also published by Routledge (2001). It makes top-quality, empirical and secondary research readily accessible to health service managers and health care professionals who are interested in research, to health service researchers and to undergraduate and postgraduate students following courses in health and health management studies.

Aileen Clarke is a Reader in Health Services Research at Barts and the London School of Medicine and Dentistry, Queen Mary, University of London. **Naomi Fulop**, Senior Lecturer in Health Services Delivery and Organisational Research; **Pauline Allen**, Lecturer in Organisational Research; **Stuart Anderson**, Senior Lecturer in Organisational Behaviour and **Nick Black**, Professor of Health Services Research are all based at the London School of Hygiene and Tropical Medicine and are involved in the national co-ordinating centre supporting the NHS research and development programme in Service Delivery and Organisation (NCCSDO).

Studying the Organisation and Delivery of Health Services

A Reader

Edited by Aileen Clarke,
Pauline Allen, Stuart Anderson,
Nick Black and Naomi Fulop

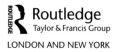

Routledge
Taylor & Francis Group

LONDON AND NEW YORK

First published 2004
by Routledge
2 Park Square, Milton Park, Abingdon, Oxfordshire OX14 4RN

Simultaneously published in the USA and Canada
by Taylor & Francis Inc
270 Madison Ave, New York, NY 10016

Routledge is an imprint of the Taylor & Francis Group

© 2004 Aileen Clarke, Pauline Allen, Stuart Anderson, Nick Black
and Naomi Fulop

Typeset in Times by Wearset Ltd, Boldon, Tyne and Wear
Printed and bound in Great Britain by The Cromwell Press,
Trowbridge, UK

All rights reserved. No part of this book may be reprinted or
reproduced or utilised in any form or by any electronic,
mechanical, or other means, now known or hereafter invented,
including photocopying and recording, or in any information
storage or retrieval system, without permission in writing from
the publishers.

Every effort has been made to ensure that the advice and
information in this book is true and accurate at the time of going
to press. However, neither the publisher nor the authors can
accept any legal responsibility or liability for any errors or
omissions that may be made. In the case of drug administration,
any medical procedure or the use of technical equipment
mentioned within this book, you are strongly advised to consult
the manufacturer's guidelines.

British Library Cataloguing in Publication Data
A catalogue record for this book is available from the British
Library

Library of Congress Cataloging in Publication Data
A catalogue record for this book has been requested

ISBN 0–415–34071–3 (hbk)
ISBN 0–415–34072–1 (pbk)

Contents

Notes on editors

Aileen Clarke worked as a GP in London before training in academic public health and health services research. She is currently a Reader at Barts and the London School of Medicine and Dentistry, Queen Mary University of London. Her research interests and publications focus on research at the individual patient level, for example, in appropriateness in health care, patient involvement in decision making, shared decision making, and the expert patient. She has also published research on performance measurement and management in health services and in women's health issues.

Pauline Allen is a lecturer in organisational research at the London School of Hygiene and a member of the National Co-ordinating Centre for NHS Service Delivery and Organisation R&D Programme. She is also qualified as a solicitor, although she no longer practises. Using economic and legal approaches, her research interests include contracts, looking at both formal and informal relationships; and professional and legal accountability. She is a co-author of the book by Fulop *et al.*, *Studying the Organisation and Delivery of Health Services*, published by Routledge in 2001.

Stuart Anderson is senior lecturer in organisational behaviour at the National Co-ordinating Centre for NHS Service Delivery and Organisation Research and Development, based in the Health Services Research Unit at the London School of Hygiene and Tropical Medicine. His principal research interests are in organisational studies in health care and in the development of organisational theory. His publications have included comparative studies of public and private provision of health care, performance measurement, and studies of the interface between primary and secondary care.

Nick Black is Professor of Health Services Research at the London School of Hygiene and Tropical Medicine. His main interests include quality improvement (particularly in surgery), the relationship between research and policy/practice, and the uses of high-quality clinical data-bases.

Naomi Fulop is Senior Lecturer in Service Delivery and Organisational Research and Director of the National Co-ordinating Centre for NHS Service Delivery and Organisation R&D Programme at the London School of Hygiene and Tropical Medicine. Her research interests are in the organisation and management of health care; implementation of health policies; relationships between organisations (mergers, integration, partnerships); and the relationship between research and policy.

Foreword

In the past decade, no Western nation on earth has taken on more seriously than the United Kingdom the difficult task of trying to improve its health care system as a whole. The mere formation of the National Health Service a half century ago was an act of vision and of deep commitment to serving an entire population with effective care and under promises of equity. But, inevitably, such a large system as the National Health Service must struggle constantly to maintain and improve its performance. The dedication of all stakeholders in the continual improvement of the National Health Service is a worthy and necessary endeavour.

I predict success, but, as in all matters affecting health care, chances of success are most enhanced by the linkage of sound and energetic leadership actions to sound and disciplined science. Among the many sciences that any health care system must harness in the effort to improve are the sciences of organisation and delivery of health care: 'health services research'.

This Reader offers a superb collection of research papers, produced by the team running the NHS Service Development and Organisation research programme in England, which can serve as a scientific guide to change agents, clinicians and managerial leaders who want to improve the care system. It is a companion volume to this group's previous popular publication: *Studying the Organisation and Delivery of Health Services: Research Methods*.

The authors have accumulated a huge variety of research papers in this Reader, involving inquiries into service delivery and organisation, and crossing many research disciplines, including history, anthropology, epidemiology and statistics. They have included both classic texts and important lesser known research that richly deserves a higher profile.

The Service Development and Organisation team is well known for its commitment to including those who actually work in health care – health care managers and professionals, as well as users of health services – in every aspect of their work. This book reflects that commitment and therefore has a strongly practical flavour. Whether you are a manager, professional, health care worker or academic, I would urge you to read this book. It will provide all of us with a deeper intellectual foundation for pursuing the important work of change and improvement in health care delivery and organisation.

Donald M. Berwick MD MPP
President and CEO
Institute for Healthcare Improvement
Clinical Professor of Pediatrics and Health Care Policy
Harvard Medical School

Acknowledgements

The editors would like to thank Don Berwick for kindly agreeing to write the foreword to this book, and Barbara Langbridge, Lydia Mounter, Olivette Stanislas and Claire Anderson for all their administrative help with the book.

The editors and publishers wish to thank the following for permission to use copyright material:

Administrative Science Quarterly
Blackwell Publishing
British Journal of Cancer
British Medical Journal
British Psychological Society
Elsevier
Journal of Nursing Scholarship
King's Fund
Lancet
Nature Publishing Group
New England Journal of Medicine
Oxford University Press
Lippincott, Williams & Wilkins
Palgrave Macmillan
Royal College of Nursing
Royal Society of Medicine Press
Sage Publications Ltd
Taylor and Francis

In many cases the authors of the articles contained in this Reader provided useful feedback to their editing and we thank them and the publishers for their co-operation.

Three of us (Pauline Allen, Stuart Anderson and Naomi Fulop) are funded by the NHS Service Delivery and Organisation R&D Programme. The programme also funded the administrative support provided to produce this book.

Introduction

There are many tensions within health services. Payers and the public are seeking improved assessment, accountability, governance and value for money (Relman 1988). Alongside these expectations there is a growing awareness of the importance of the role of the individual consumer or user of health care, and of the need for a more patient-centred and holistic approach to health care (Coulter 2002). In publicly funded health care systems, waiting lists still persist (Lingard *et al.* 2000). In countries with insurance-based systems there are still millions of uninsured and under-insured people, and managed care systems have faced severe problems (Light 2003). In the UK over the past few years, the NHS has been reorganised, and a massive programme of change has been undertaken at all levels with a major injection of new funding (Hunter 2003). There is renewed interest in health and health policy, particularly in issues relating to the workforce.

For all countries, questions such as: 'Do we need a particular service or type of health care? How should services be funded? How should services be organised? Who should receive health services? Who should deliver services?' are as pertinent now as they have ever been (Black 1997). The UK, along with many other industrialised countries, has responded to the need to answer these questions with a government-funded programme of health service delivery and organisation (SDO) research. The programme began in 1999 and is managed by a National Co-ordinating Centre based at the London School of Hygiene and Tropical Medicine.

In the light of this awareness of the importance of SDO research, the academic staff of the National Co-ordinating Centre published a book, *Studying the Organisation and Delivery of Health Services: Research Methods* in 2001 (Fulop *et al.* 2001). This described and critically considered a range of different methods for studying health services. We have now selected a range of published papers and extracts from books to produce *Studying the Organisation and Delivery of Health Services: A Reader* as a companion volume.

Until recently, research into health services has focused on health technology assessment, with its emphasis on randomised controlled trials and systematic reviews. In this Reader we have aimed to celebrate the contribution of a much wider range of methods, methodologies, disciplines and approaches. The book features 30 examples of research on how health services are organised and delivered. It is not representative of the research that has been undertaken over the last three decades; rather, it includes some classic examples of SDO research as well as some more recent real life examples selected from peer-reviewed publications or books. We have aimed to illustrate both qualitative and quantitative approaches, and primary and secondary research.

A wide range of disciplines is represented including psychology, epidemiology, sociology, history, economics, anthropology and policy studies. A range of levels of organisation of health care is also reflected within our selections. Extracts are included which relate to research at the macro or system level, meso or organisation level and micro or individual patient level. Lastly, the research reflects the work of a range of practitioners including doctors, nurses and pharmacists. However, while the Reader reflects a wide range of disciplines used in SDO research, the selection inevitably provides only a limited illustration of the depth and breadth of the work that has been conducted.

Each extract has been edited to approximately 3000 words, while reflecting the original as faithfully as possible. In each case the original version is referenced at the end of the abstract. The book is organised in six parts, around six themes. The themes were largely derived from a national 'listening exercise' in which the research needs of patients, clinicians, managers and policy makers were identified through a series of focus groups (Lomas *et al.* 2003). They reflect the themes which the NHS Service Delivery and Organisation (SDO) R&D Programme currently uses to commission its work. Each part has an introduction, which highlights the ways in which articles illustrate key methodological approaches and research issues.

We have included two parts concerned with the theme of patient- and carer-centred services: one focuses on organising services around users, largely from a health professional's perspective; the other considers user involvement in the planning and organisation of services. To some extent this is a rather artificial distinction, but one that we think is helpful in exploring the issues involved.

The six themes are:

- **Patient- and carer-centred services: organising services around the user.** Extracts from papers in this part include research on models of the chronic disease experience, continuity of care, patient satisfaction, measures of appropriateness and integrated care pathways.
- **Patient- and carer-centred services: user involvement in organising**

services. Extracts in this part include one that describes patients' view of care across the primary/secondary interface; and another that shows the range of attitudes to trade-offs between quality and quantity of life in the context of chemotherapy.

- **Workforce issues.** This part includes one paper that describes research into the roles of nurse practitioners in primary care, and a historical study of nursing recruitment and retention problems in London in the late 1890s, which shows that health care workforce problems are far from new!
- *Evaluating models of health service delivery.* This part includes a paper where a helicopter emergency medical service is evaluated, another where intensive care discharges at night are examined, and two papers that discuss stroke care from very different methodological viewpoints.
- **Change management and quality improvement.** This part includes a paper reporting an investigation of optimum and not-so-optimum contexts for change, and research into the roles of managers and the uptake of evidence.
- **Studying health care organisations.** Papers in this part include one describing collaboration between health and social care services, one involving the identification of organisational facilitators, and a classic randomised trial of alternative health insurance policies in the United States.

Our aim is to demonstrate the wealth of good quality research that has been conducted and to facilitate its availability to managers, health care professionals, health services researchers, research funders, and undergraduate and postgraduate students. We hope that this collection, *Studying the Organisation and Delivery of Health Services: A Reader*, will complement the earlier *Studying the Organisation and Delivery of Health Services: Research Methods* (Fulop *et al.* 2001), by illustrating the use of the variety of methods and methodologies described in that first volume. We hope that you enjoy the range, variety, richness and multi-disciplinarity of the research presented here as much as we do.

Aileen Clarke: Reader in Health Services Research
Pauline Allen: Lecturer in Organisational Research
Stuart Anderson: Senior Lecturer in Organisational Behaviour
Naomi Fulop: Senior Lecturer in Service Delivery and Organisation
Nick Black: Professor of Health Services Research

References

Black, N. (1997) 'Health services research: saviour or chimera?', *Lancet*, 349: 1834–6.

Coulter, A. (2002) *The Autonomous Patient*, London: Nuffield Trust.

Fulop, N., Allen, P., Clarke, A. and Black, N. (2001) *Studying the Organisation and Delivery of Health Services: Research Methods*, London: Routledge.

Hunter, D.J. (2003) 'The Wanless report and public health', *British Medical Journal*, 327: 573–4.

Light, D. (2003) 'Universal health care: lessons from the British experience', *American Journal of Public Health*, 93: 25–30.

Lingard, E.A., Berven, S., Katz, J.N.; Kinemax Outcomes Group. (2000) 'Management and care of patients undergoing total knee arthroplasty: variations across different health care settings', *Arthritis Care Research*, 13: 129–36.

Lomas, J., Fulop, N., Gagnon, D. and Allen, P. (2003) 'On being a good listener: setting priorities for applied health services research', *Milbank Quarterly*, 1: 363–88.

Relman, A.S. (1988) 'Assessment and accountability: the third revolution in medical care', *New England Journal of Medicine*, 319: 1220–2.

Part 1

Patient- and Carer-Centred Services: organising services around the user

Introduction

The need to organise health services around users, rather than arranging them for the convenience of providers, has been a theme of much health policy in recent years. There is now a diverse literature around how this might be achieved. Part 1 contains five examples illustrating this diversity.

The first paper considers whether health professionals give patients the information they want, or the information that health professionals think they need. 'Advice provided in British community pharmacies: what people want and what they get' by Hassell and colleagues explores advice-giving behaviour in community pharmacies with a view to understanding the nature and process of pharmaceutical consultations and consumers' views of the advice-giving role. It uses ethnographic methods, combining patient interviews with non-participant observation of interactions between consumers and pharmacy staff. It demonstrates that advice-giving in community pharmacies almost wholly focuses on product recommendation and use, and that this advice-giving varies according to whether consultations concern prescription or non-prescription medicines.

The second paper considers whether patients get the treatment they need, or the treatment that health professionals feel most comfortable with. 'Underuse of coronary revascularisation procedures in patients considered appropriate candidates for revascularisation', by Hemingway and others, compares the clinical outcomes of patients treated medically after angiography with those of patients who underwent revascularisation, within groups defined by ratings of the degree of appropriateness of revascularisation by an expert panel. This was a prospective study of 2552 consecutive patients undergoing coronary angiography at three London hospitals. On the basis of the ratings of an expert panel, the authors identified substantial underuse of coronary revascularisation among patients considered appropriate candidates for these procedures. Furthermore, underuse was associated with adverse clinical outcomes.

Our third paper in this section examines integrated care pathways as one mechanism for organising services around the user. In 'Integrated care pathways in stroke management' Sulch and Kalra demonstrate that an organised, goal-defined and time-specified plan of management as envisaged by the integrated care pathway approach can achieve quality outcomes at lower cost. Integrated care pathways have applications to stroke management because diagnosis is well defined, complex interdisciplinary inputs are required and there is good evidence on best practice. The authors reviewed medical, nursing, rehabilitation and health services databases to identify studies on integrated care pathways in stroke management. Of six non-randomised studies of acute stroke, five demonstrated reduced hospital stay and a reduction in costs of care. Two studies reported improved uptake of medical interventions. They concluded that integrated care pathway methodology may facilitate quality and cost improvements in stroke care, but that the evidence for this is still weak.

Our fourth paper presents a novel approach to identifying the extent to which the views of patients with chronic illnesses about their needs vary over time. 'The Shifting Perspectives Model of Chronic Illness' by Paterson is derived from a meta-synthesis of qualitative research about the reported experiences of adults with a chronic illness. The 292 primary research studies examined included a variety of interpretive research methods and were conducted by researchers from many countries and disciplines. The Shifting Perspectives Model indicates that living with chronic illness is an ongoing and continually shifting process in which an illness-in-the-foreground or wellness-in-the-foreground perspective has specific functions in the person's world. The model helps users to provide an explanation of chronically ill persons' variations in their attention to symptoms over time, sometimes in ways that seem ill-advised or even harmful to their health. It also indicates direction to health professionals about supporting people with chronic illness.

The final paper in this section considers the extent to which patient satisfaction with consultations in general practice is linked to the achievement of satisfactory continuity of care. In 'Continuity of care in general practice: effect on patient satisfaction' Hjortdahl and Lærum asked 3918 Norwegian primary care patients to rate their overall satisfaction with consultations on a six-point scale. Continuity of care was recorded as the duration and intensity of the present patient–doctor relationship, and as patients' perceptions of the present doctor being their personal doctor. An overall personal patient–doctor relationship increased the odds of the patient being satisfied with the consultation sevenfold as compared with consultations where no such relationships existed. The duration of the patient–doctor relationship had a weak link with patient satisfaction, while the intensity of contacts showed no such association. The authors concluded that personal, continuous care is linked with patient satisfaction. If patient satisfaction is accepted as an integral part of quality health care, reinforcing personal care may be one way of increasing this quality.

Organising services around the user can thus take many forms, and needs to be applied in every setting where health services are delivered. But, as this chapter shows all too clearly, simply organising services around the user does not necessarily guarantee improved patient outcomes.

Chapter 1

Advice provided in British community pharmacies: what people want and what they get

Karen Hassell, Peter Noyce, Anne Rogers, Jennifer Harris and Jane Wilkinson

Abstract

This study explored advice-giving behaviour in community pharmacies, in order to understand the nature and process of pharmaceutical consultations and consumers' views of the advice-giving role. It used an ethnographic research strategy, combining patient interviews with non-participant observation of interactions between consumers and pharmacy staff. It demonstrated that advice given in community pharmacies is almost wholly focused on product recommendation and use, but that advice-giving varied according to whether consultations concerned prescription or non-prescription medicines.

Introduction

Community pharmacies (retail chemists) operate across the interface between informal and formal primary care provided in the UK by the National Health Service. With free medical consultations and 85 per cent of patients exempt from paying prescription charges, relief from minor ailments is frequently sought from general practitioners (GPs). The British government is keen to transform this situation by making community pharmacies the first port of call for minor ailments, thus reducing GP workload and prescribing costs. Within the UK, community pharmacies dispense both medicines prescribed by GPs and those available over-the-counter, known as non-prescription medicines.

Surveys of advice provided in community pharmacies on common ailments and medicines have challenged its quality (Consumers Association 1994) and led to recommendations that further deregulation of drugs

Source: *Journal of Health Services Research and Policy*, 3.4, 1998, 219–25.

should be halted until a demonstrable improvement has occurred. While many studies have concentrated on quantifying pharmaceutical consultations and advice-giving (Smith 1992; Savage 1995) there is a paucity of work on the nature of the advice sought and provided (Tully *et al.* 1997). They have also concentrated on consultations involving the pharmacist, largely neglecting the part played by pharmacy assistants and technicians. The former tend mostly to deal with customers' general enquiries, while the main function of technicians is the dispensing of prescribed medicines. This paper uses observational data to inform the debate about the nature of pharmacy advice-giving and its content.

Methods

All pharmacies in the North West region of England were contacted to take part in the study. Maximum variation sampling (Yin 1994) was employed in the selection from among those who accepted the invitation to participate, to explore whether differences in advice-giving were affected by the type of pharmacy and the type of community in which it was located. Observations took place in ten different pharmacies. Their characteristics are shown in Table 1.1.

During the field work, staff and client interactions were observed by one researcher during the course of one week (usually six consecutive days) in each of the ten pharmacies. All interactions that involved the selling or dispensing of medicines and more general health advice were recorded verbatim using shorthand. Notes were later transcribed in full.

Based on the principles of grounded theory, two researchers examined and coded the observational data according to themes of interest to the study. The interaction episodes were coded according to whether advice had been given or not, who gave it, and whether the interaction was concerned with prescriptions, non-prescription medicines, or other general health issues. We defined 'advice' as any interaction in which someone requested or was offered guidance by any member of the pharmacy's staff in overcoming a health problem. This allowed us to look at advice in its widest context and to develop a typology grounded in the data. Data that involved advice were systematically scrutinised to determine the precise nature of the advice and the form it took. In developing the advice categories, one researcher first analysed data from two of the pharmacies. To establish the validity of the categories they were discussed and clarified with another researcher and a pharmacist. Data from the remaining eight pharmacies were then analysed. Any new categories that evolved were validated in the same way.

To improve the accuracy of the description of the behaviour that takes place in community pharmacies, several 'ideal-type' categories were developed from an analysis of all recorded advice-giving episodes. An

Table 1.1 Characteristics of pharmacy sample

Location	Type*	Pharmacist characteristics			Pharmacy setting	Per cent turnover that is NHS	Number of prescriptions dispensed per month	Pharmacy staff: type and number working full-time (ft) or part-time (pt)
1. City	Independent	White, male	Manager, aged 34 years	Qualified 10 years	Located on edge of town, on side street; high unemployment	80%	8000	6 pt pharmacy assistants (PA), 2 ft PAs
2. Rural	Small chain	White, male	Manager, aged 47 years	Qualified 24 years	Small village, affluent area	50%	1000	3 pt, 1 ft PA
3. Rural		White, female	Owner, aged 59 years	Qualified 35 years	Small village, affluent area, close to health centre	60%	2000	3 pt PA, 1 ft technician
4. Small town	Medium chain	White, male	Manager, aged 36 years	Qualified 14 years	Located in busy shopping arcade; high unemployment	50%	2200	6 pt PAs
5. Small town	Independent	White, male	Owner, aged 40 years	Qualified 18 years	Located on high street, next to GP practice	65%	4000	6 pt PAs, 1 technician
6. Large town	Small chain	White, male	Owner, aged 45 years	Qualified 18 years	Located in pedestrianised shopping precinct	70%	4000	6 pt PA, 2 locum pharmacists
7. Large town	Independent	Asian, male	Owner, aged 31 years	Qualified 10 years	One of a parade of shops, just outside city centre	65%	2500	4 pt PAs, 2 ft PAs, 1 technician, 1 driver
8. City	Chain	1 white and 1 Afro-Carribean female	Managers, 24 and 32 years	Qualified 12 and 9 years	Area of high unemployment, shop highly fortified, next to health centre	90%	6000	2 job-share pharmacists, 3 pt PAs
9. Suburb	Independent	White, male	Owner, aged 42 years	Qualified 18 years	Located inside health centre	95%	n/a	4 pt PAs, 1 ft PA, 2 technicians, 1 other pharmacist
10. Suburb	Large chain	Vietnamese female	Manager, aged 46 years	Qualified 10 years	Located in pedestrianised shopping precinct	30%	5000	1 pharmacy dispenser, 4 pt PAs, 2 ft PAs, 1 locum pharmacist

*Type: independent = 1; small chain = 5 stores or less; medium chain 6–100 stores; large chain = more than 100 stores.

interaction episode could not always be easily categorised into one discrete type, as the co-existence of more than one type of advice in one episode was common and episodes often evolved from a seemingly straightforward product demand. This indicates the often complex nature of advice in pharmacies.

In addition, an opportunistic sample of over 1000 customers was interviewed inside the pharmacies about the purpose of their visit and their use of the pharmacy. A poster was displayed in the window of each pharmacy to inform customers of the study. These interviews provided a general, quantitative view of the nature of pharmacy use. Telephone interviews with 44 customers who had been observed receiving advice, aimed at exploring the circumstances and expectations of their visits and views about the advice they had received, were also conducted. Pharmacies were located across a large geographical area, so face-to-face interviews with customers were not possible.

Results

Advice-giving episodes in community pharmacies

Sixty per cent of observed episodes were related to prescriptions (Table 1.2). Response to symptoms and general health questions each constituted 5 per cent, and non-prescription requests 29 per cent. Typically, the latter involved customers asking for information on travel precautions and smoking cessation, and included users of diagnostic services, such as

Table 1.2 Observed episodes and proportions of key activities, by pharmacy

Pharmacy	Total number of observed interactions	Prescriptions (%)	Product demands (%)	Symptom presentation (%)	General health (%)	Proportion of non-treatment episodes that were referred
P1	242	86	8	3	2	12
P2	192	61	33	2	5	5
P3	104	46	47	7	0	2
P4	283	21	64	7	8	2
P5	247	64	27	5	4	8
P6	172	41	37	6	16*	5
P7	220	49	38	10	3	12
P8	234	76	5	0	19*	2
P9	453	81	11	3	5	11
P10	232	48	41	8	3	9
Overall	2379	60	29	5	5	6

*The high figure is due to the high number of methadone and needle-exchange clients using the pharmacy.

pregnancy testing. The proportion of general health issues varied considerably between pharmacies, especially the level of service to drug misusers.

In spite of professional encouragement for pharmacists to undertake a health promotion role, there was little evidence of the provision of general advice about health and illness that was independent of the function of selling or dispensing medicines. Advice about how to stop smoking, for example, almost always centred on the non-prescription products available to facilitate this, rather than on other lifestyle changes that might accompany smoking cessation. This is not to suggest that pharmacy staff *always* sold a medicine, since there were interactions that did not result in a sale, but merely to highlight the nature of most advice as product-related.

Categories of 'advice'

We characterised the type of advice given by pharmacy staff into five main categories which help to clarify what advice means in a pharmacy context. The undifferentiated and vague term 'counselling' is often applied. Instead, the description here serves to illustrate more precisely the nature of the advice most often given or requested. In practice, it took the form of:

(a) **Product recommendation.** Example: 'Cupanol is best. It's probably a cold. Plenty of rest and give this just to bring the fever down, and plenty to drink.'

(b) **Reassurance.** Example. *Customer.* 'I want a pack of Strepsils. I'm on chemotherapy and can't take some products. I've got a bit of a sore throat this morning – will these be alright?' *Pharmacist.* 'Yes. They'll be fine.'

(c) **Instruction.** Example: 'With this you use the pessary inside and the cream outside.'

(d) **Information.** Example: 'Paracetamol will only help with the pain – not the cramp. You can take them (Buscopan and paracetamol) together'.

(e) **Referral.** Example. 'If you find you need to use them quite a bit, go to your doctor.'

Staff frequently offered unsolicited *instruction* about medication use (e.g. how much to take and when), mostly in relation to prescription medicines. In responding to symptoms, they mostly recommended which medicine to use or they *referred* a customer to another health care professional. In some circumstances they also provided *reassurance* (e.g. confirming a client's suspicion that a symptom warranted a visit to a GP). They also offered *information*. This was seen by the researchers as distinct from instruction because it involved, not the provision of guidance about how to use something, but the provision of product or professional knowledge.

The extension of 'instruction' to include 'explanation' (e.g. *why* it is necessary to take medicines with food?) was notable by its absence.

Many advice episodes also included some form of **checking (f)**. This was when pharmacy staff gathered information (such as the presence of pre-existing conditions) which enabled them to offer suitable advice (e.g. are you taking any other medication?). Although not strictly advice, *checking* was nevertheless an integral part of the advisory process.

The term 'advice' did not resonate with customers. Despite the short time between observation of the episode and the interview (two to three days), respondents often had to be reminded in some detail about the particular episode we were interested in before the interview could proceed. It may be that their visit to the pharmacy was not important enough for them to have remembered the details. However, other material from the interviews suggests that they perceive the pharmacist more in terms of their helpfulness than their clinical competence.

Advice with prescription medicines

When advice took place in interactions that involved the dispensing of prescription products, it was almost wholly characterised as instruction **(c)**; for example, directions about dosage and when to take the medicine. Occasionally advice with prescriptions also came in the form of 'information' **(d)**. The nature of most of these encounters was brief and directive. The following was typical of the exchange which took place with the handing over of prescription medicines:

> Pharmacist: Take it four times a day on an empty stomach **(c)**.
> Customer: No drinking eh?
> Pharmacist: No.
> Customer: That's OK.

The vast majority of such interactions were truncated in nature and concerned 'checking' **(f)** whether the customer knew what to do, or instructing them how to use the medicine. Many of the prescription interactions also included advice on 'finishing the course':

> Pharmacy assistant: That's a full course of antibiotics, so make sure you finish all of them, even if you're feeling better. There you go.
> Customer: Thanks, bye.

Advice with non-prescription medicines

Interactions were usually longer, more varied, and slightly more detailed than those involving prescription medicines, suggesting that pharmacy staff have a greater role, and clients more autonomy, in decisions about non-prescription medicines. When advice accompanied their provision, whether in response to the presentation of symptoms or as a result of a named product enquiry, it usually involved product recommendation **(a)**, although it occasionally included instruction **(c)**, referral **(e)**, and checking **(f)** often occurred as well.

Compared with the sale of products which, in the UK can also be bought from non-pharmacy outlets, the advice proffered when selling products restricted to pharmacies was primarily concerned with potential interactions with other products:

> Pharmacy assistant: It may cause drowsiness **(d)**. Are you on any
> other medications? **(f)**.
> Customer: No.

Official guidance from professional bodies recommends this emphasis (RPSGB 1996), such that protocols to guide pharmacy staff on appropriate questions to ask customers are now required in all pharmacies. It is likely that the rules shape the nature of many interactions over deregulated products. However, the question, following quickly after a piece of information, does not give the impression of active interest in the client's health. It appears more as a way of following rules, and suggests that adherence to protocols takes precedence over unsolicited requests for advice or giving other information. While occasionally the pharmacist referred the customer to a doctor, often without the sale of a product, there was very little evidence to suggest that pharmacy staff recommended self-care or other therapies as alternatives.

Role of customers in the encounter

Requests for non-prescription medicines were initiated by customers in one of two ways. Either they simply demanded a particular product, or they presented a condition to pharmacy staff, who responded by recommending a suitable course of action. This was usually the use of a product **(a)**, but occasionally took the form of a referral **(e)** to the GP. Other customers presented with symptoms. They often sought a product recommendation, but occasionally sought reassurance. This was sometimes about the action they intended to take, that their medication was correct, that they were taking it correctly, and that it would do no harm. Such customers asked 'is it any good?'. They seemed concerned with the effectiveness of the medication, perhaps reflecting their scepticism about the claims made in advertisements for some products.

The majority of non-life-threatening conditions fell into this category and the pharmacist's intention frequently seemed to be to sell a product that might alleviate an annoying symptom and not cause any harm. Occasionally they referred customers to their GP: 6 per cent of all non-prescription interactions involved advice to see a GP, either immediately or if their condition showed no improvement.

Product demands rather than 'response to symptoms' formed the basis of the majority of non-prescription consultations. A large proportion of the public know what they want to purchase before they reach the pharmacy, and effectively purchase the remedy in the same way as any other commodity. The pharmacy non-prescription service is very much consumer-led. As the vast majority of adults who report minor ailments have experienced the ailments before (BMRB 1987), consumers are likely to have previous experience of the product they want for their condition. They may not want to be questioned about their choice of product. In this study, these customers provided little opportunity for pharmacy staff to engage in any dialogue about the appropriateness of the product. When staff did attempt to check the suitability of the desired purchase they were occasionally met with hostility.

This creates a dilemma for pharmacy staff. Questioning everyone, they risk losing customers to other suppliers; questioning no one, they risk criticism for not checking the appropriateness of customers' purchases. Nevertheless, autonomy and being in control might be important to people who take a major role in the management of their own ailments. Conflict can arise from a mismatch between the professional ideal of what they believe their service should be about and customers' views about what they want from the service. This highlights the dangers inherent in ignoring needs identified by customers.

Discussion

Ethnography is unusual in pharmacy practice research. The advantage is that it moves away from the potentially self-serving accounts generated through self-reports of behaviour. Although the observer pursued a non-participatory and unobtrusive strategy, customers and staff were aware of her presence because of the need for staff agreement and the publicity given to the study in the pharmacy. Those under observation may have altered their usual behaviour. To minimise this source of bias, the research involved a much longer period of study in each pharmacy, comprising several periods of prolonged observation. Another limitation relates to the selection of pharmacies and consumers. Neither sampling method was random: the findings are not representative of all pharmacies or all consumers. However, since the study sought to provide insights into the process and nature of advice-giving, this was not a serious limitation.

This study illustrates the variety of forms that advice can take in a community pharmacy, and highlights the fact that the application of the term 'counselling' is a misleading way to characterise what takes place between pharmacists and their customers. Advice-giving, despite variation between pharmacies, is almost wholly focused on product recommendation and product use, with little general health advice. Overall, advice is characterised by its didactic nature, the emphasis being on checking, instruction and information, at the expense of explanation. There was little evidence to suggest that pharmacy staff engage customers in any in-depth dialogue about their health and medicine needs.

Pharmacy staff are aware of the potential danger of medicines and their prime concern is safety. The emphasis they place on checking whether the consumer is on any other medication is not surprising. However, consumers appear to be interested in the effectiveness of products. Up to now the development and mandatory implementation of protocols in pharmacies, meant to aid the process of advice-giving, has not been informed by research with actual customers (Weiss and Cantrill 1997). If their future development were to reflect such a perspective, their continued use might better facilitate interactions between practitioners and service users.

The study also revealed the extent to which the service is consumer-led. Pharmacy staff mostly respond to customer requests for named products. Criticism that pharmacists should take a more proactive role and give unsolicited advice needs to be set within this context. Consumers are increasingly encouraged to take responsibility for their own self-care. Many people using pharmacies for minor ailments view themselves as the managers of their ailment and use community pharmacies as one of several resources available. The *want* of customers for pharmacist intervention may not be great. The *need* for questions by pharmacy staff, in view of the possibility of misdiagnosis by the consumer, or risk of contraindications, may nevertheless be important.

While criticisms are predicated on the assumption that every medicine sale necessitates an intervention from pharmacy staff, in practice most pharmacy customers may be no different to patients in receipt of repeat prescriptions. Repeats account for over 80 per cent of all prescription items and nearly half of all patients receive one; contact and intervention from a GP is limited (Harris and Dajda 1996). While the pharmacy profession's defensive response to criticism is understandable, their response should be to argue – based on evidence of consumer use of pharmacies – that the scope for giving new advice about medicines and minor health problems may in reality be limited.

While customers shape the nature of the interactions they have with pharmacy staff, it is also shaped by the role and discretion pharmacists exercise over their own and their staffs' activities. With prescription medicines, pharmacy staff characteristically reinforce the prescriber's intentions. In the more open and negotiated encounters about non-prescription medicines, pharmacy staff have far more discretion and influence over the nature and outcome of the interaction, albeit still limited in scope and heavily influenced by the customer.

The finding that the term 'advice' does not resonate with many customers may be important. 'Helpfulness' appears to be what customers understand by 'advice'. While pharmacists may identify their professional role as health advisors, this notion may not be shared by the public. Although a quarter of all non-prescription medicine customers present to pharmacy staff with symptoms of minor illness, the major activity is still response to product demands. Pharmacies' function in primary care may thus be viewed more as mediator between formal services and lay users, and as resource which people can access on their own terms. The flexibility and user-friendliness of the service is valued highly. Together with the non-threatening manner in which the service is delivered, these are strengths the profession should build on.

References

BMRB (1987) *Everyday Health Care. A Consumer Study of Self-medication in Great Britain*, London: British Market Research Bureau.

Consumers' Association (1994) 'Vital checks are still not being made', *Which? Way to Health*, December: 196.

Harris, C.M. and Dajda, R. (1996) 'The scale of repeat prescribing', *British Journal of General Practice*, 46: 649–53.

RPSGB (1996) 'Council of the RPSGB has adopted standards for the sale of NPM', *Pharmaceutical Journal*, 257: 518.

Savage, I. (1995) 'Time for customer contact in pharmacies with and without a dispensing technician', *International Journal of Pharmacy Practice*, 3: 193–9.

Smith, F.J. (1992) 'A study of the advisory and health promotion activity of community pharmacists', *Health Education Journal*, 51: 68–71.

Tully, M., Hassell, K. and Noyce, P. (1997) 'Advice-giving in community pharmacies in the UK', *Journal of Health Services Research and Policy*, 2: 38–50.

Weiss, M.C. and Cantrill, J.A. (1997) 'From protocol to guideline?', *Pharmaceutical Journal*, 258: 834.

Yin, R.K. (1994) *Case Study Research: Design and Methods*, 2nd edn. London: Sage.

This article can be found complete, and unedited as 'Advice provided in British Community pharmacies: what people want and what they get' in the *Journal of Health Services Research and Policy*, Volume 3, Number 4, October 1998, pages 219–25. The authors are Hassell, K., Noyce, P., Rogers, A., Harris, J. and Wilkinson, J.

Chapter 2

Underuse of coronary revascularisation procedures in patients considered appropriate candidates for revascularisation

*Harry Hemingway, Angela M. Crook, Gene Feder,
Shrilla Banerjee, J. Rex Dawson, Patrick Magee,
Sue Philpott, Julie Sanders, Alan Wood and
Adam D. Timmis*

Abstract

Background: We compared the clinical outcomes of patients treated medically after angiography with those of patients who underwent revascularisation, within groups defined by ratings of the degree of appropriateness of revascularisation by an expert panel.

Methods: Prospective study of consecutive patients undergoing coronary angiography at three London hospitals. Before patients were recruited, a nine-member expert panel rated the appropriateness of percutaneous transluminal coronary angioplasty (PTCA) and coronary-artery bypass grafting (CABG) on a nine-point scale (1 denoted highly inappropriate, 9 highly appropriate). Ratings were then applied to a population of patients with coronary artery disease. Patients were treated without regard to ratings. A total of 2552 patients were followed for a median of 30 months after angiography.

Results: Of 908 patients with indications for which PTCA was rated appropriate, the 34 per cent who were treated medically were more likely to have angina at follow-up than those who underwent PTCA (odds ratio, 1.97; 95 per cent confidence interval, 1.29 to 3.00). Of 1353 patients with indications for which CABG was considered appropriate the 26 per cent who were treated medically were more likely than those who underwent CABG to die or have a nonfatal myocardial infarction (hazard ratio, 4.08; 95 per cent confidence interval, 2.82 to 5.93) and to have angina (odds ratio, 3.03; 95 per cent confidence interval, 2.08 to 4.42). There was a graded relation between rating and outcome over the entire scale of appropriateness (p for linear trend $= 0.002$).

Source: *New England Journal of Medicine*, 344.9, 2001, 645–54.

Conclusions: On the basis of the ratings of the expert panel, we identified substantial underuse of coronary revascularisation among patients considered appropriate candidates for these procedures. Underuse was associated with adverse clinical outcomes.

Background

Deciding which patients should undergo coronary revascularisation remains a key challenge in the management of coronary artery disease, with practice patterns varying widely (Selby *et al.* 1996). Well-designed expert panels can closely reflect the views of practising physicians (Ayanian *et al.* 1998), and methods for detecting the underuse of revascularisation are highly reproducible (Shekelle *et al.* 1998).

However, a central aspect of the validity of the appropriateness rating method remains untested (Winslow *et al.* 1988; Gray *et al.* 1990; Hilborne *et al.* 1993; Leape *et al.* 1993). If expert panels' judgements have clinical validity, patients who are treated according to their ratings should have better clinical outcomes than those who are not. In all, 22–41 per cent of patients for whom intervention was deemed not only appropriate by expert panels but also necessary, do not undergo the procedure (Kravitz *et al.* 1995, 1997; Kravitz and Laouri 1997; Laouri *et al.* 1997; Carlisle *et al.* 1999; Leape *et al.* 1999). A previous study of clinical outcomes found retrospectively that, among patients for whom revascularisation was deemed necessary, the rate of survival was higher and there was less chest pain among those who underwent revascularisation than among those who were treated medically (Kravitz *et al.* 1995).

We undertook a prospective study of clinical outcomes, the Appropriateness of Coronary Revascularization (ACRE) study. Prior judgements about the appropriateness of indications for revascularisation, determined by an expert panel, were applied to a population-based cohort of patients with coronary artery disease. The primary hypothesis was that patients classified as appropriate candidates for revascularisation, but who did not undergo the procedure, would have worse outcomes than those who did undergo it, independent of other clinical characteristics.

Methods

Appropriateness ratings

The ACRE appropriateness ratings for PTCA and CABG were determined in 1995, before the patients were recruited (Hemingway *et al.* 1999). Using the RAND–UCLA Delphi method, a nine-member expert panel rated 984 mutually exclusive indications for CABG and 995 indications for

PTCA. Specific indications were grouped into broad clinical presentations (Table 2.1) and categorised according to severity of symptoms and investigation results, including the degree of risk posed by surgery (defined according to the method of Parsonnet *et al.* (1989)), and current medication. Panellists rated the appropriateness of each procedure separately for each clinical presentation, and the median of their scores was obtained.

Median scores ranged from 1 to 9, with 1–3 considered inappropriate, 4–6 appropriateness uncertain, and 7–9 appropriate. Revascularisation was deemed inappropriate when risks were judged to exceed benefits, of uncertain appropriateness when benefits and risks were judged equal, and appropriate when benefits exceeded risks by a sufficient margin to make the procedure worth performing (Table 2.1).

Study population

A total of 3800 patients scheduled to undergo coronary angiography would be required to allow us to detect an increase of at least 60 per cent (hazard ratio ≥ 1.60) in the risk of the primary outcome (death from any cause or non-fatal myocardial infarction) among patients who had indications for which CABG was deemed appropriate but who did not undergo CABG, as compared with those who appropriately underwent CABG (90 per cent power, two-sided $P = 0.05$). Patients were eligible for inclusion in the study if they were to undergo elective or emergency coronary angiography at any of three neighbouring teaching hospitals in the City of London and the East End in 1996–1997, and if they lived within the contiguous catchment areas of the five health authorities covering the City of London, East London and Essex: 4121 eligible patients were identified (Hemingway *et al.* 2000).

Data from clinical records

Eligible patients were identified on the day of their index coronary angiography. Data were abstracted from notes by trained nurses using standardised recording forms. Details were obtained on clinical presentation (as defined by RAND), Canadian Cardiovascular Society (CCS) classification of the functional severity of angina (ranging from class I, denoting mild angina, to class IV, denoting severe angina), current medications, presence or absence of diabetes, results on exercise electrocardiography (ECG) (Campeau *et al.* 1976; Bernstein *et al.* 1992) co-existing conditions, and the physician's intended treatment plan.

Angiographic data

Angiographic findings were obtained from the case notes and were coded by a trained coder who was unaware of the clinical details. Severity of

Table 2.1 Examples of frequent indications for PTCA and CABG*

Clinical presentation	Variables used to define indications — Symptoms, therapy and ECG results	Level of operative risk	Ejection fraction (%)	No. of diseased vessels	Appropriateness category (score) — PTCA	CABG
Chronic stable angina, CCS class I or II	Submaximal medical therapy, very positive exercise ECG	Moderate	>35	1 without proximal left anterior descending artery	Uncertain (4)	Inappropriate (3)
	Any	Any	>15	3 with left main coronary artery	Inappropriate (1)	Appropriate (9)
Chronic stable angina, CCS class III or IV	Submaximal medical therapy	Moderate	>35	1 with proximal left anterior descending artery	Appropriate (7)	Uncertain (6)
	Maximal medical therapy	Low	>35	1 with proximal left anterior descending artery	Appropriate (9)	Appropriate (8)
Unstable angina	Asymptomatic with maximal medical therapy	Low or moderate	>35	Left main coronary artery, a total of 3, or 2 with proximal left anterior descending artery	Inappropriate (3)	Appropriate (9)
	Symptoms with submaximal medical therapy	Low	>35	1 or 2 without proximal left anterior descending artery	Appropriate (7)	Appropriate (7)
≤21 days after acute	Asymptomatic, very positive exercise ECG	Low or moderate	>15	2 without proximal left anterior	Uncertain (5)	Uncertain (5)
	Asymptomatic, positive exercise ECG	Low	>15	1 or 2 without proximal left anterior descending artery	Uncertain (6)	Uncertain (6)

*A total of 984 indications were rated for CABG and 995 indications for PTCA, of which 312 occurred in the study sample of 2552 patients with coronary artery disease. A total of 521 patients had indications that made them appropriate candidates for both CABG and PTCA. ECG denotes electrocardiogram. CCS class refers to the Canadian Cardiovascular Society classification of symptoms, ranging from I (mild) to IV (severe). The abnormalities on the exercise ECG were defined by RAND. Operative risk was measured by the method of Parsonnet et al. (1989).

disease was coded from 1 (no disease) to 6 (occlusion), and the number of diseased vessels was calculated (Ringqvist et al. 1983). Reliability testing was undertaken by two cardiologists who were unaware of the clinical details. There was good agreement beyond the degree expected by chance between the cardiologists and the trained coder, with weighted kappas of 0.64 and 0.63 for 209 angiograms. 2552 patients with coronary artery disease had sufficient data for us to assign a score for the appropriateness of CABG; 2503 had sufficient data to assign an appropriateness score for PTCA.

Follow-up

First revascularisation procedures performed in study patients after index coronary angiography were identified from the National Health Service national electronic information system and hospitals' logbooks using a unique identifier.

Patients were followed until death or non-fatal myocardial infarction for a median follow-up period of 30 months (range 0–36) (Tunstall-Pedoe et al. 1994).

Angina was assessed on the basis of data obtained using the CCS scale from questionnaires sent to patients 12 months after either revascularisation or angiography if no revascularisation had been performed.

Statistical analysis

Outcomes were compared between those who were treated medically, and those who underwent CABG or PTCA after angiography; comparisons were made for each procedure, within each category of appropriateness. Each patient's first revascularisation procedure after the index angiography was analysed. The independent effect of CABG or PTCA on outcomes was estimated with the use of Cox proportional-hazards models (for death and non-fatal myocardial infarction) and logistic regression (for the presence or absence of angina). The appropriateness method classifies patients on the basis of risk. We used multivariate adjustment of hazard ratios and odds ratios to reduce the possibility of residual confounding. Survival data were compared by means of Kaplan–Meier curves and the log-rank test. Proportions were compared by means of the chi-square statistic. Linear trends in the hazard ratio across categories of appropriateness were assessed with the use of a likelihood-ratio test. All analyses were performed with the use of SAS software (SAS Institute 1990).

Results

Of 2552 patients analysed, 908 had indications for which PTCA was deemed appropriate and 1353 had indications for which CABG was deemed appropriate (Table 2.2); 521 patients were deemed appropriate candidates for both procedures. PTCA was performed in 34 (6 per cent) of the 568 patients rated as inappropriate for PTCA, in 223 (22 per cent) of the 1027 patients where we rated the appropriateness of PTCA as uncertain, and in 327 (36 per cent) of the 908 patients rated as appropriate candidates (P for linear trend <0.001). For CABG, the corresponding figures were 15 (8 per cent) of 186 patients, 212 (21 per cent) of 1013 patients, and 765 (57 per cent) of 1353 patients (P for linear trend <0.001). Nine hundred and eight patients were classified as appropriate candidates for PTCA at the time of angiography: 327 (36 per cent) underwent PTCA, 273 (30 per cent) underwent CABG and 308 (34 per cent) received only medical treatment. In all, 1353 patients were classified as appropriate candidates for CABG: 765 (57 per cent) underwent CABG, 234 (17 per cent) underwent PTCA and 354 (26 per cent) received only medical treatment.

Amongst patients where PTCA was rated appropriate, stepwise logistic regression identified previous CABG, heart failure, and the presence of disease in two vessels as independent predictors for receiving only medical treatment. Among patients classified as appropriate candidates for CABG, stepwise logistic regression identified previous CABG, the presence of disease in fewer than three vessels or its absence in the left main coronary artery, a lower CCS angina class, non-use of beta-blockers, diabetes, and non-white race as independent predictors for receiving medical treatment only (Tables 2.3, 2.4 and 2.5).

Medical treatment versus PTCA

For the 584 patients undergoing PTCA, 34 (6 per cent) had indications rated as inappropriate for PTCA, 223 (38 per cent) had indications rated as uncertain and 327 (56 per cent) had indications rated as appropriate. Patients classified as appropriate candidates for PTCA but who received medical treatment were more likely to have angina at follow-up (odds ratio, 1.97; 95 per cent confidence interval, 1.29–3.00) (Table 2.3) than those who received PTCA, but the two groups were equally likely to die or have a non-fatal myocardial infarction during follow-up (hazard ratio, 0.77; 95 per cent confidence interval, 0.48–1.25) (Table 2.4).

Medical treatment versus CABG

A total of 992 patients underwent CABG: 15 (2 per cent) had indications rated as inappropriate for CABG, 212 (21 per cent) had indications

Table 2.2 Demographic and clinical characteristics of patients with indications at angiography for which revascularisation was judged appropriate, according to subsequent revascularisation status

Characteristic	All patients with coronary artery disease (n = 2552)	PTCA appropriate (n = 908)*		CABG appropriate (n = 1353)†	
		PTCA (n = 327)	Medical treatment (n = 308)	CABG (n = 765)	Medical treatment (n = 354)
Demographic					
Median age (years)	62	59	60	63	63
Female sex (%)	21	25	23	19	18
Non-white race (%)	14	12	17	14	20‡
Clinical					
Current medication (%)					
Aspirin	80	86	82	81	81
Beta-blocker	48	57	52	53	42§
Calcium antagonist	53	55	60	58	58
ACE inhibitor¶	24	21	25	21	25
Nitrate	65	73	70	70	69
Statin	22	21	25	25	23
Diabetes (%)	16	11	17‡	15	21‡
Severity of angina (%)					
CCS class I or II	48	37	47	41	45
CCS class III or IV	52	63	53‡	59	55
Previous myocardial infarction (%)	51	53	58	44	52‡
Abnormal exercise ECG (%)	80	86	87	89	84
Angiographic findings (%)					
1 diseased vessel	42	76	67	9	22
2 diseased vessels	29	24	33	24	32
3 diseased vessels or left main coronary artery	30	<1	0‡	67	46§
Diffuse disease	16	7	12‡	20	23
Impaired left ventricular function (%)	30	16	25‡	28	30
Heart failure (%)	14	7	15§	11	16‡
Previous PTCA or stenting (%)	8	16	10‡	5	7
Previous CABG (%)	10	6	19§	5	19§
Operative risk (Parsonnet score)‖					
Median	6	4	5	6	6
Interquartile range	3–10	1–7	3–8‡	3–10	3–11
Co-existing condition (%)					
Stroke or peripheral arterial disease	8	5	8	9	11
Non-cardiovascular condition	37	37	40	38	40

See page 23 for footnote.

rated as uncertain and 765 (77 per cent) had indications rated as appropriate. Patients classified as appropriate for CABG but who received medical treatment were more likely than those who received CABG to have angina at follow-up (odds ratio, 3.03; 95 per cent confidence interval, 2.08–4.42) (Table 2.3) and to die or have a non-fatal myocardial infarction during the follow-up period (hazard ratio, 4.08; 95 per cent confidence interval, 2.82–5.93) (Table 2.4). The risk of death or non-fatal myocardial infarction was 21 per cent with medical treatment and 6 per cent among those who underwent CABG ($P < 0.001$ by the log-rank test) (Figure 2.1).

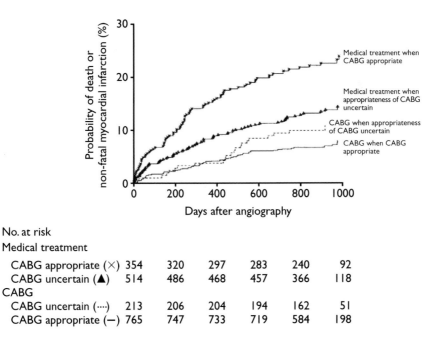

No. at risk						
Medical treatment						
CABG appropriate (×)	354	320	297	283	240	92
CABG uncertain (▲)	514	486	468	457	366	118
CABG						
CABG uncertain (····)	213	206	204	194	162	51
CABG appropriate (—)	765	747	733	719	584	198

Figure 2.1 Risk of death or non-fatal myocardial infarction in different appropriateness and treatment groups.

*Of these, 635 patients underwent PTCA or medical treatment; the remaining 273 underwent CABG.
†Of these, 1119 patients underwent CABG or medical treatment; the remaining 234 underwent PTCA.
‡$P < 0.05$ for the comparison with the subgroup that received PTCA or CABG.
§$P < 0.01$ for the comparison with the subgroup that received PTCA or CABG.
¶ACE denotes angiotensin-converting enzyme.
‖Operative risk was measured according to the method of Parsonnet et al. (1989). RAND defined scores lower than 9 as low risk, scores of 9–18 as moderate risk, and scores higher than 18 as high risk.

Table 2.3 Presence of angina at 12 months of follow-up, according to treatment received and appropriateness category*

Appropriateness category	Angina at follow-up (no. with angina/total no.)		Odds ratio (95% CI)	Odds ratio†
	Medical treatment	Revascularisation		
PTCA				
Inappropriate	56/110	9/14	0.73 (0.22–2.42)	
Uncertain	172/317	67/142	2.15 (1.34–3.44)	
Appropriate	143/205	114/210	1.97 (1.29–3.00)	
CABG				
Inappropriate	49/70	6/8	0.82 (0.15–4.40)	
Uncertain	189/348	60/136	2.23 (1.40–3.55)	
Appropriate	137/208	213/547	3.03 (2.08–4.42)	

*The odds ratios compare the odds of having angina at follow-up for patients treated medically with the odds for patients who underwent PTCA or CABG. For patients with indications rated appropriate or uncertain, the odds ratios have been adjusted for age, sex, race, use or non-use of beta-blockers, presence or absence of diabetes, history with respect to myocardial infarction, Canadian Cardiovascular Society angina class, number of diseased vessels, presence or absence of diffuse disease, presence or absence of impaired left ventricular function, presence or absence of heart failure, history with respect to revascularisation and Parsonnet score (which measures operative risk). For patients with indications rated inappropriate, the odds ratios have been adjusted for age. CI denotes confidence interval.
†Odds ratios are indicated by the solid circles (and their 95 per cent confidence intervals by the horizontal lines) on a logarithmic scale. An odds ratio of 1.0 indicates no difference in the effects of revascularisation and medical therapy with respect to angina at follow-up. Values > 1.0 indicate a beneficial effect of revascularisation over medical treatment and values < 1.0 indicate a beneficial effect of medical treatment over revascularisation.

Table 2.4 Incidence of death from any cause or non-fatal myocardial infarction at 2.5 years of follow-up, according to treatment received and appropriateness category*

Procedure and category	Death from any cause (no. who died/total no.)			Death from any cause or non-fatal MI (no. with event)			Hazard ratio for death from any cause or non-fatal MI†
	Medical treatment	Revascularisation	Hazard ratio (95% CI)	Medical treatment	Revascularisation	Hazard ratio (95% CI)	
PTCA							
Inappropriate	48/170	4/34	2.16 (0.78–6.02)	54	5	2.00 (0.80–4.94)	
Uncertain	60/486	13/223	1.78 (0.96–3.30)	73	23	1.29 (0.79–2.09)	
Appropriate	20/308	18/327	0.90 (0.45–1.78)	35	40	0.77 (0.48–1.25)	
Total	128/964	35/584		162	68		
CABG							
Inappropriate	13/109	3/15	0.65 (0.18–2.28)	18	3	0.87 (0.26–2.97)	
Uncertain	53/514	19/212	1.66 (0.95–2.86)	70	22	1.69 (1.02–2.78)	
Appropriate	68/354	42/765	4.96 (3.27–7.51)	81	55	4.08 (2.82–5.93)	
Total	134/977	64/992		169	80		

Medical treatment better — PTCA better
TAKE IN ARTWORK
0.40 1.00 2.00 4.00

Medical treatment better — CABG better
0.20 0.40 1.00 2.00 6.00

*The hazard ratios compare the likelihood of the outcomes in patients treated medically with the likelihood in patients treated with PTCA or CABG. For patients with indications rated appropriate or uncertain, the hazard ratios have been adjusted for age, sex, race, use or non-use of beta-blockers, presence or absence of diabetes, history with respect to myocardial infarction, Canadian Cardiovascular Society angina class, number of diseased vessels, presence or absence of diffuse disease, presence or absence of impaired left ventricular function, presence or absence of heart failure, history with respect to revascularisation and Parsonnet score (which measures operative risk). For patients with indications rated inappropriate, the hazard ratios have been adjusted for age. CI denotes confidence interval, and MI myocardial infarction.

†Hazard ratios are indicated by the solid circles (and their 95 per cent confidence intervals by horizontal lines) on a logarithmic scale. A hazard ratio of 1.0 indicates no difference in the effects of revascularisation and medical treatment in terms of death or non-fatal myocardial infarction at follow-up. Values >1.0 indicate a beneficial effect of revascularisation over medical treatment and values <1.0 indicate a beneficial effect of medical treatment over revascularisation.

Table 2.5 Incidence of death from any cause or non-fatal myocardial infarction at 2.5 years of follow-up, according to receipt of medical treatment or CABG, within five categories of appropriateness*

5-Level appropriateness category (range of ratings)	Death from any cause or non-fatal MI (no. with event/total no.)	Hazard ratio (95% CI)	P value	Hazard ratio[†]
1–2	13/68	0.80 (0.18–3.67)	0.78	
3–4	38/293	0.78 (0.27–2.27)	0.65	
5–6	62/489	1.94 (1.09–3.44)	0.023	
7–8	80/623	3.27 (2.01–5.33)	<0.001	
9	56/496	5.58 (3.13–9.96)	<0.001	

Medical treatment better ← → CABG better

0.20 0.40 1.00 2.00 4.00 10.00

*The hazard ratios compare the likelihood of death from any cause or non-fatal myocardial infarction in patients treated medically with that in patients undergoing CABG. For patients with indications rated 3–9, the hazard ratios have been adjusted for age, sex, race, use or non-use of beta-blockers, presence or absence of diabetes, history with respect to myocardial infarction, Canadian Cardiovascular Society angina class, number of diseased vessels, presence or absence of diffuse disease, presence or absence of impaired left ventricular function, presence or absence of heart failure, history with respect to revascularisation and Parsonnet score (which measures operative risk). For patients with indications rated 1 or 2, the hazard ratios have been adjusted for age. CI denotes confidence interval, and MI myocardial infarction. In other analyses, ratings of 1–3 indicate the inappropriateness of revascularisation, 4–6 uncertain appropriateness and 7–9 appropriateness.

[†]Hazard ratios are indicated by the solid circles (and their 95 per cent confidence intervals by the horizontal lines) on a logarithmic scale. A hazard ratio of 1.0 indicates no difference in the effects of CABG and medical treatment with respect to the composite endpoint at follow-up. Values >1.0 indicate a beneficial effect of CABG over medical treatment and values <1.0 indicate a beneficial effect of medical treatment over CABG. P for linear trend = 0.002.

Dose–response relationship

The effect on the primary outcome of not undergoing CABG, as compared with undergoing CABG, was greatest for patients whom we classified as the most appropriate candidates for CABG (those with a rating of 9), but it remained significant in the groups defined by ratings of 7 or 8 and 5 or 6 (P for linear trend across the five groups = 0.002) (Table 2.5).

Discussion

In this study medical treatment was common among patients with indications for whom revascularisation had been deemed appropriate by the expert panel. Over 2.5 years of follow-up, these medically treated patients had higher mortality and a higher prevalence of angina than patients who underwent revascularisation. The findings of this prospective study provide strong evidence that ratings of appropriateness have clinical validity in measuring underuse of revascularisation after angiography. Our use of the appropriateness scale enabled us to identify underuse of revascularisation both among appropriate candidates and among patients with indications for whom revascularisation was rated as of uncertain appropriateness.

The increase in the risk of adverse outcomes associated with medical treatment was greatest among patients classified as the most appropriate candidates for CABG (patients with a rating of 9). However, these effects were not confined to the patients for whom CABG was rated as appropriate. Among patients to whom we assigned a rating of 5 or 6 (usually considered 'uncertain'), there were also significant effects, with a hazard ratio intermediate in magnitude between that for patients rated as appropriate and that for patients rated as inappropriate. Previous studies have restricted the definition of underuse to the subgroup of patients for whom revascularisation is judged not only appropriate but also necessary. The graded risk–benefit relation across categories of appropriateness in our study suggests that this definition is too narrow.

The better outcomes among patients for whom revascularisation was deemed appropriate or uncertain were independent of a large number of clinical variables. Furthermore, they were not explained by differences in medical treatment; among the patients whom we rated as appropriate candidates for CABG we found no difference at follow-up in the use of aspirin, beta-blockers or statins between those who underwent CABG and those who were treated medically. The effects tended to be consistent for mortality, non-fatal myocardial infarction and angina status.

One-third of the patients whom we rated as appropriate candidates for PTCA and one-quarter of those whom we rated as appropriate candidates for CABG were treated medically; these rates are in line with previous estimates that 22–41 per cent of necessary invasive procedures are not performed (Kravitz et al. 1995; Kravitz and Laouri 1997; Laouri et al. 1997; Carlisle et al. 1999; Leape et al. 1999). Observational studies cannot exclude unmeasured factors, and cardiologists and surgeons may choose to perform revascularisation in patients destined to do well for other reasons. Preference of the patient is unlikely to be a major factor, since willingness to consider revascularisation is a precondition for undergoing angiography.

Our findings raise a fundamental question about clinical decision making in that the explicit, quantified judgements of an expert panel may be a better guide to the proper use of coronary revascularisation than the variable decisions of individual clinicians.

Acknowledgements

Supported by grants from the Health Authorities of East London and the City, North Essex, Barking and Havering, and Redbridge and Waltham Forest; the North Thames National Health Service Research and Development Program (RFG 258); the British Heart Foundation (PG/97216); Guidant; and Boston Scientific.

We are indebted to the patients for their participation in this research.

Source information

From the Department of Research and Development, Kensington & Chelsea and Westminster Health Authority (H.H., A.M.C., S.P., J.S.); the Department of Epidemiology and Public Health, University College London Medical School (H.H.); the Department of General Practice and Primary Care, St Bartholomew's and the Royal London School of Medicine and Dentistry (G.F.); and the Cardiac Directorate, Barts and the London National Health Service Trust (S.B., J.R.D., P.M., A.W., A.D.T.) – all in London.

References

Ayanian, J.Z., Landrum, M.B., Normand, S.L.T, Guadagnoli, E. and McNeil, B.J. (1998) 'Rating the appropriateness of coronary angiography – do practicing physicians agree with an expert panel and with each other?', *New England Journal of Medicine*, 338: 1896–904.

Bernstein, S.J., Laouri, M., Hilborne, L.H. *et al.* (1992) *Coronary Angiography: A Literature Review and Ratings of Appropriateness and Necessity*, Santa Monica, CA: RAND.

Campean, L. (1976) 'Grading of angina pectoris', *Circulation*, 54: 522–3.

Carlisle, D.M., Leape, L.L., Bickel, S., Bell, R., Kamberg, C., Genovese, B.,

French, W.J., Kaushik, V.S., Mahrer, P.R., Ellestad, M.H., Brook, R.H. and Shapiro, M.F. (1999) 'Underuse and overuse of diagnostic testing for coronary artery disease in patients presenting with new-onset chest pain', *American Journal of Medicine*, 106: 391–8.

Gray, D., Hampton, J.R., Bernstein, S.J., Kosecoff, J. and Brook, R.H. (1990) 'Audit of coronary angiography and bypass surgery', *Lancet*, 335: 1317–20.

Hemingway, H., Crook, A.M., Dawson, J.R., Edelman, J., Edmondson, S., Feder, G., Kopelman, P., Leatham, E., Magee, P., Parsons, L., Timmis, A.D. and Wood, A. (1999) 'Rating the appropriateness of coronary angiography, coronary angioplasty and coronary artery bypass grafting: the ACRE study', *Journal of Public Health Medicine*, 21: 421–9.

Hemingway, H., Crook, A.M., Feder, G., Dawson, J.R. and Timmis, A. (2000) 'Waiting for coronary angiography: is there a clinically ordered queue?' *Lancet*, 355: 985–6.

Hilborne, L.H,. Leape, L.L., Bernstein, S.J., Park, R.E., Fiske, M.E., Kamberg, C.J., Roth, C.P. and Brook, R.H. (1993) 'The appropriateness of use of percutaneous transluminal coronary angioplasty in New York State', *Journal of the American Medical Association*, 269: 761–5.

Kravitz, R.L., Laouri, M., Kahan, J.P., Guzy, P. Sherman, T., Hilborne, L. and Brook, R.H. (1995) 'Validity of criteria used for detecting underuse of coronary revascularization', *Journal of the American Medical Association*, 274: 632–8.

Kravitz, R.L. and Laouri, M. (1997) 'Measuring and averting underuse of necessary cardiac procedures: a summary of results and future directions', *The Joint Commission Journal on Quality Improvement*, 23: 268–76.

Laouri, M., Kravitz, R.L., French, W.J., Yang, I., Milliken, J.C., Hilborne, L., Wachsner, R. and Brook, R.H. (1997) 'Underuse of coronary revascularization procedures: application of a clinical method', *Journal of the American College of Cardiology*, 29: 891–7.

Leape, L.L., Hilborne, L.H., Bell, R., Kamberg, C. and Brook, R.H. (1999) 'Underuse of cardiac procedures: do women, ethnic minorities and the uninsured fail to receive needed revascularisation?', *Annals of Internal Medicine*, 130: 183–92.

Leape, L.L., Hilborne, L.H., Park, R.E., Bernstein, S.J., Kamberg, C.J., Sherwood, M. and Brook, R.H. (1993) 'The appropriateness of use of coronary artery bypass graft surgery in New York State', *Journal of the American Medical Association*, 269: 753–60.

Parsonnet, V., Dean, D. and Bernstein, A.D. (1989) 'A method of uniform stratification of risk for evaluating the results of surgery in acquired adult heart disease', *Circulation*, 79 (Suppl I): I–3–I–12.

Ringqvist, I., Fisher, L.D., Mock, M., Davis, K.B., Wedel, H., Chaitman, B.R., Passamani, E., Russell, R.O., Jr, Alderman, E.L., Kouchoukas, N.T., Kaiser, G.C., Ryan, T.J., Killip, T. and Fray, D. (1983) 'Prognostic value of angiographic indices of coronary artery disease from the Coronary Artery Surgery Study (CASS)', *Journal of Clinical Investigation*, 71: 1854–66.

SAS Institute (1990) *SAS User's Guide*, version 6, Cary, NC: SAS Institute.

Selby, J.V., Fireman, B.H., Lundstrom, R.J., Swain, B.E., Truman, A.F., Wong, C.C., Froelicher, E.S., Barron, H.V. and Hlatky, M.A. (1996) 'Variation among hospitals in coronary-angiography practices and outcomes after myocardial infarction in a large health maintenance organization', *New England Journal of Medicine*, 335: 1888–96.

Shekelle, P.G., Kahan, J.P., Bernstein, S.J., Leape, L.L., Kamberg, C.J. and Park, R.E. (1998) 'The reproducibility of a method to identify the overuse and underuse of medical procedures', *New England Journal of Medicine*, 338: 1888–95.

Tunstall-Pedoe, H., Kuulasmaak, K., Amouyel, P., Arveiler, D., Rajakangas, A.M. and Pajak, A. (1994) 'Myocardial infarction and coronary deaths in the World Health Organization MONICA Project: registration procedures, event rates, and case-fatality rates in 38 populations from 21 countries in four continents', *Circulation*, 90: 583–612.

Winslow, C.M., Kosecoff, J.B., Chassin, M., Kanouse, D.E. and Brook, R.H. (1988) 'The appropriateness of performing coronary artery bypass surgery', *Journal of the American Medical Association*, 260: 505–9.

A complete, unedited version of this article can be found as 'Underuse of coronary revascularization procedures in patients considered appropriate candidates for revascularization' in the *New England Journal of Medicine* (2001) Volume 344, Number 9, pages 645–54. The authors are Hemingway, H., Crook, A.M., Feder, G., Banerjee, S., Rex Dawson, J., Magee, P., Philpott, S., Sanders, J., Wood, A. and Timmis, A.D.

Chapter 3

Integrated care pathways in stroke management

David Sulch and Lalit Kalra

Abstract

Background: An organised, goal-defined and time-specified plan of management as envisaged by the integrated care pathway approach can achieve quality outcomes at lower cost. Integrated care pathways may have applications to stroke management because diagnosis is well defined, complex interdisciplinary inputs are required and there is good evidence on best practice.

Method: We reviewed medical, nursing, rehabilitation and health services databases to identify studies on integrated care pathways in stroke management. Criteria for inclusion were: use of a care pathway or similar methods in acute or rehabilitation settings, randomised studies or non-randomised comparisons with concurrent or historical controls and some form of outcome assessment.

Results: We identified six non-randomised studies of acute stroke. One used concurrent controls; the rest used historical controls. Only one study investigated stroke rehabilitation and this used a quasi-randomised controlled design. Five studies in the acute setting demonstrated reduced hospital stay. A reduction in costs of care was reported in all five studies that examined costs. Two studies reported improved uptake of medical interventions. No difference in length of hospital stay, costs or functional status was seen in the rehabilitation study.

Conclusions: Integrated care pathway methodology may facilitate quality and cost improvements in stroke care, but evidence is weak and uncertainty exists. Further evidence is needed before implementation in practice.

Source: *Age and Ageing*, 29, 2000, 349–52.

Introduction

The provision of high-quality stroke care presents several challenges. Co-ordinated care by specialist staff is associated with reductions in mortality, dependence and length of stay (Stroke Unit Trialists Collaboration 1997). There is increasing pressure to incorporate emerging research evidence into clinical practice and introduce management practices which stream-line the process of care to increase effectiveness or produce cost savings. One way of achieving these objectives is to introduce 'integrated care pathways', a project network technique, which is gaining increasing popularity in health care delivery.

Project network techniques were first used in the American space programme and then in industry to manage complex processes. This methodology has been extended to patient care involving interdisciplinary interventions because it improves communication and co-ordination without necessarily changing the clinical practice of individual disciplines (Pearson *et al*. 1995). It involves the development of a project network diagram, which charts the order of activities and the nature of relationships between different activities that must be completed within a given time. It provides the interdisciplinary team with prompts to initiate certain investigations, referrals and treatments at pre-ordained intervals and checks to ensure that the patient is progressing in the expected manner.

Deviations from the expected path of care are termed variances, which are useful for early identification and resolution of problems affecting outcome or the time required to achieve this outcome. Integrated care pathways are also referred to as care pathways, critical pathways, anticipated pathways of recovery, managed care pathways or practice guidelines in different settings (Pearson *et al*. 1995; James *et al*. 1997; Weingarten *et al*. 1998).

Development of a care pathway is an interdisciplinary task. Steps in its development include formation of a team of appropriate professionals, research to determine current practice and identify evidence for best practice, and production of a preliminary pathway. This pathway is then implemented in a target group of patients to assess applicability and refine interventions before production of the final agreed pathway.

The success of integrated care pathway methodology depends on the quality of implementation. This has been facilitated by using care pathways with the case management system of health care (Aubert *et al*. 1998), in which a health care professional designated as the 'case manager' oversees the patient's episode of care using a care pathway as the template for timely provision of appropriate care. This professional is usually an experienced nurse who initiates investigations, requests referrals and prescribes medication within the constraints of the pathway but without need for prior medical consultation (Aubert *et al*. 1998).

Here, we present a review of the literature on the role of integrated care pathways in stroke management, with emphasis on evidence for their effectiveness and implications for use in clinical practice.

Methods

We searched the MEDLINE, CINAHL, Best Evidence, Cochrane and Ovid Nursing Collection databases from 1966. In view of the variety of names given to care pathways, we searched for the terms 'case management', 'care pathway', 'critical path', 'management model' 'anticipated recovery' and 'practice guidelines'. We combined these with the terms 'stroke or cerebrovascular'. In addition, we combined the latter term with the terms 'pathway or guidelines' to identify papers with other alternative names for their care pathways. We searched the ACP Journal Club and Evidence Based Medicine databases using the terms 'pathway', 'guidelines' and 'stroke or cerebrovascular'. We scrutinised the reference lists of any papers identified in this way for other relevant papers which we might have missed on the initial search.

Reports which described the effects of introducing a care pathway for the management of acute stroke or rehabilitation in any setting were eligible. We included papers if outcome following the introduction of the pathway was assessed and compared with control data. The control data could be obtained either prospectively by a randomised method or from historical controls treated on the unit before introduction of the pathway. This strategy was necessary because of the paucity of well-designed randomised controlled studies. The key outcome measures were length of stay, cost of episode, functional outcome (such as Functional Independence Measure or Barthel index), discharge destination and uptake of investigations or interventions deemed relevant to patient care. The pathway had to include a plan for medical and nursing interventions and instructions on access to other members of the interdisciplinary team as a minimum requirement.

Results

In the search we identified seven papers on the use of integrated care pathways in stroke management meeting the predetermined criteria for inclusion in the review (Table 3.1).

Acute stroke

Six papers describe the effect of introducing integrated care pathways in acute stroke care (Table 3.1, papers 1–6). Patients were admitted to acute units for the initial medical management and investigation before being transferred to rehabilitation facilities or discharged home.

Table 3.1 Papers identified following literature search

No.	Paper	Setting	Type of pathway	Controls	Reduction in length of stay	Resource use
1	Anon. CVA (cerebrovascular accident) pathway cuts across seven hospital units. *Hospital Case Management* 1998; 6: 33–4.	Acute	5-day 'cross unit' pathway	Historical	1.6 days	Not analysed
2	Bowen, J., Yaste, C. Effect of a stroke protocol on hospital costs of stroke patients. *Neurology* 1994; 44: 1961–4.	Acute	Protocol including emergency department algorithm, nursing 'critical path' and admission orders	Historical and concurrent – not randomised	From 6.7 to 5.5 days	32%
3	Odderson, I.R., McKenna, B.S. A model for management of patients with stroke during the acute phase. Outcome and economic implications. *Stroke* 1993; 24: 1823–7.	Acute	Admission orders, swallow screen, referrals to other disciplines	Historical	From 10.9 to 7.3 days	14.60%
4	Ross, G., Johnson, D., Kobernick, M. Evaluation of a critical pathway for stroke. *Journal of the American Osteopath Association* 1997; 97: 269–72, 275–6.	Acute	Medical algorithm	Historical	From 7.5 to 6.3 days	15%
5	Summers, D., Soper, P.A. Implementation and evaluation of stroke clinical pathways and the impact on cost of stroke care. *Journal of Cardiovascular Nursing* 1998; 13: 69–87.	Acute	Care path introduced on new stroke unit	Historical	–	Yes
6	Wentworth, D.A., Atkinson, R.P. Implementation of an acute stroke program decreases hospitalization costs and length of stay. *Stroke* 1996; 27: 1040–3.	Acute	Path developed around standing stroke orders	Historical	From 7.0 to 4.6 days	23%
7	Falconer, J.A., Roth, E.J., Sutin, J.A. et al. The critical path method in stroke rehabilitation: lessons from an experiment in cost containment and outcomes improvement. *Quality Review Bulletin* 1993; 19: 8–16.	Rehabilitation	Critical path managed by trained team	Concurrent, randomised	None: 35.6 (15.5) days vs 32.3 (15.4) days in controls	None

A non-randomised controlled design was used in one study (paper 2); the others compared outcomes with historical controls on the unit before introduction of the integrated care pathway. Two integrated care pathways were biased towards medical care and focus on investigations (computerised tomography scanning, carotid Doppler examinations) and interventions (prescription of aspirin, deep vein thrombosis prophylaxis, swallow screening) (papers 2 and 4). The other four papers describe a more integrated multidisciplinary approach with less of a medical bias (papers 1, 3, 5 and 6). Only one study includes times for social work review (paper 3).

The main effect of integrated care pathway management is to reduce length of hospital stay for the acute episode compared with historical or concurrent controls. The largest reduction (36%) is reported by Wentworth and Atkinson (paper 6): their length of stay decreased from 7 to 4.6 days, with the greatest reductions occurring in the fourth year of introduction of the care pathway in patient care. Five papers report a cost analysis, showing a reduction in costs for the acute episode of between 14 and 32% (papers 2, 3, 5 and 6). Two papers report improved uptake of medical interventions (papers 2 and 4). Bowen and Yaste (paper 2) demonstrated an increased frequency of carotid Doppler examinations and deep vein thrombosis prophylaxis. Ross *et al.* (paper 4) reported improvement in the speed with which investigations are undertaken, but the total number of tests performed did not increase.

Odderson and McKenna (paper 3) reported a reduced frequency of complications such as aspiration pneumonia (reduced by 63%) and urinary tract infections (reduced by 38%) but these did not achieve statistical significance. This is the only study which includes a specific requirement to undertake a swallow screen within 24 hours of admission. None of the studies show an improvement in functional outcome or an increase in the proportion of patients being discharged home from the acute unit following the introduction of the integrated care pathway.

Stroke rehabilitation

Only one study evaluated integrated care pathway methodology in stroke rehabilitation (paper 7). A multidisciplinary integrated care pathway was used with well defused medical, nursing and therapy interventions at designated time points which were specified in advance. Patients up to 120 days after acute onset were included. Randomisation was subject to referred patterns as well as bed availability, resulting in imbalance between the intervention ($n = 53$) and control limbs ($n = 68$). The main outcome measures (length of stay, hospital charges and functional status) showed no differences between the integrated care pathway and the control group (Table 3.1). There were no differences in motor and cognitive scores or patient satisfaction scales between the two groups.

Discussion

The interdisciplinary nature of stroke management in acute and rehabilitation phases is well suited to care pathway methodology. Despite the firm evidence on the benefits of co-ordinated care (Stroke Unit Trialists Collaboration 1997), the National Sentinel Audit of Stroke Care has shown deficiencies in clinical assessment, rapidity of and access to investigations, acute management, and provision of information to patients and relatives across the UK (Rudd *et al.* 1999). Recent studies have shown the advantages of early initiation of therapy and increased intensity of therapy input (Langhorne *et al.* 1996) in improving outcome in stroke patients, but these are not widely implemented in practice. Since the main expense of stroke care is the 'hotel cost' associated with inpatient care, any saving on length of stay will have important resource implications. Although integrated care pathways can address these issues, the important question is whether evidence supports their widespread implementation.

The quality of evidence is limited by methodological problems in published studies. Most studies have been undertaken in small samples of patients and may not be generalisable. Nearly all are open to bias because of the historical nature of comparisons, lack of randomisation and the possibility of observer preferences in reporting outcome. The development of pathways has been described in great detail, but little information is provided on their implementation, which may have affected outcome. The number of variances from the pathway and the number of patients showing such variances have not been described, and it is not clear how these were dealt with in the analysis of data.

Care pathways for the acute phase are relatively easy to produce and are exemplified by the algorithmic style of the studies (Table 3.1, papers 2, 4 and 6). Most acute studies have not used clinically relevant measures (such as mortality, prevention of complications and successful implementation of secondary prevention interventions) but concentrated on cost issues, such as completeness of investigations and reductions in the length of stay. These pathways are geared towards earlier transfer of the patients out of the acute unit, and eventual outcome in terms of residual disability or destination of discharge has not been evaluated. It is also not known whether the improved efficiency of care on the acute unit eventually leads to an overall reduction in hospital stay, or whether the costs of care are merely transferred from the acute to rehabilitation settings.

It is even harder to draw conclusions on the use of pathways in rehabilitation. The only reported study took patients up to three months after their stroke, a time at which most of the gains produced by early, effective and co-ordinated multidisciplinary care would have occurred (Table 3.1, paper 7). The inherent assumption in integrated care pathway methodology, that care can be standardised, may not be true for stroke rehabilitation. Many of the therapy inputs need to be individualised and can vary between patients and even within patients from day to day. Interdisciplinary practice is well established on rehabilitation units, and integrated care pathways may make little further contribution. Outcome of stroke rehabilitation is not only determined by the processes of care but is also influenced by external factors, such as patient/carer expectations and services provided by other agencies that may not share the priorities or timescales of the treating unit. Against this background, the integrated care pathway process may be seen as time-consuming but contributing little to changing team focus or priorities, which will continue to be dictated by patient need and professional assessments.

There is considerable enthusiasm to introduce management techniques from non-stroke settings into stroke management to improve quality of care and reduce costs of services provided (May 1995). Although the theoretical advantages of such methods are clear, the benefits may be less than expected because of patient variability, pre-existing practice or dependence on external factors. Our review of the literature suggests that integrated care pathway methodology may have a role in stroke management but the evidence is weak and there is much uncertainty. Further randomised controlled trials are needed before implementation of this technique in stroke patients.

References

Aubert, R.E., Herman, W.H., Waters, J., Moore, W., Sutton, D., Peterson, B.L., Bailey, C.M. and Koplan, J.P. (1998) 'Nurse case management to improve glycemic control in diabetic patients in a health maintenance organization', *Annals of Internal Medicine*, 129: 605–12.

James, P.A., Cowan, T.M., Graham, R.P., Majeroni, B.A., Fox, C.H. and Jaen, C.R. (1997) 'Using a clinical practice guideline to measure physician practice: translating a guideline for the management of heart failure', *Journal of American Board of Family Practice*, 10: 206–12.

Langhorne, P., Wagenaar, R. and Partridge, C. (1996) 'Physiotherapy after stroke: more is better?', *Physiotherapy Research International*, 1: 75–88.

May, A. (1995) 'Over hyped and over here', *Health Services Journal*, 3: 14.

Pearson, S.D., Goulart-Fisher, D. and Lee, T.H. (1995) 'Critical pathways as a strategy for improving care: problems and potential', *Annals of Internal Medicine*, 123: 941–8.

Rudd, A.G., Irwin, P., Rutledge, Z., Lowe, D., Wade, D., Morris, R. and Pearson, M.G. (1999) 'National Sentinel Audit of Stroke: a tool for raising standards of care', *Journal of the Royal College of Physicians London*, 33: 460–4.

Stroke Unit Trialists Collaboration (1997) 'Collaborative systemic review of the randomised trials of organised inpatient (stroke unit) care after stroke', *British Medical Journal*, 314: 1151–8.

Weingarten, S., Riedlinger, M.S., Sandhu, M., Bowers, C., Ellrodt, A.G., Nunn, C., Hobson, P. and Greengold, N. (1998) 'Can practice guidelines safely reduce hospital length of stay? Results from a multicenter interventional study', *American Journal of Medicine*, 105: 33–40.

A complete, unedited version of this article can be found as Sulch, D. and Kalra, L., 'Integrated care pathways in stroke management' in *Age and Ageing* (2000) Volume 29, pages 349–52.

Chapter 4

The Shifting Perspectives Model of Chronic Illness

Barbara L. Paterson

Abstract

Purpose: To present the Shifting Perspectives Model of Chronic Illness, which was derived from a metasynthesis of 292 qualitative research studies.

Design: The model was derived from a metasynthesis of qualitative research about the reported experiences of adults with a chronic illness. The 292 primary research studies included a variety of interpretive research methods and were conducted by researchers from numerous countries and disciplines.

Methods: Metastudy, a metasynthesis method developed by the author in collaboration with six other researchers consisted of three analytic components (meta-data-analysis, metamethod and metatheory), followed by a synthesis component in which new knowledge about the phenomenon was generated from the findings.

Findings: Many of the assumptions that underlie previous models, such as a single, linear trajectory of living with a chronic disease, were challenged. The Shifting Perspectives Model indicated that living with chronic illness was an ongoing and continually shifting process in which an illness-in-the-foreground or wellness-in-the-foreground perspective has specific functions in the person's world.

Conclusions: The Shifting Perspectives Model helps users provide an explanation of chronically ill persons' variations in their attention to symptoms over time, sometimes in ways that seem ill-advised or even harmful to their health. The model also indicates direction to health professionals about supporting people with chronic illness.

Source: *Journal of Nursing Scholarship*, 33.1, 2001, 21–6.

Introduction

The Shifting Perspectives Model is a model of chronic illness that arose from the synthesis of qualitative research findings. This model allows users to extend the contributions of previous attempts to describe the experience of chronic illness, and offer new understanding about why people with chronic illness may manifest behaviours that at first glance seem ill-advised and even harmful. Many paradoxes that occur in living with a chronic illness, as well as some unintended outcomes when people with chronic illness attempt to use the health care system, are revealed.

Research design

The data for this paper were derived from a metasynthesis, or a meta-study, of 292 qualitative research reports pertaining to chronic physical illness. Metastudy is a systematic analytic and synthesis research method (Thorne and Paterson 1998). It is an interpretive qualitative research approach in the constructivist paradigm in which the researcher's role is to understand how people construct knowledge about the phenomenon under study (Guba and Lincoln 1994). Metastudy researchers analyse and synthesise what has been reported by researchers as findings, research design and theoretical perspectives in qualitative research reports (primary research) in a substantive area to identify similarities and differences among them and to generate new or expanded theory about the phenomenon under study. The two phases or components of metastudy are analysis and synthesis. Traditionally, qualitative researchers who have attempted metasynthesis have focused entirely on the analysis of primary research findings, but in metastudy, analysis and synthesis are separate. To analyse in a metastudy is to identify commonalities, differences, patterns and themes in a body of qualitative research. Synthesis extends beyond analysis as the analytical findings are used to identify the 'truths' that primary researchers have held in their interpretation of research data and their choice of research design and theoretical frameworks. In synthesising qualitative research new understandings of the phenomenon under study are generated.

The three aspects of the analytic component of metastudy are meta-data-analysis, metamethod and metatheory (see Table 4.1).

In the analytic phase, each primary research report was reviewed by at least three members of the research team, using a standardised appraisal form. If consensus was not achieved in the review, we met with other members of the research team to arrive at a defensible decision.

Sandelowski (1997) noted that the challenge for metasynthesists is to maintain the integrity of primary research studies while at the same time avoiding producing so much detail that 'no usable synthesis is produced'

Table 4.1 Analytical components of metastudy

Meta-data-analysis

(a) Translating the findings of primary research study into metaphors that explain them
(b) Comparing and contrasting the metaphors in research reports with other studies, as a whole or in subgroups (e.g. all those that pertain to a particular ethnic or age group), noting the similarities and differences between key metaphors
(c) Determining how the key metaphors of each study relate to those of other accounts and hypothesising about the nature of the relationships between metaphors in various studies

Metamethod

(a) Appraising, according to agreed-upon criteria, the research design, the role of researcher(s), sampling procedures and data collection procedures of each research report
(b) Depicting historical cultural and disciplinary trends regarding the research questions, methodological orientations, researcher roles, sampling procedures and data collection procedures that characterise the body of qualitative research in the field of study

Metatheory

(a) Reviewing each report to identify the theoretical perspective used and the emergent theory
(b) Identifying the major cognitive paradigms or schools of thought that underlie each theory
(c) Identifying the assumptions underlying each theory
(d) Examining the historical development of each theory, including significant markers
(e) Determining how the context may have influenced the choice of theoretical frameworks
(f) Evaluating the quality of the selected theory according to agreed-upon criteria

---

(p. 130). A high quality metasynthesis provides sufficient information for readers to track sources and decisions, but is focused on the synthesis of the primary research.

Selection criteria

The metastudy project included research reports in nursing, medicine, social science and allied health that were identifiable as a qualitative, interpretive research investigation and were reported from January 1980 to January 1996 in refereed journals, research-based books, or theses in which (a) the researchers investigated the experience of living with a chronic illness from the perspective of the person with the disease, (b) participants had a chronic physical illness, (c) reports provided evidence of the data trail and (d) demographic profiles of participants were provided.

The Shifting Perspectives Model

Previous researchers have described living with chronic illness as a phased process in which the person follows a predictable trajectory. The implication is that an end goal exists and it can be reached only if the person has lived with the disease long enough to progress through previous stages. In contrast, the Shifting Perspectives Model shows living with chronic illness as an ongoing, continually shifting process in which people experience a complex dialect between themselves and their 'world'. The experience of chronic illness is depicted as ever-changing perspectives about the disease that enable people to make the most of their experience.

People with chronic illness live in 'the dual kingdoms of the well and the sick' (Donelly 1993, p. 6). The measure of wellness is determined by comparing the experience to what is known and understood about illness and vice versa. Consequently, the perspective of chronic illness contains elements of both illness and wellness. Perspectives of chronic illness are illustrated in the schematic representation of the Shifting Perspectives Model as illness in the foreground or wellness in the foreground (see Figure 4.1). Each perspective is depicted by overlapping circles in which either illness or wellness takes precedence. As the reality of the illness experience and its personal and social context changes, the people's perspectives shift in the degree to which illness is in the foreground or background of their 'world'. Whether the illness is as significant and present as the individual perceives is irrelevant.

Illness in the foreground

The illness-in-the-foreground perspective is characterised by a focus on the sickness, suffering, loss and burden associated with living with a chronic illness; the chronic illness is viewed as destructive to self and

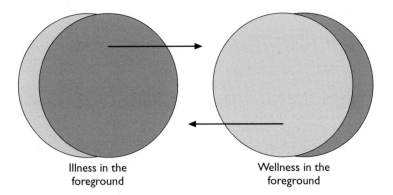

Illness in the foreground

Wellness in the foreground

Figure 4.1 The Shifting Perspectives Model of Chronic Illness.

others. People who assume this perspective tend to be absorbed in their illness experience and often have difficulty attending to the needs of their significant others. The most common depiction of this perspective occurs in newly diagnosed people who often express being overwhelmed by the disease.

The diagnosis of a chronic disease or the onset of new disease-related symptoms forces a person to attend to the illness. Focus on illness helps a person to learn about and to reflect on the disease to come to terms with it. For example, people with spinal cord injury must see themselves as having a disability before they can come to terms with having a disability (Carpenter 1994). In cases with few objective indicators of pathology, such as chronic pain, focusing on symptoms assists the person to provide evidence to others that the illness is real.

Wellness in the foreground

The wellness-in-the-foreground perspective includes an appraisal of the chronic illness as an opportunity for meaningful change in relationships with the environment and others. The person attempts to create consonance between self-identity and the identity that is shaped by the disease, the construction of the illness by others, and by life events (Fife 1994). For example, Stuifbergen and colleagues (1990) reported that participants in their research described their health as good or excellent, despite significantly impaired physical functioning.

In the wellness-in-the-foreground perspective, the self, not the diseased body, becomes the source of identity. People gain this perspective in many ways, particularly by learning as much as they can about the disease, creating supportive environments, developing personal skills such as negotiating, identifying the body's unique patterns of response, and sharing their knowledge of the disease with others. The wellness-in-the-foreground perspective allows people with chronic illness a means of mediating the effects of the disease. They shift from 'a victim of circumstances to creator of circumstances' (Barroso 1995, p. 44).

Shifting from wellness to illness in the foreground

The major factor that has been identified as fostering a shift in perspective from wellness to illness in the foreground is the perception of a threat to control. Signs of disease progression, lack of skill to manage the disease, disease-related stigma, and interactions with others that emphasise dependence and hopelessness are common threats to control. Any threat to control that exceeds the person's threshold of tolerance will cause a shift in perspective from wellness to illness in the foreground. Raleigh (1992) determined that some people with cancer experienced such periods of transition when symptoms grew worse or when they received discouraging news about their disease. Life incidents and situations also can result in people with chronic illness shifting perspective from wellness to illness in the foreground. For example, mothers in one study (Primomo 1989) indicated that their children's emotional or physical crises were often sufficient to make their own chronic illness seem overwhelming and their future bleak.

Some of the strategies people use to sustain a wellness-in-the-foreground perspective can actually result in shift to the illness-in-the-foreground perspective. Self-help groups can accentuate the sickness focus because they may require that the person focus on the sickness to participate in group discussion. People with chronic illness learn to select people with whom they can share their experiences in ways that will not be detrimental to their preferred perspective.

Shifting from illness to wellness in the foreground

The return to a wellness-in-the-foreground perspective from the focus on sickness has been referred to by researchers as 'bouncing back' with renewed hope and optimism (Dewar and Morse 1995). Returning to a wellness-in-the-foreground perspective may require people to reframe the situation so that it appears less daunting or to locate resources for dealing with the situation. Or they may have to consciously disengage from attention to their illness.

The initial change in perspective from illness in the foreground to wellness in the foreground is either gradual or the result of a sudden awareness. Researchers generally assume that the change is related to the duration of the illness. Loomis and Conco (1991) determined that because participants had chronic illness for many years, their tendency was to place 'health in the foreground and illness in the background' (p. 170). However, research reports are not clear about how the duration of the disease, and the experience of living with it, contribute to shifts to a wellness-in-the-foreground perspective. Limited evidence exists in this research that health care professionals and others can assist people with chronic illness to shift to a wellness perspective. Paterson and Sloan (1994) described how people with diabetes actively sought practitioners who would support the wellness-in-the-foreground perspective. Others have noted that a significant other or a person with the same disease was often a major influence on people with chronic illness to make a shift towards a wellness perspective (Raleigh 1992; Remien *et al.* 1995).

The paradoxes that arise

The Shifting Perspectives Model shows several paradoxes in the chronic illness experience. The major paradox of living in the wellness-in-the-foreground perspective of chronic illness is that, although the sickness is distant, the management of the disease must be foremost; that is, the illness requires attention in order not to have to pay attention to it. For people without a chronic illness, living life as normally as possible means the flexibility to be spontaneous in one's activities and behaviour. People with chronic illness, however, have to plan and anticipate even minor activities of daily life; spontaneity must be curtailed so that they can participate in the experiences they value.

Another paradox is that people who find meaning, hope and quality of life by maintaining a wellness-in-the-foreground perspective are often required to assume an illness-in-the-foreground perspective if they are to receive health care services. Social and health care structures and policies may reinforce an illness-in-the-foreground perspective, such as requiring that people who still wish to work instead take disability and unemployment benefits (Crossley 1998).

The illness-in-the-foreground perspective is a self-absorbing process that may further alienate a person from others. People who attend to their illness in an absorbed way may be regarded as hypochondriacs. Consequently, people may perceive that they have lost the support of others and, as a result, the powerlessness and suffering of the illness experience are reinforced. A further paradox is that in order to manage the disease so that it may be kept in the background, people with chronic illness consult practitioners and others who may convey that the person is helpless, thereby emphasising their dependency and sickness.

Discussion

According to the Shifting Perspectives Model, perspectives of chronic illness are not right or wrong but instead reflect people's needs and situations. The role of health care professionals becomes, therefore, to assist people with chronic illness to identify and understand their perspectives about the illness. In turn, practitioners must be committed to hearing what people see as important in health care (Lindsey 1993). Although people with chronic illness may assume one predominant perspective, it is not a static entity.

The terms 'acceptance' and 'denial' of illness as they are traditionally used by health care professionals have little or no meaning for those with chronic illness. The Shifting Perspectives Model of chronic illness indicates the need for understanding statements of optimism and pessimism, not as failing to understand the reality of the disease, but as indicators of the person's perspective.

Researchers have tended to view an irregular trajectory of chronic illness as solely based on periods of exacerbation and remission of distressing symptoms. The body of related research does not support such a conclusion. Pakenham, Dadds and Terry (1996), for example, reported little difference between asymptomatic, newly diagnosed and longstanding, symptomatic participants with HIV/AIDS regarding their emotional and existential issues of living with the disease. The Shifting Perspectives Model indicates additional factors such as social context and life events that may influence perspectives of chronic illness.

Many health care professionals are caught in a tradition of 'rehabilitating' people with chronic illness by assisting them to accept the limitations imposed by their disease. Such an approach might be counterproductive.

Conclusions

The Shifting Perspectives Model of Chronic Illness indicates a dialectical, constantly shifting perspective in which either illness or wellness is in the foreground. This model indicates that researchers and clinicians extend the focus on chronic illness from how it affects the person's well-being to a conceptualisation of the person's perspective of the illness in a larger sociocultural and psychological context. The model has reframed many aspects of living with a chronic illness. For example, what may have been interpreted as an excessive fixation on the body can now be seen as a functional response to a need or desire in living with chronic illness. The model also indicates the individuation of the chronic illness experience. It indicates reasons as to why people vary in their attention to symptoms and it directs practitioners to support persons with either perspective.

References

Barroso, J. (1995) 'Self-care activities of long-term survivors of acquire immunodeficiency syndrome', *Holistic Nursing Practice*, 10: 44–53.

Carpenter, C. (1994) 'The experience of spinal cord injury: the individual's perspective – implications for rehabilitation practice', *Physical Therapy*, 74: 614–29.

Crossley, M. (1998) '"Sick role" or "empowerment"? The ambiguities of life with an HIV positive diagnosis', *Sociology of Health and Illness*, 20: 507–31.

Dewar, A.L. and Morse, J.M. (1995) 'Unbearable incidents: failure to endure the experience of illness', *Journal of Advanced Nursing*, 22: 957–64.

Donnelly, G.E. (1993) 'Chronicity: concept and reality', *Holistic Nursing Practice*, 8: 1–7.

Fife, B.L. (1994) 'The conceptualization of meaning in illness', *Social Science and Medicine*, 38: 309–16.

Guba, E.G. and Lincoln, Y.S. (1994) 'Competing paradigms in qualitative research', in N.K. Denzin and Y.S. Lincoln (eds) *Handbook of Qualitative Research*, Thousand Oaks, CA: Sage.

Lindsey, A.E. (1993) Health within illness: Experiences of the chronically ill disabled. Unpublished doctoral dissertation, University of Victoria, Victoria, BC, Canada.

Loomis, M.E. and Conco, D. (1991) 'Patients' perceptions of health, chronic illness, and nursing diagnosis', *Nursing Diagnosis*, 2: 162–70.

Pakenham, K.I., Dadds, M.R. and Terry, D.J. (1996) 'Adaptive demands along the HIV disease continuum', *Social Science and Medicine*, 42: 245–56.

Paterson, B.L. and Sloan, J. (1994) 'A phenomenological study of the decision-making experience of individuals with long-standing diabetes', *Canadian Journal of Diabetes Care*, 18: 10–19.

Primomo, J. (1989) Patterns of chronic illness management, psychosocial development, family and social environment and adaptation among diabetic women. Unpublished doctoral dissertation, University of Washington, Seattle, WA, USA.

Raleigh, E.D.H. (1992) 'Sources of hope in chronic illness', *Oncology Nurses Forum*, 19: 443–8.

Remien, R.H., Carballo-Dieguez, A. and Wagner, G. (1995) 'Intimacy and sexual risk behaviour in serodiscordant male couples', *AIDS CARE*, 7: 429–38.

Sandelowski, M. (1997) "To be of use:' enhancing the utility of qualitative research', *Nursing Outlook*, 45: 125–32.

Stuifbergen, A.K., Becker, H.A., Ingalsbe, K. and Sands, D. (1990) 'Perceptions of health among adults with disabilities', *Health Values*, 14: 18–26.

Thorne, S. and Paterson, B. (1998) 'Shifting perspectives of chronic illness. Image', *Journal of Nursing Scholarship*, 30: 173–8.

A complete, unedited version of this article can be found as Paterson, B., 'The Shifting Perspectives Model of Chronic Illness' in the *Journal of Nursing Scholarship* (2001) Volume 33, Number 1, pages 21–6.

Chapter 5

Continuity of care in general practice: effect on patient satisfaction

Per Hjortdahl and Even Lærum

Abstract

Objective: To evaluate the influence of continuity of care on patient satisfaction with consultations.

Design: Direct and episodic specific evaluation of patient satisfaction with recent consultation.

Setting and subjects: A representative sample of 3918 Norwegian primary care patients were asked to evaluate their consultations by filling in a questionnaire. The response rate was 78 per cent.

Main outcome measures: The patient's overall satisfaction with the consultation was rated on a six-point scale. Continuity of care was recorded as the duration and intensity of the present patient–doctor relationship and as patients' perception of the present doctor being their personal doctor or not.

Results: Multivariate analysis indicated that an overall personal patient–doctor relationship increased the odds of the patient being satisfied with the consultation sevenfold (95% confidence interval 4.9 to 9.9) as compared with consultations where no such relationships existed. The duration of the patient–doctor relationship had a weak but significant association with patient satisfaction, while the intensity of contacts showed no such association.

Conclusion: Personal, continuous care is linked with patient satisfaction. If patient satisfaction is accepted as an integral part of quality health care, reinforcing personal care may be one way of increasing this quality.

Source: *British Medical Journal*, 304, 1992, 1287–90.

Introduction

Patient satisfaction is important. Evidence has accumulated that care which is less satisfactory to the patient is associated with non-compliance with treatment and return appointments and a poor understanding and retention of medical information. (Fitzpatrick 1991a). Patient satisfaction also reflects the technical competence of doctors (Roter *et al.* 1987) and satisfaction may be directly related to improvement in the health status of patients (Fitzpatrick *et al.* 1983).

Ware and Snyder (1975) have identified four independent factors, of which continuity of care is one that explains most of the variation in satisfaction.

Continuity has commonly been viewed quantitatively as a succession of visits to the same provider (Freeman 1984). However, Banahan and Banahan (1981) described it mainly as a qualitative phenomenon that may occur between patient and physician. In their view, continuity of care can best be characterised as a mutual attitudinal contract in which patients perceive a dependency on the physician for some or all of their primary health care needs and the physician accepts a responsibility for these needs.

As part of a larger assessment of the patient–doctor relationship (Hjortdahl and Borchgrevink 1991) the present study was undertaken to evaluate the influence of continuity of care on patient satisfaction in an unselected population of patients in primary care. Our hypothesis is that continuous, personal doctoring increases patient satisfaction.

Subjects and methods

A random sample of 133 Norwegian general practitioners agreed to record 30 consecutive surgery consultations, with patients of all ages. The physician recorded the age and sex of the patient, main reason for the encounter, and duration and intensity of the doctor–patient relationship. At the end of each consultation the doctor handed the patient a sealed envelope, asking the patient to take it home, read it, and follow the included instructions. In consultations with children the accompanying adults were asked to complete the questionnaire.

The envelope contained an explanation of the study, an assurance that their physician would not see the answer, and a two-page, self-explanatory questionnaire pertaining to the present patient–doctor relationship and satisfaction with the consultation they had just finished. A stamped, self-addressed envelope was included for return of the questionnaire directly to the department of general practice in Oslo. The questionnaire was anonymous and no effort was made to reach non-responders. Each questionnaire and doctor's recording were given similar numbers, and basic information about the non-responders could be obtained from the doctors' recordings. The participating physicians were not informed about either the content of the envelope they gave to the patients or the nature of the questionnaire.

Patient's perception of continuity of care was recorded on two dimensions. Longitudinal care was noted as the duration of the relationship and intensity (the number of encounters with the doctor during the previous 12 months). In Norway, patients are free to change primary care physicians at will. The relationship that may develop is usually unspoken and frequently unconscious. During the pilot phase it was found that the common phrase 'having a personal doctor' best captured the qualitative dimension of continuity of care, and the following response alternatives were given: today's doctor was not my personal doctor; or, today's doctor was the personal doctor for some, for most, or for all of my health problems.

Satisfaction was recorded as the answers to ten questions pertaining to the doctor's communicative skills and technical proficiency, and with the answer to one general question relating to overall satisfaction with the consultation. Possible responses ranged through six steps: very great, great, fair, somewhat, slight, and no satisfaction, with a separate category for uncertain. As each of the ten specific responses correlated to a large degree with the overall response (coefficients between 0.74 and 0.83) this global evaluation was used in the final analysis. Respondents were dichotomised into 'very satisfied', including those who had indicated very great or great satisfaction, and 'less satisfied' for the remainder.

The main reason for the encounter as noted by the physician was coded by the authors in accordance with the new *International Classification of Primary Care (ICPC)* (Lamberts and Wood 1987). The doctor's availability to patients was recorded as the average hours per week in clinical practice.

Multiple logistic regressions (Hosmor and Lemeshow 1989) were used to evaluate the relative importance of continuity of care for patient satisfaction, and factors related to patient, doctor and reason for encounter were controlled for. The doctor's age, stability and availability were continuous variables, and the others were categorical.

Results

The 133 participating physicians recorded 3918 out of a possible 3990 consultations. The patients' age, sex and morbidity patterns were closely compatible with those in a previous representative survey (Rutle 1983). In all, 3044 (78%) of the questionnaires were returned. No significant differences were observed in age, sex or morbidity pattern between responders and non-responders. There was, however, a somewhat higher proportion of new patients among the non-responders (15% vs 9%, $P < 0.001$), and a greater usage of emergency and unscheduled appointments among non-responders (26% vs 21%, $P < 0.004$).

Mean age of the respondents was 39 (range 0–98) years and among the participating physicians 38 (30–70) years. The doctors had been in general practice in the same geographical area for an average of seven (0–40) years. They did a mean of 27 (12–45) hours of clinical work a week.

The results showed that 1652 (54%) of all patients considered the present doctor to be their regular doctor for all their primary health care needs, 1032 (34%) named him or her as their regular doctor for some of their health needs and 357 (12%) did not feel any personal relationship had been established with the present doctor. For 232 (8%) the patient encounter was with a new doctor, while 1032 (34%) had known him or her for more than five years (Table 5.1).

Table 5.2 shows the multivariate relation between continuity of care

Table 5.1 Influence of the doctor–patient relationship on patient satisfaction with the consultation

	Overall satisfaction with present consultation			Total
	Very great/ great	*Fair/ somewhat*	*Slight/ none at all*	
Today's doctor was:				
Not my personal doctor	230 (64)	108 (30)	19 (5)	357 (99)
My personal doctor for:				
Some of my health problems	142 (68)	54 (26)	12 (6)	208 (100)
Most of my health problems	644 (78)	170 (21)	10 (1)	824 (100)
All of my health problems	1495 (90)	146 (9)	11 (1)	1652 (100)
Total	2511 (82)	478 (16)	52 (2)	3041 (100)
Duration of doctor–patient relationship (time since first encounter)				
First contact today	185 (77)	46 (19)	10 (4)	241 (100)
<3 months	135 (75)	45 (25)	0	180 (100)
3–12 months	287 (78)	74 (20)	6 (2)	367 (100)
1–5 years	1008 (83)	191 (16)	19 (2)	1218 (101)
>5 years	893 (87)	122 (12)	17 (2)	1032 (101)
Total	2508 (82)	478 (16)	52 (2)	3038 (100)
Intensity of doctor–patient relationship (no. of encounters in last 12 months)				
Present encounter only	378 (78)	88 (18)	16 (3)	482 (99)
2–3	788 (80)	177 (18)	15 (2)	980 (100)
4–5	431 (86)	63 (13)	9 (2)	503 (101)
6–10	608 (85)	101 (14)	8 (1)	717 (100)
≥11	299 (85)	48 (14)	5 (1)	352 (100)
Total	2504 (82)	477 (16)	53 (2)	3034 (100)

Results are numbers (row percentages).

Table 5.2 Influence of continuity of care on patient satisfaction with consultation, evaluated by multiple logistic regression, adjusting for patient-, doctor- and consultation-related factors

	No.	Odds ratio (95% confidence interval)	P value	Estimate (SE)
Factors related to continuity of care				
Today's doctor was:				
Not my personal doctor	357	1.00		
My personal doctor for:				
Some of my health problems	207	1.48 (0.99–2.19)	0.060	0.39 (0.20)
Most of my health problems	821	2.62 (1.87–3.64)	0.001	0.96 (0.17)
All of my health problems	1644	6.95 (4.89–9.90)	0.001	1.94 (0.18)
Duration of doctor–patient relationship (time since first encounter)				
First contact today	241			
<3 months	179	1.03 (0.66–1.61)	0.915	0.03 (0.23)
3–12 months	366	1.24 (0.91–1.71)	0.173	0.22 (0.16)
1–5 years	1215	1.32 (0.92–1.86)	0.129	0.27 (0.18)
>5 years	1028	1.85 (1.07–3.19)	0.026	0.61 (0.28)
Intensity of doctor–patient relationship (no. of encounters in past 12 months)				
Present encounter only	485			
2–3	979	1.03 (0.71–1.50)	0.889	0.03 (0.19)
4–5	502	1.10 (0.75–1.59)	0.631	0.09 (0.19)
6–10	715	1.20 (0.79–1.79)	0.400	0.17 (0.21)
≥11	351	1.27 (0.83–1.96)	0.268	0.24 (0.22)
Factors related to patient				
Age (years)				
≥15	193	1.00		
16–69	2266	1.08 (0.72–1.64)	0.721	0.08 (0.21)
≥70	570	1.04 (0.65–1.67)	0.879	0.04 (0.24)
Sex				
Female	2024	1.00		
Male	1005	0.99 (0.80–1.23)	0.937	−0.01 (0.11)
Factors related to doctor				
Age (years)		1.0 (0.99–1.03)	0.727	0.01 (0.01)
Sex				
Female	835	1.00		
Male	2194	0.92 (0.71–1.18)	0.334	−0.09 (0.13)
Stability of doctor in practice (years)		0.99 (0.97–1.01)	0.334	−0.01 (0.01)
Location of practice				
Major cities	450	1.00		
Towns	1120	1.05 (0.77–1.44)	0.749	0.05 (0.16)
Rural area	1459	0.95 (0.71–1.28)	0.731	−0.05 (0.15)

Table 5.2 continued

	No.	Odds ratio (95% confidence interval)	P value	Estimate (SE)
Type of practice				
Solo practitioner	770	1.00		
Dual partnership	785	1.05 (0.77–1.44)	0.750	0.05 (0.16)
Group practice	1474	0.95 (0.71–1.28)	0.733	−0.05 (0.15)
Reimbursement				
Set salary	1099	1.00		
Fee for service	1930	1.38 (1.10–1.78)	0.011	0.32 (0.13)
Availability (clinical hours per week)		1.03 (1.01–1.05)	0.004	0.03 (0.01)
Factors related to consultation				
Type				
Scheduled	2395	1.00		
Unscheduled	341	0.91 (0.68–1.23)	0.558	−0.09 (0.15)
Emergency	293	0.82 (0.59–1.14)	0.235	−0.20 (0.17)
Type of illness				
Somatic or non-psychosocial	2755	1.00		
Psychosocial	274	0.54 (0.40–0.74)	0.010	−0.61 (0.16)
Duration of problem				
New	1053	1.00		
Follow-up	698	1.15 (0.87–1.51)	0.326	0.14 (0.14)
Chronic	955	1.41 (0.95–2.08)	0.090	0.34 (0.20)
Preventive or other	323	1.08 (0.82–1.41)	0.618	0.07 (0.14)

and satisfaction with the consultation, adjusted for patient- and doctor-related factors associated with the consultation and illness. An overall personal patient–doctor relationship increased the odds of the patient being satisfied with the consultation sevenfold as compared with consultations where no such relationships existed. When the doctor was considered responsible only for some of the needs the odds of being satisfied increased by 50% as compared with new relationships, and it was two and a half times as great if the doctor was considered responsible for most of the patient's primary care needs. The duration of the patient–doctor relationship in itself showed a weak but significant association with patient satisfaction, taking as much as five years to develop. The intensity of contacts showed a lesser, not significant association with patient satisfaction.

No significant associations were found between the age or gender of the patient or doctor and satisfaction with the consultation, or the stability or location of the practice, or the type of partnership (Table 5.2). The patient had, however, a significantly increased chance of being satisfied with doctors on a fee for service system as compared with salaried doctors.

There was a significant relation between the doctor's availability, as measured by hours of curative practice a week, and patient satisfaction with the consultation. A doctor spending 40 hours a week at the office had an 82% increased chance of patients being satisfied with the consultation as compared with a doctor working only 20 curative hours a week. Patients with psychosocial reasons for their encounter showed significantly less satisfaction with their consultations than patients with somatic problems.

Discussion

The sevenfold odds ratio shown in the present study is substantial and suggests a close linkage between personal care and patient satisfaction. There may be several explanations for this finding. It may be an artefact of study design. In spite of the high response rate and the representativeness of the sample, response bias may have influenced the result, in that non-responders tend to be less satisfied (Harris 1978).

Personal care and satisfaction are related cognitive constructs that may be mixed by the respondents. To reduce the possibility of measuring the same thing the constructs were evaluated through independent questions and on separate pages of the questionnaire. From interviews with respondents in the pilot phase we believe that this source of error did not have a great role.

In this study we used an approach that was both direct and specific to the episode to evaluate patient satisfaction. These are generally accepted methods of eliciting patient satisfaction but tend to give high ratings (Pascoe 1983; Fitzpatrick 1991b). As shown in Table 5.1, 82% of the patients were to a large degree satisfied with their primary care encounter. The cut-off point between satisfied and less satisfied, between two and three on the six-point scale we used, was arbitrary. As 76–84% levels of satisfaction have been found in most other studies (Hall and Dornan 1988), this seems to be a valid demarcation.

A major reason for the strong link between personal care and patient satisfaction may be found in an understanding of the psychosocial mechanisms underlying satisfaction (Pascoe 1983). In the present setting satisfaction may be understood as the patients' reaction to a conscious or subconscious standard, set before and usually influenced by a subjective average of past experiences in similar situations (Pascoe 1983). With continuity of care and accumulated knowledge about the specific physician and consultation setting, the patient's standards may be set more realistically and major discrepancies between expectation and experience may be less common, thus increasing the likelihood of satisfaction. The personal connections that frequently develop in an ongoing patient–doctor relationship (McWhinney 1989) may widen the latitudes of acceptance around the patient's standard, increasing the chance of satisfaction.

In addition to continuity leading to increased satisfaction, satisfaction ratings predict what patients will do next time they need health services (Marquis *et al.* 1983). In all primary health care systems, incompatibility may cause patients to use their 'exit' options and change doctors (Hirschman 1970); some of the increase in satisfaction that takes place over time, as seen in Table 5.2, may be related to this. Unsatisfied patients who often change doctors have short patient–doctor relationships. After trial and error the patient may find a doctor fitting his or her own style and standard, causing the significant increase in satisfaction found with longitudinal care.

Patients with psychosocial reasons for the encounter showed significantly less satisfaction with their consultations than patients coming for other, usually somatic reasons. This may be due to the possibility that patients with psychosocial problems actually get inferior care. Psychosocial problems may be more time-consuming, complex and difficult for the physician to handle than somatic problems, or the patients may have unrealistic expectations of help (Pascoe 1983). The patient–doctor relationship and continuity of care are integral parts in both diagnosis and treatment for patients with psychosocial problems (Murphy 1989); it seems important therefore to evaluate further why these patients are less satisfied with their consultations.

The present study shows a link between personal, continuous care and patient satisfaction. If patient satisfaction is accepted as an integral part of quality health care, reinforcing personal care may be one way of increasing this quality.

References

Banahan, B.F. and Banahan, B.F. III. (1981) 'Continuity as an attitudinal contract', *Journal of Family Practice*, 12: 767–8.

Fitzpatrick, R. (1991a) 'Surveys of patient satisfaction. II. Designing a questionnaire and conducting a survey', *British Medical Journal*, 302: 1129–32.

Fitzpatrick, R. (1991b) 'Surveys of patient satisfaction. I. Important general considerations', *British Medical Journal*, 302: 887–9.

Fitzpatrick, R., Hopkin, A. and Harvard-Watts, O. (1983) 'Social dimensions of healing: a longitudinal study of outcomes of medical management of headaches', *Social Science and Medicine*, 17: 501–10.

Freeman, G.K. (1984) 'Continuity of care in general practice: a review and a critique', *Family Practice*, 1: 245–52.

Hall, J.A. and Dornan, M.C. (1988) 'Meta-analysis of satisfaction with medical care: description of research domain and analysis of overall satisfaction levels', *Social Science and Medicine*, 27: 637–44.

Harris, R. (1978) 'Improving patient satisfaction through action research', *Journal of Applied Behavioural Science*, 14: 382–99.

Hirschman, A.O. (1970) *Exit, Voice and Loyalty: Responses to Decline in Firms, Organizations and States*, Cambridge, MA: Harvard University Press.

Hjortdahl, P. and Borchgrevink, C.F. (1991) 'Continuity of care: influence of general practitioners' knowledge about their patients on use of resources in consultations', *British Medical Journal*, 303: 1181–4.

Hosmor, D.W. and Lemeshow, S. (1989) *Applied Logistic Regression*, New York: Wiley.

Lamberts, H. and Wood, M. (1987) *ICPC: International Classification of Primary Care*, Oxford: Oxford University Press.

McWhinney, I.R. (1989) *A Textbook of Family Medicine*, New York: Oxford University Press.

Marquis, M.S., Davies, A.R. and Ware, I.E. (1983) 'Patient satisfaction and change in medical care provider: a longitudinal study', *Medical Care*, 21: 821–9.

Murphy, M. (1989) 'Somatisation: embodying the problem', *British Medical Journal*, 298: 1331–2.

Pascoe, G.C. (1983) 'Patient satisfaction in primary health care: a literature review and analysis', *Evaluation and Program Planning*, 6: 185–210.

Roter, D., Hall, J. and Katz, N. (1987) 'Relations between physicians' behaviours and analogue patients' satisfaction, recall, and impressions', *Medical Care*, 25: 437–51.

Rutle, O. (1983) *Pasienten fram i lyset – analyse av legekontaktar I primæhelsetenesta* [Getting the patient into the limelight: an analysis of encounters in primary health care], Oslo: Staten Intitutt for Folkehelse (Report No. 1/1983).

Ware, J. and Snyder, M. (1975) 'Dimensions of patient attitudes regarding doctors and medical services', *Medical Care*, 13: 669–79.

This article can be found complete, and unedited as Hjortdahl, P. and Lærum, E., 'Continuity of care in general practice: effect on patient satisfaction', in the *British Medical Journal*, Volume 304, May 1992, pages 1287–90.

Part 2

Patient- and Carer-Centred Services: user involvement in organising services

Introduction

The importance of patient involvement in most aspects of health care is increasingly recognised. In the UK NHS, the 'expert patient' programme has been running for a number of years and has trained many people in how to become an expert in their own disease. In a similar programme, the DAFNE (Dose Adjustment for Normal Eating) trial is testing a new approach to diabetes management, which trains people with type 1 diabetes to take greater control of their condition. This programme is described by the organisation Diabetes UK, as a programme which 'teaches people how to adjust their insulin doses to fit with their own lifestyle, rather than having to bend what they do and eat to a preset insulin regimen'. There are also now substantial programmes of research and development into decision aids which allow people to take decisions about their own care. Nearly 500 decision aids are listed in the Cochrane Database of Decision Aids, covering a wide variety of diseases and interventions, from warts and acne to prostate cancer screening and breast cancer surgery. In the United States and Canada, the Foundation for Informed Decision Making and the Ottawa Health Decision Center (OHDEC) at the Ottawa Health Research Institute have led the way in designing and collating information about decision aids. And the World Wide Web allows unprecedented access to health information, which is widely used.

Despite all this effort, many patients feel unable to communicate with their health carers. Studies of compliance with medication suggest that high proportions simply do not take medicines at the times or in the doses in which they are prescribed. And although measured satisfaction with health services has until recently appeared to be uniformly high, more sophisticated measures now demonstrate that dissatisfaction is also high among some groups of patients. There has been an approach to 'user involvement' which suggests that it is invariably a good thing. However, newer approaches incorporate an awareness that while there may be variation in the extent of desire to be involved in decisions about one's own care, the aim is an outcome which accurately reflects the values and preferences of the user not the carer.

In this section we look at user involvement and user's views of health care in a variety of different settings. Preston and colleagues highlight the importance of identifying patients' feelings about their clinical and personal progress and describe some of the issues involved in negotiating health care across boundaries. In a qualitative study of 33 patients who had recent experience of hospital care, they found that people identified 'getting in' to the health care system, 'fitting in', 'knowing what's going on' and 'continuity' as the important issues for making progress in the system. Sadly the last theme that they identified was 'limbo' where some patients felt let down, unable to make progress and as though they may have been forgotten. As one patient in this paper describes, 'the system rolls on whether you're there or not ... '.

In their article on chemotherapy for lung cancer, Silvestri and colleagues describe the sophisticated awareness which people bring to trade-offs between life expectancy and reductions in quality of life due to chemotherapy. They used vignettes to undertake time trade-off studies on the length of time people with lung cancer would buy in exchange for different chemotherapy regimens with differing side effects and toxicity. They found substantial variation in choices based in heuristic approaches adopted by patients and report one patient who chose chemotherapy for a week's survival benefit. He hypothesised that a 'cure' might appear in that week and he 'wouldn't want to miss that!'.

In a systematic review of decision aids for patients facing health treatment decisions, O'Connor and colleagues considered randomised controlled trials of interventions providing structured and specific information on treatment options and outcomes. They concluded that decision aids improve knowledge, reduce decisional conflict and stimulate patients to be more active in decision making. However, the evidence on whether decision aids actually improve health outcomes is still not clear. And there is now some debate as to whether decision aids should be expected to improve health outcomes rather than the 'fit' of the individual treatment pattern to the individual patient's views.

Brown and colleagues describe other methods for improving the 'fit' of the individual treatment pattern to the individual patient's views. In particular they found that a prompt sheet for the cancer consultations nearly doubled the number of questions that patients asked compared with a control group. The prompt sheet includes such questions as, 'What kind of cancer have I got?', 'Will my sexual life be affected by my treatments?' and 'If we get rid of the cancer, what are the chances of it coming back?'.

These articles all take the individual patient as their unit of consideration but there are potential problems with this approach for health systems. It is not clear how to balance the contributions of the evidence base, the epidemiology of different conditions, the patient's own values and preferences (patient choice) and the health system's resource constraints. What might represent best practice at a population level in this context of enhanced user involvement?

In the final paper, Ann Bowling describes involving users – the public – in the health care rationing debate in the UK. She asked a random sample of the population to prioritise types of health care. She found that age was important: life-saving treatments for children were ranked in first place while life-saving treatments for those over 75 years of age were ranked much lower. Health promotion was given a middle to low ranking. She suggests that 'if the public's values seem to conflict with firm medical evidence on effectiveness or ... be prejudiced against certain groups, then open debate and the provision of sound information ... is even more essential'.

Chapter 6

Left in limbo: patients' views on care across the primary/ secondary interface

Carolyn Preston, Francine Cheater, Richard Baker and Hilary Hearnshaw

Abstract

Objectives: To discover the views of patients about their experiences across the interface between primary and secondary health care, including referral from general practitioners, outpatient and inpatient care, discharge and aftercare.

Design: A qualitative study involving individual and focus group interviews of patients and interviews of carers.

Subjects: 33 patients who had attended at least one outpatient appointment or had been an inpatient between two and four months previously, and eight carers of patients with chronic conditions.

Setting: Three acute hospitals and one community health service in Leicestershire.

Main outcome measures: Common themes in the views of patients and carers towards their experiences of care.

Results: Five themes emerged. The first four were: 'getting in' (access to appropriate care), 'fitting in' (orientation of care to the patient's requirements), 'knowing what's going on' (provision of information), and 'continuity' (continuity of staff and co-ordination and communication among professionals). The fifth theme was limbo (difficulty in making progress through the system), which was influenced by failures in care relation to the other four themes.

Conclusions: The concept of progress is central to patients' view of care. It involves both progress through the health care system and progress towards recovery or adjustment to an altered health state. Patients' views on how well they progress through the health care system may be an appropriate indicator for monitoring health care performance.

Source: *Quality in Health Care*, 8, 1999, 16–21.

Introduction

One reason for the reforms of health systems in different countries has been the need to control costs by ensuring that patients' care is managed effectively but in the least expensive settings. In the National Health Service (NHS) in the UK, costs are controlled to some degree through general practitioners' (GP) 'gate-keeping' function, although this can create problems of disjunction between primary and secondary care services. In the UK, there has been increased interest in improving co-ordination across the interface between primary and secondary care.

At the same time, the health service is seeking to become more responsive to the views of patients. However, methods of assessing patients' views have been criticised. Often measures are not based on the values and experiences of the patients themselves (Avis *et al.* 1995) and may exaggerate the importance of amenities such as food or facilities at the expense of more important issues such as outcome and relationship with professionals (Scott and Smith 1994; Cleary and Edgman-Levitan 1997). The lack of an accepted theory to explain what 'patient satisfaction' means to the patient and its implications for health care present a particular problem because it is difficult to access the validity of a measure when it is not clear what is being measured (Wensing *et al.* 1994; Baker 1997). Thus, before developing a measure of patients' views, the variety of those views and the relationships between them should be identified.

Although many studies of aspects of patient satisfaction in different health settings have been undertaken, the systematic investigation of patients' experiences of pathways of care, through the health care system, is comparatively limited. In one such survey in the UK, an instrument originally developed in the USA was used (Bruster *et al.* 1994), but patients in the UK experience a different health care system and may have different perspectives.

In this paper, we describe a study to identify and describe patients' views about their experiences of the health care system. It was the first stage of a project to develop a new instrument to measure patients' views across the interface. The findings in this paper were used to generate a pool of items for inclusion in the instrument. To avoid making assumptions about patients' views, we undertook a qualitative study.

Methods

Focus groups and interviews

Focus groups and interviews were the methods of data collection. The purpose of focus groups is to 'determine the perceptions, feelings, and manner of thinking of consumers about products, services or opportunities' (Krueger 1990). Their advantage is that they enable participants to discuss and compare experiences, allowing exploration of different points of view, often leading to the generation of additional information or unanticipated topics for discussion. When attendance at a focus group was not possible, participants were offered an interview in their own home.

Selection of participants

Lists of patients who had attended their first outpatient appointment, or had been discharged from the hospital two and four months before, were obtained from the registers of three acute hospitals and one provider of community health services in Leicestershire. Seven GPs also provided lists of patients they had referred to outpatient departments between four and six months previously. Lists included basic details including age, sex, and the speciality which the patient attended or was referred to. From these, we selected a smaller, random sample and undertook purposeful sampling to recruit patients who might hold a range of views about their care. Patients were selected to ensure that they were from a wide range of clinical specialities and there was a mix of men and women and different age groups. We had limited information about patients' socioeconomic background but postcodes were used as a guide in selecting a range of patients (the range of Jarman scores (Jarman 1985) of patients' practices reflected this, although these may be an insensitive measure of individual patient's socioeconomic status). Patients less than 16 years of age, emergency admissions or those attending accident and emergency (which usually involves self-referral), maternity services and those receiving palliative care were excluded. Before inviting patients to take part, GPs were asked to exclude those who were too ill.

A sample of carers of relatives with chronic health conditions including respiratory disease, renal disease and psychiatric conditions (who met the study criteria), unrelated to the patient participants, was also identified through three local carers' groups.

Letters to recruit patients were translated into Gujerati or Hindi when appropriate, and an interpreter and single sex groups were also offered. A topic guide was developed and assessed in a pilot group. It contained open questions and prompts relating to what happened and how the patient felt in relation to progress through the health system. The topic guide was also used in the individual patient interviews, and in modified form in the care interviews. The groups were moderated by one researcher with a second as an assistant (Krueger 1990). All interviews were undertaken by Carolyn Preston. Groups and interviews were continued until no new ideas emerged. All group and individual interviews were tape recorded.

Analysis

All tapes were fully transcribed. Transcripts were analysed using the constant comparative method (Strauss and Corbin 1990) to generate themes and concepts that consistently emerged within the data. Two researchers independently developed coding schemes, and any differences between them were resolved through discussion. All transcripts were then coded to support analysis, using Ethnograph (v3.0) to assist data handling. Five main themes were identified. Throughout data analysis all four researchers conferred regularly and checked the original transcripts for inconsistencies and alternatives to ensure that the process of analysis and interpretations was consistent (Baker *et al.* 1999).

Results

Six focus groups involving 28 patients were held, and five patients and eight carers were interviewed in their own homes. The findings are presented under the five main themes that emerged from the analysis of the qualitative data of both the patients and carers. The themes are labelled in the words frequently used by patients/carers to describe their experiences.

(1) Getting in

This theme comprised responses about gaining access to appropriate care, and included obtaining appointments, being referred, hospital admission procedures and receiving after-care. When access was fully negotiated, patients talked not only of gaining entry to the health care system but also being able to make progress through it.

Patients and carers identified various factors that facilitated or delayed access and their subsequent progress through the system. For example, the attitudes of reception staff in practices and outpatient clinics were often identified as presenting barriers, the consequences of which made patients feel 'in the way' or 'a nuisance'.

Good patient–doctor relationships were associated with fewer barriers to referral. Patients were generally less confident about being referred, or receiving appropriate treatment, when they were unable to see their personal doctor, or when the relationship with their GP was poor. The need for their problems to be recognised as legitimate was viewed by patients as essential, determining the speed with which they gained access to care. Delays in referral and treatment were often associated with chronic health problems (for example, persistent back pain), stigmatising conditions (for example, mental illness or alcohol dependency), and problems thought to be of psychological or social origin. For some patients this led to a mismatch between their expectations and the actions of their doctor:

'It's all subjective, pain in the back, so you feel that perhaps they don't believe you if they can't see it or feel it.' (patient)

Gaining access to the appropriate care was often accompanied by feelings of intense relief, even in circumstances when quite serious conditions had been diagnosed. Being successful at 'getting in' affirmed patients' legitimacy to investigation and treatment, and enabled them to begin to make progress through the health system:

'I was in a lot of pain and was not really noticed until the person who took me said "I think he's having a heart attack" – "oh right we'll look at you in a minute, not half an hour". They did the tests and said "yes you are having a heart attack". I was quite relieved at this stage, I thought "Oh good, I'm glad I'm not wasting your time!"' (patient)

(2) Fitting in

This theme was concerned with the extent to which health care settings and routines took account of the needs of patients and the extent to which the patient had to 'fit in' with the service. If doctors, nurses and other staff were perceived as caring and responsive to an individual patient's needs, respondents talked about being comfortable, confident, and the system 'fitting in' with their requirements. Responses also reflected a desire for care to be provided in ways that preserved dignity and privacy, which in turn increased confidence.

When care was perceived to be impersonal and organised according to the routines of staff or the organisation, patients commonly described feeling anxious, insignificant and powerless. In these situations, patients described having to fit in with a system that appeared to take no account of them as people:

'I think you feel a bit like an accessory, the system rolls on whether you're there or not ... as a patient I thought the system was there because of you, not you there because of the system' (patient)

Patients'–carers' and staff relationships were influenced by the organisational context in which they interacted. Relationships with GPs were often built up over a period of time, and, consequently, respondents often felt that they had access to information and had some degree of participation in decisions about their care. In comparison, relationships with hospital doctors tended to be viewed as more impersonal, interactions being of limited duration and presenting fewer opportunities for sharing information and participating in decisions about care.

(3) Knowing what's going on

Patients and carers wanted understandable and consistent information, presented in an honest and sympathetic way. Not knowing what to expect produced feelings of uncertainty and anxiety. This was most evident when patients were waiting for the results of investigations or for a diagnosis to be confirmed. When appropriate, timely information was provided, patients were reassured, gained confidence, and felt they had some degree of control over what happened to them.

When information was lacking, patients and carers often described feelings of 'being stuck' in the system and unable to make progress:

> 'When I came to the (hospital) they didn't have anyone come and see you. Nobody knew what to expect, and ... that was distressing people more than anything else, they knew they were going in for major surgery, but they didn't know what to expect at all.' (patient)

The quality of staff–patient relationships was a major factor influencing the accessibility of information, as described in the theme 'fitting in'. Patients and carers tended to find it easier to obtain information from their GPs, whereas in hospital settings barriers to communication were related to perceptions of lack of staff time and inequality in status between hospital consultants and their patients.

Lack of information perpetuated patients' feelings of an imbalance in status and power, and reduced their sense of being involved in their own care.

When information was not readily given, or perceived to be inadequate, patients or carers often used strategies to find out more, including preparing lists of questions to ask during their consultations, arguing with doctors or other staff, and getting others, particularly those with inside knowledge of the NHS, to act for them.

(4) Continuity

Continuity was achieved through receiving care from a particular professional throughout the care process, and receiving consistent, co-ordinated care from different staff working together. Seeing the same professional made patients feel that there was someone who was interested in them and would take time to listen. Patients recognised that continuity could facilitate the progress of treatment because the professional had sufficient background information and knowledge of their case.

When care was provided across different settings, communication and co-ordination were crucial. Lack of consistency across settings was a frequent source of problems; for example, patients receiving conflicting information from their GP and the consultant. This could prevent patients making progress and could result in reduced confidence in care providers, increasing anxiety, and feelings of not being valued as individuals. The co-ordination of different services, and the degree to which care continued across interfaces, were important preconditions for the smooth progress of patients through the system. Sometimes GPs were not informed of outcomes of their patients' treatment or care:

> '*Separate clinics don't talk to each other or ring each other. Waiting weeks to see a consultant to be told "I don't know why you've been referred to me . . . ". It can make you feel very insignificant.*' (patient)

(5) Limbo

Limbo described a state in which patients felt they were not making progress and were unable to take action to progress onwards through the system. Limbo was precipitated by poor experiences in any of the four other themes. The main features that characterised the feeling of limbo were: an indefinite period of waiting, with uncertainty about what to expect or what would happen next; a feeling of being unimportant and insignificant; and a feeling of powerlessness and loss of control over what was happening.

Limbo was most often experienced as patients moved from one stage of care to another across interfaces or between professionals, or when awaiting the results of investigations or decisions about their management. At these times, they could experience feelings of discomfort and uncertainty which were exacerbated by lack of information or failures of continuity.

Relationship between the themes

The central issue which emerged from the views of patients and carers is the concept of progress. Patients perceive themselves as making progress through the health care system, which begins with care from the GP and goes on to include outpatient, inpatient and after-care. From the patient's perspective, however, progress is more than a temporal sequence of events within a system; it also includes the patient's passage from illness to recovery, or if recovery is not possible, psychological and social adjustment to an altered state of health. Failures within the system may not only delay the patient's clinical progress but may also have consequences for psychological progress, one feature of which can be the feelings associated with limbo, such as anxiety and powerlessness. In contrast, efficient progress through the system leads to feelings of confidence and reassurance. The theme patients identified as limbo reflects their psychological or emotional reaction to the extent of their progress.

Failures in any of the first four themes can cause progress through the system to be delayed, and can also have a negative impact on psychological progress, giving rise to feelings of limbo. For example, patients' progress through the system can be obstructed by failures in co-ordination of the system, and delayed by obstructive receptionists or failure of the GP to recognise that referral is required. Even where progress through the system is not obstructed, however, lack of information or poor relationships with health care staff may cause patients to feel that they are failing to make any progress. Also, lack of information or poor relationships with staff can leave patients and carers feeling powerless to challenge failures in the system. Those patients who felt able to take action to resume their progress through the system and escape from limbo often relied on their carer or a friend to act on their behalf.

Discussion

We investigated the views of a group of patients and carers of their recent experiences of the health care system. We identified five common themes underlying these views and developed a preliminary model to describe the relationship between them. Other studies that have examined patients' views of their health care in different settings have identified themes which are similar to those of this study (Ware *et al.* 1978; Delbanco 1992; Aharonay and Strasser 1993; Wensing *et al.* 1994; Barr 1995; Hall and Dornan 1998). For example, themes relating to access to services (getting in), orientation of care to the patient's needs (fitting in), information and communication (knowing what's going on) and continuity of care were identified in both hospital and primary care. In this study these four themes emerged consistently, suggesting that regardless of setting, these dimensions of care are of central importance to patients. In our study, patients were asked about experiences through the health care system as a whole, which provided an insight into how experiences at one stage of care related to experiences at later stages. In particular, this study identified that poor experiences associated with any of the four themes could lead to feelings of 'limbo', a state in which patients perceived that their progress through the system was prevented or delayed.

This study was qualitative and cannot identify the numbers of patients that had particular views. Nevertheless, the model has practical implications for health providers in primary and secondary care. The findings indicate that patients experience care across the interface as a clinical and personal path or journey in which they make progress towards a particular goal. The needs of each patient in reaching their goal may be different, and the actions of professionals or organisation of the system, or both, can assist or obstruct that progress. Rather than simply focusing on clinical progress, health professionals should check whether their patients feel they are making progress, and consider what steps may be needed to promote it. For example, some patients may require additional information, some may need the professional to listen to their concerns about their illness, and some may require organisational arrangements to ensure continuity. Health professionals also need to recognise the interdependency of their roles within the health system as a whole if patients are to avoid the fragmented care that frequently leads to limbo.

The findings also suggest that services should be organised to avoid system failures that cause patients to feel in limbo. The identification of the most appropriate organisational structures for delivering care should be investigated in studies that include measurement of patients' views. Measures that concentrate on amenities such as food and cleanliness, however, will not provide information about issues of central concern to patients. Even asking for factual reports about accessibility or continuity may fail to identify patients' feelings about their clinical and personal progress.

Acknowledgements

We are grateful to all the patients and carers who took part and the staff who facilitated access.

The study was funded by the NHS R&D programme (primary/secondary interface) project reference 01-26.

References

Aharonay, L. and Strasser, S. (1993) 'Patient satisfaction: what we know about and what we still need to explore', *Medical Care Review*, 50: 49–79.

Avis, M., Bond, M. and Arthur, A. (1995) 'Satisfying solutions? A review of some unresolved issues in the measurement of patient satisfaction', *Journal of Advanced Nursing*, 22: 316–22.

Baker, R. (1997) 'Pragmatic model of patient satisfaction in general practice: progress towards a theory', *Quality in Health Care*, 6: 201–4.

Baker R., Preston, C., Cheater, F. and Hearnshaw, H. (1999) 'Measuring patients' attitudes to care across the primary/secondary interface: development of the patient career diary', *Quality in Health Care Volume*, 8: 154–61.

Barr, D. (1995) 'The effects of organizational structure on primary care outcomes under managed care', *American College of Physicians*, 122: 353–9.

Bruster, S., Jarman, B., Bosanquet, N., Weston, D., Erens, R. and Delbanco, T.L. (1994) 'National survey of hospital patients', *British Medical Journal*, 309: 1542–9.

Cleary, P.D. and Edgman-Levitan, S. (1997) 'Health care quality. Incorporating consumer perspectives', *Journal of the American Medical Association*, 278: 1608–12.

Delbanco, T.L. (1992) 'Enriching the doctor-patient relationship by inviting the patient's perspective', *Annals of Internal Medicine*, 116: 414–18.

Hall, J.A. and Dornan, M.C. (1998) 'What patients like about their medical care and how often they are asked: a meta-analysis of the satisfaction literature', *Social Science and Medicine*, 27: 935–9.

Jarman, B. (1985) 'Underprivileged areas', in D.J.P. Gray (ed.) *The Medical Annual*, Bristol: Wright.

Krueger, R.A. (1990) *Focus Groups: A Practical Guide for Applied Research*, Newbury Park: Sage Publications.

Scott, A. and Smith, R.D. (1994) 'Keeping the customer satisfied: issues in the interpretation and use of patient satisfaction surveys', *International Journal of Quality in Health Care*, 6: 353–9.

Strauss, A. and Corbin, J. (1990) *Basics of Qualitative Research. Grounded Theory Procedures and Techniques*, Newbury Park: Sage Publications.

Ware, J.E., Davies-Avery, A. and Stewart, A.L. (1978) 'The measurement and meaning of patient satisfaction', *Health and Medical Care Services Review*, 1: 1–7.

Wensing, M., Grol, R. and Smits, A. (1994) 'Quality judgments by patients on general practice care: a literature analysis', *Social Science and Medicine*, 38: 45–53.

A complete, unedited version of this article can be found as Preston, C., Cheater, F., Baker, R. and Hearnshaw, H., 'Left in limbo: patients' views on care across the primary/secondary interface' in *Quality in Health Care* (1999) Volume 8, pages 16–21.

Chapter 7

Preferences for chemotherapy in patients with advanced non-small cell lung cancer: descriptive study based on scripted interviews

Gerard Silvestri, Robert Pritchard and H. Gilbert Welch

Abstract

This paper determined how patients with lung cancer valued the trade-off between the survival benefit of chemotherapy and its toxicity. It involved scripted interviews that included three hypothetical scenarios with 81 patients previously treated with chemotherapy. The study found that the minimum survival threshold for accepting the toxicity of chemotherapy varied widely. Many patients would not choose chemotherapy for a likely survival benefit of three months, but would if it improved quality of life.

Introduction

Lung cancer is a common disease that is difficult to treat successfully. In the United States each year about 178,000 people are diagnosed with lung cancer and about 160,000 die of the disease, making it the leading cause of cancer-related mortality (Parker *et al.* 1997). In the UK the death rate from lung cancer is similarly high, and it is even higher in eastern Europe and Russia. Most patients have non-small cell lung cancer and the majority of them have metastatic disease – either at the time the disease is diagnosed or during the course of their illness (Ginsberg *et al.* 1993). Median survival is only about four months in untreated patients with metastatic non-small cell lung cancer (Grilli *et al.* 1993).

Several meta-analyses concluded that chemotherapy is effective in the treatment of metastatic non-small cell lung cancer (Souquet *et al.* 1993; Marino *et al.* 1994). The impact of chemotherapy on survival is limited, however; median survival is improved by about 1.5–3 months. Based on

Source: *British Medical Journal*, 317, 1998, 771–5.

these data some authors advocate chemotherapy as standard treatment for all patients with metastatic non-small cell lung cancer. Other authors are more cautious in their interpretation in the absence of additional information on quality of life and the informed preferences of patients for the expected effects of treatment. Although most patients in the UK with metastatic non-small cell lung cancer are not considered for cytotoxic chemotherapy, many such patients are in the USA.

Although patient preferences have been systematically examined in breast cancer (Richards *et al.* 1995), little is known about how lung cancer patients value the potential benefits and risks of chemotherapy. Therefore, we assessed the treatment preferences of a group of patients who recently completed a course of chemotherapy for non-small cell lung cancer. We determined the minimum survival benefit necessary before they would accept a treatment regimen with its associated toxicity.

Subjects and methods

Subjects

All study subjects had advanced (stage III or IV) non-small cell lung cancer diagnosed histologically and had received at least one cycle of cis-platinum-based chemotherapy (with or without radiotherapy). To ensure that responses were not influenced by recently experienced side effects, subjects were interviewed at least one month after completion of chemotherapy. Subjects with known or suspected brain metastases were excluded.

The subjects were recruited from three practice settings: the cancer centre at the Medical University of South Carolina, two departments of veteran affairs medical centres (White River Junction, VT and Charleston, SC), and two community office practices (Hilton Head, SC and Charleston, SC).

Interview structure

Each interview followed the same format. Subjects were initially asked five questions about their understanding of treatment options before chemotherapy and their experience during chemotherapy. In addition they were asked to rate their overall quality of life during chemotherapy as either excellent, very good, good, fair, or poor. They were then given three scenarios, each describing the same hypothetical patient: a woman with advanced metastatic lung cancer who has been told by her physician that she has an incurable illness and an expected survival without treatment of approximately four months. The scenarios were presented in the following order.

- **Scenario 1: mild toxicity** – In this scenario chemotherapy was described as producing mild side effects and as being well tolerated. The side effects lasted several days after the treatment cycle and comprised nausea, fatigue and occasional diarrhoea. The benefits of treatment were not discussed.
- **Scenario 2: severe toxicity** – In this scenario chemotherapy was described as producing severe side effects and included the potential need for hospitalisation and a 1 per cent chance of death. The side effects lasted several days after the treatment cycle, but were more numerous than in the first scenario: fatigue and weakness, poor appetite, mouth sores, diarrhoea, infection and fever. Again, the benefits of treatment were not discussed.

Subjects were asked to choose the minimum survival benefit required to accept chemotherapy for the treatment of metastatic lung cancer in these two scenarios. As in previous studies of patient preferences for cancer treatment, a modification of the time trade-off approach was used (Yellen *et al.* 1994; McQuellon *et al.* 1995). Briefly, after hearing the scenario the subject was asked: 'If you were this patient would you agree to this standard treatment if it added one week to your life?'. If the answer was 'no' the question was repeated substituting one month for one week. The process was repeated using different survival durations (3, 6, 12, 18 and 24 months) until the subject judged the benefit to be of sufficient importance to warrant the side effects.

- **Scenario 3: supportive care versus chemotherapy** – In this scenario the benefit of treatment was made explicit. The hypothetical patient is offered the choice between supportive care (average survival four months) and chemotherapy (average survival seven months). She is told that supportive care addresses a patient's comfort needs (and may include radiation) and that its goal is to alleviate pain and other symptoms associated with cancer. She is told about both the mild and severe side effects of chemotherapy and that her chance of experiencing severe side effects is 20 per cent. After this scenario the subject was asked: 'If you were this patient which would you choose, supportive care or chemotherapy?'. In addition, subjects were asked: 'If you were this patient would you take this treatment if it did not prolong your life but significantly reduced the pain and other symptoms that might be related to your cancer?'. Finally, to determine their willingness to be randomised to either supportive care or chemotherapy, subjects were asked: 'Would you allow a flip of the coin to determine which therapy you would receive?'.

Analysis

For scenarios 1 and 2 we recorded the shortest survival duration at which each subject chose chemotherapy. We then constructed a cumulative distribution of the percentage of subjects choosing chemotherapy as a function of the additional survival offered by chemotherapy (Figure 7.1).

Because we only provided seven discrete survival categories (1 week, and 1, 3, 6, 12, 18 and 24 months) we were unable to determine precisely the survival duration at which each subject was indifferent to the choice presented. To estimate this threshold value for each subject we averaged the longest survival duration for which chemotherapy was rejected with the shortest survival duration for which chemotherapy was accepted. For example, if a subject rejected chemotherapy when offered 6 months' survival benefit and accepted chemotherapy when offered 12 months' survival benefit then the threshold value was 9 months. This survival threshold was used both to characterise patient subgroups (Table 7.1) and to stratify the proportion choosing best supportive care in scenario 3 (Figure 7.2).

Three subjects rejected chemotherapy even when offered 24 months' survival benefit in the mild toxicity scenario (scenario 1), as did six subjects in the severe toxicity scenario (scenario 2). Because we did not ask about periods longer than 24 months we do not have the survival duration for which chemotherapy is acceptable in these individuals, and thus we are unable to estimate the threshold value. For the purposes of the statistical

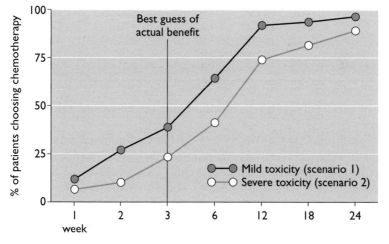

Figure 7.1 Treatment preferences for 81 patients who had had chemotherapy for lung cancer. Relation between additional survival offered and percentage of patients choosing chemotherapy is shown for mild toxicity (scenario 1) and severe toxicity (scenario 2).

Table 7.1 Responses to three scenarios by patient subgroups (*P* values are for differences across subgroups)

Patient subgroup	No. (%) of patients	Median survival threshold for accepting chemotherapy (months)		Percentage of patients choosing supportive care: scenario 3
		Scenario 1 (mild toxicity)	Scenario 2 (severe toxicity)	
All patients	81 (100)	4.50	9.00	78.00
Age (years)				
<60	31 (38)	2.00	4.50	65.00
60–70	30 (37)	4.50	9.00	87.00
>70	20 (25)	4.50	9.00	85.00
P value		0.14	0.01	0.07
Sex				
Men	54 (67)	4.50	9.00	74.00
Women	27 (33)	4.50	9.00	85.00
P value		0.23	0.32	0.28
Treatment setting				
University cancer centre	29 (36)	9.00	9.00	86.00
Community practice	29 (36)	2.00	9.00	72.00
Veterans' medical centre	23 (28)	4.50	4.50	74.00
P value		0.19	0.10	0.39
Self-assessed quality of life during chemotherapy				
Excellent	8 (10)	4.50	6.80	87.00
Very good	23 (28)	4.50	9.00	70.00
Good	22 (27)	3.30	4.50	68.00
Fair	15 (19)	4.50	9.00	87.00
Poor	13 (16)	9.00	15.00	92.00
P value		0.01	0.01	0.31

tests we arbitrarily assigned 24 months as the threshold value for these patients.

We used the Kruskal–Wallis test for the two nominal subgroups (sex, treatment setting) and the non-parametric test of trend for the two ordered subgroups (age, quality of life), to compare median survival thresholds (scenarios 1 and 2) across patient subgroups. We used the χ^2 test for the nominal subgroups and χ^2 test of trend for the ordered subgroups (including the subgroups in Figure 7.2) for differences across patient subgroups in scenario 3. All analyses were performed with STATA 4.0 (College Station, TX, USA).

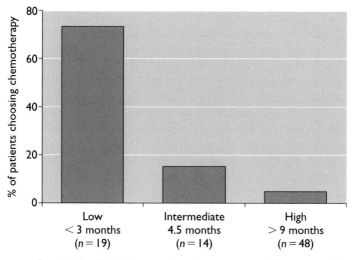

Survival threshold for accepting chemotherapy with severe toxicity

Figure 7.2 Percentage of patients choosing chemotherapy instead of supportive care (scenario 3) stratified by their imputed survival threshold for accepting chemotherapy for severe toxicity (scenario 2). (χ^2 test of trend $P < 0.001$.) Overall, 78% of the patients chose supportive care.

Results

The 81 patients, all of whom had received chemotherapy for their lung cancer, agreed to discuss and therefore reconsider decisions for various survival durations. Although a few patients found the process difficult, all patients who started the survey were able to finish it. Generally we were able to solicit the responses to the three scenarios in less than 20 minutes per patient, although longer discussions often ensued.

Figure 7.1 shows the treatment preferences for the 81 patients in the scenarios including side effects: mild toxicity (scenario 1) and severe toxicity (scenario 2). The figure is a cumulative distribution of the percentage of patients choosing chemotherapy as a function of the survival benefit offered. As expected, for any given level of survival a higher proportion of patients chose chemotherapy in the mild toxicity scenario. Most surprising was the heterogeneity of the expressed preferences. In the setting of severe toxicity, for example, five (6 per cent) patients would choose chemotherapy for only 1 week's survival benefit while nine (11 per cent) would not choose the treatment even when offered 24 months' survival benefit. In both scenarios, however, less than half the patients would choose chemotherapy given the best guess of benefit – three months' additional survival.

Table 7.1 details the responses to the three scenarios and considers various patient subgroups. Overall, the median survival threshold for accepting chemotherapy was 4.5 months for mild toxicity and 9 months for severe toxicity. As might be expected, elderly patients tended to demand greater benefit before accepting chemotherapy – a trend which was significant when severe toxicity was presented. Sex and treatment setting had little relation to these thresholds. There was, however, a significant trend with self-assessed quality of life during chemotherapy: patients reporting lower quality of life during chemotherapy had higher thresholds for accepting chemotherapy.

When offered the choice between supportive care and chemotherapy (scenario 3), only 18 (22 per cent) patients chose chemotherapy. Figure 7.2 displays their responses stratified by the survival threshold imputed from scenario 2. As expected, patients with lower survival thresholds in scenario 2 were more likely to choose chemotherapy when offered a direct choice. Although only 18 (22 per cent) subjects chose chemotherapy for three months' improvement in survival, the majority ($n = 55$, 68 per cent) would choose chemotherapy if it substantially reduced symptoms without prolonging life.

The patients had strong views on chemotherapy. One patient who chose chemotherapy for only one week's survival benefit theorised that the cure for lung cancer could be discovered during that week – he wouldn't want to miss the opportunity to be cured, however remote. Conversely, a second patient who did not choose chemotherapy even when offered 24 months' survival benefit said that she had lived a full and productive life and would not want anything to interfere with the quality of time she had left. The resolve of these patients was also evidenced by our finding that only 14 (17 per cent) were willing to be randomised between supportive care and chemotherapy.

Discussion

Patients previously treated with chemotherapy vary considerably in their attitudes towards this treatment for advanced lung cancer. For some patients, even two years' survival benefit did not constitute a fair trade-off for the toxicities associated with chemotherapy. Other patients required very little, if any, increase in survival for chemotherapy to seem worthwhile. Most patients, however, expected more in return from chemotherapy than the best estimate of three months' survival benefit. Furthermore, when given the choice between chemotherapy and supportive care only a quarter of patients would choose chemotherapy if its benefit was only to prolong survival.

These results seem at odds with the care these patients previously received. All patients were treated with chemotherapy, so why would only a quarter of them make the same decision again? This disparity may reflect either problems with our method for assessing patient preferences or problems in the initial decision making process.

How patient preferences are assessed clearly matters. Several methods are available for assessing patient preferences, including the time trade-off and standard gamble (Sox *et al.* 1988). Although it is clear that different methods will often yield different results (Read *et al.* 1984; Nord 1992; Stiggelbout *et al.* 1994) it is less clear if any method accurately captures the patients' real attitudes toward different outcomes (Kassirer 1994). We did not use the classic time trade-off technique and our scenarios were not designed to elicit formal patient utilities for discrete health states. Rather, the scenarios were designed to be easily understood. We wanted to approximate what patients with metastatic lung cancer might be told by their physician and to allow a simple expression of their treatment preference. It is possible that our results would be different had we used a different method.

We are confident, however, that our approach for assessing patients' attitudes towards the trade-off between survival and toxicity was at least understood by the patients. The patients' responses were consistent. Each patient's survival threshold either remained stable or increased as the toxicity of treatment increased. In other words, no patient chose chemotherapy in scenario 2 (severe toxicity) for less survival time than they did in scenario 1 (mild toxicity). And although patients may have not understood in scenario 3 that chemotherapy can include the services of supportive care, there was a direct relation between the survival thresholds imputed from the first two scenarios and the choice of treatment in scenario 3.

The correct units for expressing the benefits of treatment may also matter. In our scenarios the benefits were expressed as an average gain in survival. And while it is true that for most patients chemotherapy improves survival in metastatic non-small cell lung cancer by no more than several months in the majority of patients, the use of averages may hide the fact that a few patients may benefit substantially. Since the framing of benefits can have important consequences on the choice of treatment (McNeil *et al.* 1982), it is possible that if we expressed the benefits of treatment differently we would have got different results. Whether the expression of a small chance of a big gain would have meaningfully changed our results is the subject of future investigation.

There may be other information besides toxicity, survival and quality of life that patients with terminal illnesses consider important when thinking about complex decisions. For example, fear of alienating family members or acting to maximise the chance of reaching some future landmark event (for example, a son or daughter's wedding) may overshadow quantitative estimates of survival. These types of considerations are not easily dealt with in our scenario-based decision making.

There may also be problems in the initial decision making process. Firstly, patients may have been unaware that there was a choice between supportive care and treatment with chemotherapy. Only a quarter of our subjects could recall having supportive care discussed as an option when they were originally diagnosed with advanced lung cancer. Secondly, it is possible that the patients were not properly informed about the risks and survival benefits of chemotherapy – either because the benefits of chemotherapy were portrayed as overly optimistic or because patients misunderstood or chose to ignore information about the expected size of the survival benefit. We did not, however, interview patients at the time of the initial decision. Had we done so our results may have been different (Slevin *et al.* 1990). Alternatively our results may simply reflect the patients' recent experience with chemotherapy – 'knowing what I know now, I wouldn't make the same choice'.

Implications

Our results have several important implications. The finding that most patients would not choose chemotherapy for a survival benefit of three months suggests that from the patient's perspective best supportive care is a realistic treatment option worthy of discussion. Yet there was also striking variation in the patients' willingness to accept cancer treatment that was potentially toxic. This finding, which has been seen in similar studies (Brundage *et al.* 1997) reinforces the notion that for patients there is no right or wrong answer. When different patients value alternative treatment options differently, clinical rules or protocols based on average preferences will not be effective in helping patients select the treatment they actually want. And while guidelines may be useful tools for synthesising the scientific evidence used to formulate clinical decisions, they cannot obviate the need for good compassionate clinical decision making that is responsive to patients' values.

But patients also care about more than survival when faced with difficult choices. Although most of the patients who participated in this study would not choose chemotherapy for a survival benefit of threee months, the majority would if it improved the symptoms of their cancer. Adequately informing patients about the benefits of chemotherapy therefore requires better information about the impact of chemotherapy, compared with an untreated control group, on the quality of life of patients with advanced lung cancer. It also requires a better understanding of what other information is important to patients facing these types of decisions.

Conclusion

In 1997 between 80,000 and 100,000 patients in the USA will have to decide about having chemotherapy for the treatment of advanced non-small cell lung cancer. Because the survival benefit is modest and the toxicities real, the decision is extremely difficult. Choosing the proper treatment for cancer patients requires that they are fully aware of the merits of chemotherapy. Our results suggest that some patients may not be getting what they want.

References

Brundage, M.D., Davidson, J.R. and Mackillop, W.J. (1997) 'Trading treatment toxicity for survival in locally advanced non-small cell lung cancer', *Journal of Clinical Oncology*, 15: 330–40.

Ginsberg, R., Kris, M. and Armstrong, J. (1993) 'Cancer of the lung: non-small cell lung cancer', in J.V. DeVita, S. Hellman and S. Rosenberg (eds) *Cancer: Principles and Practice of Oncology*, Philadelphia: JB Lippincott, 673–723.

Grilli, R., Oxman, A. and Julian, J. (1993) 'Chemotherapy for advanced non-small cell lung cancer: how much benefit is enough?', *Journal of Clinical Oncology*, 11: 1866–72.

Kassirer, J. (1994) 'Incorporating patients' preferences into medical decisions', *New England Journal of Medicine*, 330: 1895–6.

McNeil, B., Pauker, S., Sox, H. and Tversky, A. (1982) 'On the elicitation of preferences for alternative therapies', *New England Journal of Medicine*, 306: 1259–62.

McQuellon, R.P., Muss, H.B., Hoffman, S.L., Russell, G., Craven, B. and Yellen, S.B. (1995) 'Patient preferences for treatment of metastatic breast cancer: a study of women with early breast cancer', *Journal of Clinical Oncology*, 13: 858–68.

Marino, P., Pampallona, S., Preatoni, A., Cantoni, A. and Invernizzi, F. (1994) 'Chemotherapy vs supportive care in advanced non-small cell lung cancer: results of a meta-analysis of the literature', *Chest*, 106: 861–5.

Nord, E. (1992) 'Methods for quality adjustment of life years', *Medical Decision Making*, 34: 559–69.

Parker, S., Tong, T., Bolden, S. and Wingo, P. (1997) 'Cancer statistics, 1997', *CA: A Cancer Journal for Clinicians*, 47: 5–27.

Read, J., Quinn, R., Berwick, D., Finebergh, H.F. and Weinstein, M. (1984) 'Preferences for health outcomes. Comparison of assessment methods', *Medical Decision Making*, 4: 315–29.

Richards, M.A., Ramirez, A.J., Degner, L.F., Fallowfield, L.J., Maher, E.J. and Neuberger, J. (1995) 'Offering choice of treatment to patients with cancer: a review based on symposium held at the 10th annual conference of the British Psychosocial Oncology Group, December 1993', *European Journal of Cancer*, 31A: 112–16.

Slevin, M.L., Stubbs, L., Plant, H.J., Wilson, P., Gregory, W., Armes, P.J., *et al.* (1990) 'Attitudes to chemotherapy; comparing views of patients with cancer with those of doctors, nurses, and general public', *British Medical Journal*, 300: 1458–60.

Souquet, P.J., Chauvin, F., Boissel, J.P., Cellerino, R., Cormier, Y., Ganz, P.A., *et al.* (1993) 'Polychemotherapy in advanced non-small cell lung cancer: a meta-analysis', *Lancet*, 342: 19–21.

Sox, H., Blatt, M., Higgins, M. and Marton, K. (1988) *Medical Decision Making*, Boston: Butterworths.

Stiggelbout, A.M., Kiebert, G.M., Kievit, J., Leer, J.W., Stoter, G. and de Haes, J.C. (1994) 'Utility assessment in cancer patients: adjustment of time trade-off scores for the utility of life years and comparison with standard gamble scores', *Medical Decision Making*, 14: 82–90.

Yellen, S., Cella, D. and Leslie, W. (1994) 'Age and clinical decision-making in oncology patients', *Journal of the National Cancer Institute*, 86: 1766–70.

This article can be found complete, and unedited as Silvestri, G., Pritchard, R. and Welch, H.G., 'Preferences for chemotherapy in patients with advanced non-small cell lung cancer: descriptive study based on scripted interviews', in the *British Medical Journal* (1998) Volume 317, pages 771–5.

Chapter 8

Decision aids for patients facing health treatment or screening decisions: systematic review

Annette M. O'Connor, Alaa Rostom, Valerie Fiset, Jacqueline Tetroe, Vikki Entwistle, Hilary Llewellyn-Thomas, Margaret Holmes-Rovner, Michael Barry and Jean Jones

Abstract

Objective: To conduct a systematic review of randomised trials of patient decision aids in improving decision making and outcomes.

Design: We included randomised trials of interventions providing structured, detailed, and specific information on treatment or screening options and outcomes to aid decision making. Two reviewers independently screened and extracted data on several evaluation criteria. Results were pooled by using weighted mean differences and relative risks.

Results: 17 studies met the inclusion criteria. Compared with the controls, decision aids produced higher knowledge scores (weighted mean difference = 19/100, 95% confidence interval 14 to 25); lower decisional conflict scores (weighted mean difference = −0.3/5, −0.4 to −0.1); more active patient participation in decision making (relative risk = 2.27, 95% confidence interval 1.3 to 4); and no differences in anxiety, satisfaction with decisions (weighted mean difference = 0.6/100, −3 to 4), or satisfaction with the decision making process (2/100, −3 to 7). Decision aids had a variable effect on decisions. When complex decision aids were compared with simpler versions, they were better at reducing decisional conflict, improved knowledge marginally, but did not affect satisfaction.

Conclusions: Decision aids improve knowledge, reduce decisional conflict, and stimulate patients to be more active in decision making without increasing their anxiety. Decision aids have little effect on satisfaction and a variable effect on decisions. The effects on outcomes of decisions (persistence with choice, quality of life) remain uncertain.

Source: *British Medical Journal*, 319, 1999, 731–4.

Introduction

Practice guidelines for difficult decisions recommend that patients understand the probable outcomes of options; consider the personal value they place on benefits versus risks; and participate with their practitioners in deciding about treatment (Eddy 1992). Decision aids or shared decision making programmes have been developed as adjuncts to counselling from practitioners. We conducted a systematic overview of the trials of decision aids to determine whether they improved decision making and outcomes for patients facing treatment or screening decisions.

Methods

We searched the following electronic databases: Medline (1966–April 1998), Embase (1980–November 1998), Psyc INFO (1979–March 1998), CINAHL (1983–February 1998), Aidsline (1980–1998), Cancer Lit (1983–April 1998) and the Cochrane Controlled Trials Register (1998, Issue 4). Additional studies were searched for in our personal files and the contents lists of *Health Expectations* (1998), *Medical Decision Making* (January–March 1986 to January–March 1998) and *Patient Education and Counselling* (January 1995–February 1998).

We included randomised controlled trials comparing decision aids to controls or alternative interventions. Participants were 14 years and over who were deciding about screening or treatment options. Decision aids were defined as interventions designed to help people make specific and deliberative choices among options by providing information on the options and outcomes relevant to a patient's health. The aid may also have included information on the disease or condition, probabilities of outcomes tailored to personal health risk factors, an explicit exercise to clarify values, information on others' opinions, and guidance or coaching in the steps of decision making and communicating with others.

Evaluation of outcomes depends on the framework used to develop the decision aids. To ascertain whether the decision aids achieved their objectives, we examined a broad range of positive or negative effects on decision making processes and outcomes of decisions.

Two reviewers screened each study and extracted data independently using standardised forms. Inconsistencies were resolved by discussion and consensus. Missing data were obtained from the authors when possible.

The results of the studies were described individually and pooled when similar measures were used. We used RevMan v3.1 (Mulrow and Oxman 1997) to estimate a weighted treatment effect (with 95% confidence intervals). We used weighted mean differences for continuous measures to calculate pooled relative risks for dichotomous outcomes. Heterogeneity was tested with a χ^2 test ($\alpha = 0.10$). If clinically and statistically appropriate, heterogeneous data were analysed with a random effects model.

Results

We identified 10,387 unique citations from the electronic databases and nine studies from personal files and contacts. Of these, 500 citations focused on patient decision making and 17 met our inclusion criteria (Table 8.1).

The decision aids focused on 11 screening or treatment decisions. All aids included information on the clinical problem in addition to information on the options and outcomes. Over half included outcome probabilities, examples of others, and guidance in the steps of decision making. A quarter included a values clarification exercise.

Compared with usual care (Table 8.2), decision aids improved average knowledge scores for the options and outcomes by 13 to 25 points out of 100 (weighted mean difference = 19, 95% confidence interval 14 to 25). Compared with simpler interventions, more intensive decision aids improved average knowledge scores by 0.9 to 6 points (weighted mean difference 3, 0.7 to 5).

Decision aids had a positive impact on decisional conflict in three of four studies (Table 8.3) with reductions ranging from 0.2 to 0.4 out of 4 (weighted mean difference = 0.3, 0.1 to 0.4).

Three studies evaluated satisfaction with the decision making process and satisfaction with the decision using similar interventions, designs and measures (Table 8.1, papers 1, 2 and 11). One study found that decision aids improved satisfaction with the decision making process (paper 1), but the pooled difference was not significant (weighted mean difference = 2, −3 to 7). There were no significant differences between usual care and decision aids in satisfaction with the decision in either the individual trials or in the pooled studies (weighted mean difference = 0.6, −3 to 4). Two other studies that used different measures also found no significant differences in satisfaction with the decision (Table 8.1, papers 10 and 14).

Fourteen studies assessed the effect of decision aids on the decision made by the participants (Table 8.4). In trials examining decisions about major surgery, decision aids reduced the preference for the more intensive treatment by 21–42% (relative risk = 0.74, 95% confidence interval 0.6–0.9).

In three studies decision aids showed a consistent trend in increasing the proportion of participants assuming a more active role in decision making compared with usual case controls (pooled relative risk = 2.27, 1.3–4) (Table 8.1, papers 4, 5 and 11).

We were unable to combine the results of some studies because of lack of information on standard deviations. One study found that decision aids

Table 8.1 Papers meeting the inclusion criteria

1. Barry MJ, Cherkin DC, Chang YC, Fowler FJ, Skates S. A randomized trial of a multimedia shared decision-making program for men facing a treatment decision for benign prostatic hyperplasia. *Disease Management and Clinical Outcomes* 1997; 1: 5–14.
2. Bernstein SJ, Skarupski KA, Grayson CE, Starling MR, Bates ER, Eagle KA. A randomized controlled trial of information-giving to patients referred for coronary angiography: effects on outcomes of care. *Health Expectations* 1998; 1: 50–61.
3. Clancy CM, Cebul RD, Williams SV. Guiding individual decisions: a randomized, controlled trial of decision analysis. *American Journal of Medicine* 1988; 84: 283–8.
4. Davison BJ, Degner LF. Empowerment of men newly diagnosed with prostate cancer. *Cancer Nursing* 1997; 20: 187–96.
5. Davison BJ, Kirk P, Degner LF, Hassard TH. Information and patient participation in screening for prostate cancer. *Patient Education and Counselling* 1999; 37: 255–63.
6. Flood AB, Wennberg JE, Nease RFJ, Fowler FJJ, Ding J, Hynes LM. The importance of patient preference in the decision to screen for prostate cancer. Prostate Patient Outcomes Research Team. *Journal of General Internal Medicine* 1996; 11: 342–9.
7. Herrera AJ, Cochran B, Herrera A, Wallace B. Parental information and circumcision in highly motivated couples with higher education. *Pediatrics* 1983; 71: 233–4.
8. Lerman C, Biesecker B, Benkendorf JL *et al.* Controlled trial of pretest education approaches to enhance informed decision-making for BRCA1 gene testing. *Journal of the National Cancer Institute* 1997; 89: 148–57.
9. Maisels JM, Hayes B, Conrad S, Chez RA. Circumcision: the effect of information on parental decision making. *Pediatrics* 1983; 71: 453–4.
10. Michie S, Smith D, McClennan A, Marteau TM. Patient decision making: an evaluation of two different methods of presenting information about a screening test. *British Journal of Health Psychology* 1997; 2: 317–26.
11. Morgan MW. A randomized trial of the ischemic heart disease shared decision making program: an evaluation of a decision aid. Master's thesis, University of Toronto, 1997.
12. O'Connor AM, Tugwell P, Wells GA *et al.* Randomized trial of a portable, self-administered decision aid for postmenopausal women considering long-term preventive hormone therapy. *Medical Decision Making* 1998; 18: 295–303.
13. Phillips C, Hill BJ, Cannac C. The influence of video imaging on patients' perceptions and expectations. *Angle Orthodontist* 1995; 65: 263–70.
14. Rothert ML, Holmes-Rovner M, Rovner D *et al.* An educational intervention as decision support for menopausal women. *Research in Nursing and Health* 1997; 20: 377–87.
15. Street RLJ, Voigt B, Geyer CJ, Manning T, Swanson GP. Increasing patient involvement in choosing treatment for early breast cancer. *Cancer* 1995; 76: 2275–85.
16. Thornton JG, Hewison J, Lilford RJ, Vail A. A randomised trial of three methods of giving information about prenatal testing. *British Medical Journal* 1995; 311: 1127–30.
17. Wolf AM, Nasser JF, Schorling JB. The impact of informed consent on patient interest in prostate-specific antigen screening. *Archives of Internal Medicine* 1996; 156: 1333–6.

Table 8.2 Effect of decision aids on patient's knowledge of options and outcomes

Decision	Decision aid		Comparison group		Weight	Mean difference (95% CI)**
	No. of patients	Mean (SD)* knowledge score	No. of patients	Mean (SD) knowledge score		
Compared with usual care						
Benign prostate disease (15)	104	75 (45)	123	54 (45)	14.1	21 (9 to 33)
Ischaemic heart disease (25)	86	75 (17)	94	62 (17)	29.4	13 (8 to 18)
Ischaemic heart disease (16)	61	83 (16)	48	58 (16)	26.4	25 (19 to 31)
BRCA1 gene test (22)	122	69 (19)	164	49 (21.7)	30.1	20 (15 to 25)
Total (random effects $\chi^2 = 9.6$ (df = 3), Z = 6.85)	373	–	429	–	100.0	19 (14 to 25)
Compared with less intensive decision aid						
Hormone therapy (28)	83	87 (11)	87	84 (12)	47.4	3 (−0.4 to 6)
Hormone therapy (26)	81	75 (20)	84	71 (21)	14.3	4 (−2 to 10)
Prenatal screen (24)	67	88 (15)	88	87 (16)	24.7	0.9 (−4 to 6)
Mastectomy (29)	30	83 (12)	30	76 (14)	13.5	6 (−0.3 to 13)
Total (fixed effects $\chi^2 = 1.8$ (df = 3), Z = 2.54)	261	–	289	–	100.0	3 (0.7 to 5)

Knowledge tests regarding options and outcomes were specific to the decision and were scored from 0 (0% items correct) to 100 (100% items correct).
*(SD) standard deviation.
**(95% CI) 95% confidence interval.

Table 8.3 Effect of decision aids on decisional conflict

Decision	Decision aid		Comparison group		Weight	Mean difference (95% CI)**
	No of. patients	Mean (SD)* conflict score	No. of patients	Mean (SD) conflict score		
Compared with usual care						
Prostate specific antigen test (19)	50	1.8 (0.5)	50	2.2 (0.7)	27.5	−0.4 (−0.7 to −0.2)
Ischaemic heart disease (25)	86	2.1 (1.5)	94	2.1 (1.5)	8.1	0.0 (−0.4 to 0.4)
Compared with less intensive decision aid						
Hormone therapy (28)	83	2.6 (1.0)	89	3.0 (1.0)	17.8	−0.4 (−0.7 to −0.1)
Hormone therapy (26)	81	2.1 (0.6)	84	2.3 (0.6)	46.6	−0.2 (−0.4 to −0.02)
Total (fixed effects $\chi^2 = 3.89$ (df = 3), Z = 4.3)	300	—	317	—	100.0	−0.3 (−0.4 to −0.1)

Decisional conflict ranges theoretically from 1 (strong agreement that one is certain, informed, clear about values, and supported in decision making) and 5 (strong disagreement). Scores above 2.5 are associated with decision delay and those below 2 are associated with decision implementation. A negative mean difference means that the decision aid had a positive benefit.

*(SD) standard deviation.

**(95% CI) 95% confidence interval.

Table 8.4 Effect of decision aids on patients' decisions

Decision	Decision aid		Comparison intervention		Weight	Relative risk (95% CI)**
	No. of patients	% choosing option	No. of patients	% choosing option		
Major surgery						
Coronary revascularisation (16)	61	41.0	48	58.0	26.4	0.7 (0.5 to 1.0)
Coronary revascularisation (25)	86	59.0	94	76.0	57.2	0.79 (0.6 to 1.0)
Prostatectomy (15)	104	5.0	123	8.0	6.2	0.74 (0.3 to 2)
Mastectomy (29)	30	24.0	30	42.0	10.1	0.58 (0.3 to 1.0)
Total (fixed effects $\chi^2 = 0.73$ (df = 3), Z = 3.18)	281	–	295	–	100.0	0.74 (0.6 to 0.9)
Circumcision of newborn boys						
Maisels et al. (23)	23	91.3	28	96.4	67.3	0.95 (0.8 to 1.1)
Herrara et al. (21)	56	84.0	47	87.0	32.7	1.07 (0.9 to 1.3)
Total ($\chi^2 = 0.02$ (df = 1), Z = 0.76)	79	–	75	–	–	0.96 (0.85 to 1.07)
Testing for prostate specific antigen						
Davison and Degner (19)	50	48.0	50	38.0	31.1	1.26 (0.8 to 2)
Flood et al. (20)	103	11.7	93	22.6	21.8	0.52 (0.3 to 1.0)
Wolf et al. (31)	103	60.2	102	76.5	47.2	0.79 (0.6 to 0.9)
Total (random effects $\chi^2 = 5.56$ (df = 2), Z = 0.91)	256	–	245	–	100.0	0.83 (0.6 to 1.3)
Other screening						
BRCA1 gene test (22)	122	69.7	164	65.2	38.0	1.07 (0.9 to 1.3)
Amniocentesis (30)	441	37.0	431	34.1	62.0	1.08 (0.9 to 1.3)
Total (fixed effects $\chi^2 = 0.02$ (df = 1), Z = 1.15)	563	–	595	–	100.0	1.08 (0.95 to 1.22)
Other						
Hepatitis B vaccine (17)	753	23.4	263	13.3	–	1.76 (1.3 to 2.5)
Dental surgery (27)	37	85.0	37	70.3	–	1.19 (0.9 to 1.5)
Hormone therapy (26)*	81	13.6	84	15.5	–	0.88 (0.4 to 1.8)

*Comparison between more intensive and less intensive decision aids.
**(95% CI) 95% confidence interval.

significantly reduced the decline in quality of life after treatments for benign prostatic hypertrophy (paper 1), but a study focusing on treatments for ischaemic heart disease showed no difference (paper 2). Four studies showed that the use of decision aids did not affect patients' anxiety (papers 4, 5, 10, 16). One study found that patients receiving a decision aid with detailed outcome descriptions and probabilities had more realistic expectations (accurate perceptions of the probabilities of outcomes) than those who did not have this information included (paper 12).

Discussion

Despite the variability in decisions, interventions and measurement, the trials were consistent in showing that decision aids do a better job than usual care in improving patients' knowledge about options, reducing their decisional conflict, and stimulating patients to take a more active role in decision making without increasing their anxiety. Decision aids had a variable effect on decisions and virtually no effect on satisfaction. The effects on the outcomes of decisions (such as quality of life) are still uncertain. When compared with simpler versions, more intensive decision aids reduced decisional conflict, and improved knowledge marginally.

Knowledge, comfort and empowerment

The largest and most consistent benefit of decision aids over usual care is better knowledge of options and outcomes. The 19% improvement in scores is clinically important because the scores of people in the usual care group were inadequate for informed decision making and they often made different decisions. These results suggest that doctors' usual methods may not be good enough for informing patients about these complex, value-laden decisions. Patients need to comprehend the options and outcomes in order to consider and communicate the personal value they place on the benefits versus the harms.

Decision aids help patients to feel more comfortable with their choices, as shown by the reduced decisional conflict scores. Patients uniformly feel more informed about options, and in some cases (notably primary care settings) feel clearer regarding personal values and supported in decision making. The improvement is one to two thirds of a standard deviation. Cross-sectional studies suggest that this shift places more patients in the zone where they are more likely to follow through their decisions. However, the effect of reduced decisional conflict on persistence with choices needs to be established prospectively.

Decision aids also increased active participation in decision making.

Altering choices

The variable effect of decision aids on patients' decisions may be due to several reasons. Firstly, most studies were underpowered to detect important differences. Secondly, some of the 11 options may have been under-used at baseline and others overused. This would influence the direction of effect once patients became informed and involved in decision making. Thirdly, patients may react differently to the outcomes being considered in the different decisions. Some decisions may be driven predominantly by the probabilities of outcomes and others by the values for outcomes. For example, the aids seem to have a small effect on decisions about major surgical procedures. This may be because patients have inflated perceptions of the probability of benefit and do not understand the probabilities of risks and uncertainties in evidence of effectiveness. When given better knowledge of the outcomes and their associated probabilities, fewer patients may decide that the benefits outweigh the risks.

Satisfaction

The studies showed no effect on satisfaction with decision making. This may be because it is difficult to show improvements in satisfaction when control ratings are already quite high and when choices are inherently difficult because of competing benefits and risks. Furthermore, once the decision is made, people may find it more psychologically comforting to say that they are satisfied than to entertain doubts about what they chose (Gruppen *et al.* 1994).

Further research

The small differences between simpler and more complex versions of decision aids indicate a need to establish the essential ingredients in decision aids and to identify the patients who are most likely to benefit from more complex versions.

There are several gaps in research. Few studies examined the effects on persistence with choices or health outcomes. We also know little about doctors' views about decision aids, the effect on patient–doctor interactions, and cost-effectiveness. More trials are needed to gain a better understanding of what types of decision support work with which types of patients. Baseline predisposition towards choices, preference for participation in decision making, age, sex, ethnicity and education may all have a bearing on the effectiveness of decision aids. Future reviews would be aided if investigators used standard search terms (such as 'shared decision making') and gave structured reports of the composition of decision aids and comparison interventions. Moreover, people who develop and use decision aids need to reach a consensus on a minimum set of criteria for evaluating their effects.

Acknowledgements

Contributors: all authors contributed to the design of the protocol, the interpretation of results, and the revision and final approval of the final paper. A.O'C. led the team and J.T. co-ordinated the project. A.O'C., M.H-R., A.R., V.F., and J.T. pilot tested the data extraction forms. A.R., V.F., and J.T. screened studies and extracted data. A.R., J.T., and A.O'C. analysed the results. The Cochrane Consumers and Communication Review Group (editor Alex Jadad) provided peer review and advice regarding the research protocol. Marie O'Donnell from the University of Aberdeen Health Services Research Unit assisted with literature searching. A.O'C. is the study guarantor.

Funding: the overview was supported by a group grant from the Medical Research Council of Canada. At the time of the study A.O'C. was funded by the Ontario Ministry of Health, V.E. held a special research fellowship from the Leverhulme Trust and H.L-T. was a national health scholar funded by Health Canada's National Health Research Development Program. The Cochrane Library holds updates of this systematic review. The website maintained by the authors (www.ohri.ca) allows access to an inventory of over 400 decision aids.

References

Eddy, D.M. (1992) *A manual for assessing health practices and designing practice policies: the explicit approach*. American College of Physicians.

Gruppen, L.D., Margolin, J., Wisdom, K. and Grum, C. (1994) 'Outcome bias and cognitive dissonance in evaluating treatment decisions', *Academic Medicine*, 10 (Suppl): S57–S59.

Mulrow, C.D. and Oxman, A. (1997) *How to Conduct a Cochrane Systematic Review*, Version 3.0.2, Oxford: Cochrane Collaboration.

A complete, unedited version of this article can be found as 'Decision aids for patients facing health treatment or screening decisions: systematic review' in the *British Medical Journal* (1999) Volume 319, pages 731–4. The authors are O'Connor, A.M., Rostom, A., Fiset, V., Tetroe, J., Entwistle, V., Llewellyn-Thomas, H., Holmes-Rovner, M., Barry, M. and Jones, J.

Chapter 9

Promoting patient participation in the cancer consultation: evaluation of a prompt sheet and coaching in question-asking

R. Brown, P.N. Butow, M.J. Boyer and M.H.N. Tattersall

Abstract

Objective: Active participation in the medical consultation has been demonstrated to benefit aspects of patients' subsequent psychological well-being. We investigated two interventions promoting patient question-asking behaviour. The first was a question prompt sheet provided before the consultation, which was endorsed and worked through by the clinician. The second was a face to face coaching session exploring the benefits of, and barriers to, question-asking, followed by coaching in question-asking behaviour employing rehearsal techniques.

Method: 60 patients with heterogeneous cancers, seeing two medical oncologists for the first time, were randomly assigned to one of three groups: two intervention groups and one control group. Sociodemographic variables and anxiety were assessed prior to the intervention which preceded the consultation. The consultations were audiotaped and subsequently analysed for question-asking behaviour. Anxiety was assessed again immediately following the consultation. Questionnaires to assess patient satisfaction, anxiety and psychological adjustment were sent by mail two weeks following the consultation.

Results: Presentation and discussion of the prompt sheet significantly increased the total number of questions asked and the number of questions asked regarding tests and treatment. Coaching did not add significantly to the effects of the prompt sheet. Psychological outcomes were not different among the groups.

Conclusion: A question prompt sheet addressed by the doctor is a simple, inexpensive and effective means of promoting patient question asking in the cancer consultation.

Source: *British Journal of Cancer*, 80, 1999, 242–8.

Introduction

An examination of trends in clinician behaviour in Western cultures over three decades reveals a move away from a paternalistic style, characterised by providing minimal information to patients (Oken 1961). Previously, doctors usually withheld detailed information regarding cancer diagnosis, prognosis and treatment options in the belief that such information would cause the patient excessive fear, anxiety and loss of hope, thus worsening patient outcomes (Oken 1961; Mosconi *et al.* 1991; Girgis and Sanson-Fisher, 1995). Various reasons have been offered to account for this shift in clinician behaviour, including: (1) an increased fear of litigation among physicians, (2) the publication of guidelines for the disclosure of diagnoses (Reiser 1980), (3) more effective therapies for cancer patients through technological advancement and (4) a change in public opinion regarding patients' rights to medical information and full disclosure (Thomasma 1983).

Western cancer patients who are informed of their diagnosis are increasingly unwilling to adopt a traditional, passive role in the medical consultation. Patients commonly now seek information to enable them to make decisions about treatment, to understand prognostic issues and to be clear about treatment side effects (Roter 1977; Tattersall *et al.* 1994). Patient advocacy groups have endorsed a consumeristic philosophy, which portrays the physician as a service provider. Self-help groups have been established which provide support and training for patients and their carers, who also often pursue a more active role in the medical consultation (Levin *et al.* 1976; Green *et al.* 1977; Cassileth *et al.* 1980; Tattersall *et al.* 1994).

Patients who actively participate are able to change the focus of the consultation and influence the duration and the amount of information provided (Kaplan *et al.* 1996). Research has demonstrated a relationship between the active pursuit of information and involvement in treatment decisions, and improved psychological adjustment and increased patient satisfaction (Korsch *et al.* 1968; Kupst *et al.* 1975; Bertakis *et al.* 1991; Butow *et al.* 1994). The direction of causality, however, is unclear. Patient activity may cause such beneficial outcomes or, alternatively, well-adjusted patients who are satisfied with their care may ask more questions.

Patients may not be asking questions for a variety of reasons. These reasons include, (a) an unwillingness to appear ignorant, (b) lack of knowledge about the illness and not knowing which questions to ask, (c) patient belief in an expert authority and (d) unease about communication with a person of a perceived higher status (Roter 1977). Conversely, some physicians may feel uncomfortable answering patients' questions because it reduces their control over the consultation.

The current study investigated the effects of providing a question prompt sheet that the physician endorsed and discussed, and the added effect of an individualised method of coaching patients in question-asking behaviour. The aims of this study were: (a) to evaluate two interventions designed primarily to influence physician–patient communication and to increase question-asking behaviour and (b) to investigate the impact of increased question-asking on psychological outcome measures.

Methods

Consecutive patients seeing two medical oncologists for the first time at a tertiary referral teaching hospital in Sydney, Australia, were invited to participate in the study. One patient refused to participate. Thirty-one females and 29 males, with an average age of 53.1 years were recruited (Table 9.1).

Patients were informed of the purpose and the requirements of the study and permission was sought to audiotape the consultation. Eligible patients were randomly allocated to one of three groups of equal size. Group 1 – standard practice consultation. Group 2 – participants were provided with a question prompt sheet (QPS) which contained a structured list of 17 questions commonly asked by patients of their medical oncologist. The questions were derived from a content analysis of 20 taped consultations and consultation with four experts: two medical oncologists and two psychologists experienced in cancer research. These questions were grouped according to their content using a method of categorisation described by Ley *et al.* (1973). The categories include questions concerning diagnosis, tests, treatment, prognosis, psychosocial issues and support services available (Figure 9.1). The doctor endorsed the prompt sheet and, towards the end of the consultation, went through each category eliciting and answering questions according to a standard protocol. Group 3 – participants received the QPS plus an interactive coaching session immediately before the consultation, with a research psychologist.

Before the consultation and the introduction of the interventions, all participants completed a short questionnaire measuring anxiety. The consultations were audiotaped to allow analysis of information presented in the consultation and collation of the number of questions asked by patients. One of us listened to each audiotape and counted patient questions within each category of the QPS. The category subtotals were summed to calculate a total number of questions asked by each patient.

Immediately following the consultation, anxiety was assessed. Seven to ten days after the consultation, participants were mailed questionnaires to assess satisfaction with the consultation, anxiety and psychological adjustment to cancer. Anxiety was measured using the Spielberger State Anxiety Scale (SSAS) (Spielberger 1983) which is a widely used scale measuring situational anxiety. Patient satisfaction with the consultation

Table 9.1 Demographic and disease characteristics of sample (*n* = 60)

	Control group (n = 20)	QPS group (n = 20)	QPS + coach group (n = 20)	Total sample (n = 60)
Age (years)				
Mean	53.1	52.8	52.9	53
Range	32–71	17–71	29–77	17–77
Gender				
Female	11 (55%)	9 (45%)	11 (55%)	31 (52%)
Male	9 (45%)	11 (55%)	9 (45%)	29 (49%)
Education level				
Completed ≤10 years High School	11 (45%)	10 (50%)	12 (60%)	33 (55%)
Completed High School (12 years)	2 (10%)	1 (5%)	3 (15%)	6 (10%)
Tertiary non-university	3 (15%)	1 (5%)	2 (10%)	6 (10%)
Tertiary University	4 (20%)	8 (40%)	3 (15%)	15 (25%)
Occupation				
Professionals	11 (55%)	12 (60%)	9 (45%)	32 (53%)
Trades people	2 (10%)	0	5 (25%)	7 (12%)
Clerks and sales	3 (15%)	3 (15%)	3 (15%)	9 (15%)
Labourers	2 (10%)	4 (20%)	2 (10%)	8 (13%)
Home duties/students	2 (10%)	1 (5%)	1 (5%)	4 (7%)
Marital status				
Single	2 (10%)	3 (15%)	3 (15%)	8 (12%)
Married	15 (75%)	12 (60%)	15 (75%)	42 (70%)
Divorced/separated	2 (10%)	3 (15%)	1 (5%)	6 (10%)
Common law	0	1 (5%)	1 (5%)	2 (3%)
Widowed	1 (5%)	1 (5%)	0	2 (3%)
Type of cancer				
Breast	6 (30%)	5 (25%)	5 (25%)	16 (27%)
Lung	2 (10%)	4 (20%)	1 (5%)	7 (12%)
Testes	1 (5%)	3 (15%)	0	4 (7%)
Prostate	4 (20%)	1 (5%)	2 (10%)	7 (12%)
Colorectal	0	1 (5%)	5 (25%)	6 (10%)
Other	7 (35%)	6 (30%)	7 (35%)	20 (33%)
Stage				
Loco-regional	11 (55%)	11 (55%)	7 (35%)	29 (48%)
Metastasis	9 (45%)	9 (45%)	13 (65%)	31 (52%)
Estimated prognosis				
≤1 year	8 (40%)	8 (40%)	6 (30%)	22 (37%)
1–5 years	9 (45%)	7 (35%)	10 (50%)	26 (43%)
Normal life expectancy	3 (15%)	5 (25%)	4 (20%)	12 (20%)
Time since diagnosis				
≤2 months	11 (55%)	11 (55%)	13 (65%)	35 (58%)
>2 months	9 (45%)	9 (45%)	7 (35%)	25 (42%)

How to make the most of your time with the doctor

Most people who see their doctor for the first time have questions and concerns. Often these get forgotten in the rush of the moment, only to be remembered later. To help you make the most of your time with the doctor we have compiled a list of questions people often ask. We suggest that you tick those you want to ask and then write down any other specific questions you have in the space provided.

You can keep this sheet with you when you see the doctor. You may find that the doctor answers your questions without you even asking, but this sheet can serve as a checklist so that you know that you have covered everything that is important to you.

Questions people often ask

1   What kind of cancer do/did I have?
2   Where is the cancer at the moment? Has it spread?
3   What symptoms will the cancer cause?
4   Will I need any more tests
5   If so, will they hurt?
6   What will they tell us?
7   What treatment will I need?
8   Does the treatment have any side effects? If so, what can be done about them?
9   What should I do or not do while having treatment?
10   How long will it be before I know my treatment is working?
11   Will my family be affected by my cancer?
12   Will my work be affected?
13   Will my sexual life be affected?
14   What will the outcome be? Will I get better?
15   If we get rid of the cancer, what are the chances of it coming back?
16   Do members of my family have a greater risk of getting cancer?
17   Are there services available to help me cope with this illness?

Write any other questions you have in the space below:

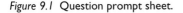

Figure 9.1 Question prompt sheet.

was assessed during the follow-up phase using a 25-item Likert scale adapted from Roter (1977) and Korsch *et al.* (1968). This scale assessed satisfaction with: (1) the amount and quality of information presented, (2) the communication skills demonstrated by the doctor and (3) the level of patient participation in the consultation.

The internal reliability of this scale in a sample of 80 patients enrolled in a similar study was high (Cronbach's Alpha = 0.91). Psychological adjustment to the diagnosis of cancer was measured using the Mental Adjustment to Cancer Scale (MAC) (Watson *et al.* 1988). This scale has been used in previous studies and has shown good reliability and sensitivity.

Results

An exploration of demographic and disease variables between the three experimental groups revealed no major imbalances (Table 9.1).

Impact of prompt sheet and coaching on question-asking

Patients in the control group asked a median of 8.5 questions (IQR, 5–21.5), the prompt sheet group 15 (IQR, 10.7–26.7) and the coaching group 13 (IQR, 8–27.7). As there was no significant difference in the number of questions asked between participants receiving a QPS and those who received coaching in addition to the prompt sheet, the two groups were combined. All subsequent analysis was conducted comparing the control group with the combined intervention groups that had received a prompt sheet. The results indicated that the prompt sheet increased question-asking significantly ($P = 0.043$).

An analysis of the number of questions asked in each of the question categories, according to the provision of a prompt sheet or not, was then conducted. The result demonstrated that patients with a prompt sheet asked significantly more questions (median = 1; IQR, 0–3) than patients in the control group (median = 0; IQR, 0–1.75) regarding tests ($P = 0.048$). Differences between the groups in questions asked about other topics were not statistically significant.

On the assumption that the interventions may have prompted non-active patients to ask at least one question, rather than increasing the total number of questions asked, the patients were grouped according to whether they had asked no questions, or one or more questions. In this analysis, the treatment category was significant ($P = 0.024$), while in other topic areas results were non-significant. There was also a tendency for more patients in the intervention groups 27/40 (67.5 per cent) than those in the control group 9/20 (45 per cent), to ask at least one question about prognosis.

Impact of prompt sheet on anxiety, satisfaction and psychological adjustment to cancer

Anxiety

Anxiety was not affected by the use of a prompt sheet (Table 9.2). To assess differences among groups on the extent to which anxiety changed following the consultation, change scores were computed between the immediate pre-consultation and immediate post-consultation measurements. Independent samples *t*-tests conducted on these scores to investigate differences among groups were non-significant. Kruskall–Wallis

Table 9.2 Mean scores according to psychosocial measures between the control and prompt sheet groups

	Control group (n = 20)		Combined QPS + coach groups (n = 40)		P value
	Mean	SD	Mean	SD	
Anxiety					
Pre-consultation	46.4	5.5	47	7.5	0.772
Immediate post-consultation	48.5	6.1	47.2	7.9	0.540
Change scores	1.947	5.892	0.25	7.7476	0.389
Psychological adjustment (MAC subscales)					
Fighting spirit	50	5.1	49.7	5.5	0.882
Helpless/hopeless	9.5	3.3	9.9	2.9	0.658
Satisfaction	Median	IQR	Median	IQR	0.705
	108	100–109	107	97–113.5	

one-way ANOVAs used to assess the relationship between question-asking and anxiety scores, both immediately following the consultation and one week post-consultation, were non-significant.

Satisfaction

While the scores on the satisfaction scale exhibited considerable variability (52–124), the distribution was significantly skewed with most people reporting high satisfaction with the consultation. A Mann–Whitney U-test used to explore differences in satisfaction between the combined intervention group and the control group was non-significant, indicating that increased question-asking was not associated with total satisfaction with the consultation (Table 9.2).

Psychological adjustment

Differences in psychological adjustment between the control and the prompt sheet produced non-significant results indicating that the prompt sheet did not significantly affect fighting spirit or the patients' sense of helplessness/hopelessness (Table 9.2).

Discussion

Our results indicate that patients who were provided with a prompt sheet asked significantly more questions in general than those without and, in particular, asked more questions about tests and treatment. The addition of a complex coaching intervention to the simpler prompt sheet did not increase further the number of questions asked. Our results support those of Roter (1977) and Butow et al. (1994).

Patients in the current sample asked far more questions overall than patients in the previous studies. The current patients were more highly educated and in more prestigious occupations than the general population, which may account for an increase in the number of questions asked. However, it is also possible that the endorsement of the prompt sheet by the clinician and discussion of the selected questions encouraged patients to ask a greater number of questions than previous samples.

The fact that significant differences were detected in the number of questions asked about tests and treatment in particular, suggests that patients benefit most from additional encouragement to explore these areas.

The failure of the coaching intervention

The coaching intervention addressed the model proposed by Roter (1977); however, discussion of the benefits of, and barriers to, question-asking did not translate to increased question-asking, or to increase the patient's sense of control over the consultation. The role-playing technique, based on rehearsal of a behaviour prior to a stressful event, did not cause patients to ask more questions in the consultation. As the differences between groups were so small it is unlikely that insufficient power is to blame for this result. Perhaps a ceiling in the desired question-asking had been achieved by the doctor-endorsed QPS. Alternatively, an intervention such as this may need to be conducted on more than one occasion in order to produce a substantial change in assertive behaviour.

Psychological outcomes

Patients' anxiety levels did not change measurably as a result of the provision of the prompt sheet, indicating that this intervention can be used by patients without increasing their distress. Anxiety also remained stable over the trial period in all three groups. This result is at odds with the literature (Derogatis et al. 1983; Molleman et al. 1984). However, anxiety levels may have been stable in this sample, as approximately 40 per cent of patients had known of their diagnosis for three or more months prior to the study consultation. Similarly, perhaps psychological adjustment to the diagnosis and treatment of cancer is influenced by such a complex array of factors that short-term interventions, such as those employed in the present study, would not have impact.

Satisfaction with the consultation was similarly unaffected by the interventions studied. Perhaps cancer patients overlook characteristics of the oncologist or features of the consultation with which they are dissatisfied more than general practice patients with less severe illnesses, as cancer patients must rely heavily on the knowledge and skills of their oncologist and need to believe that their oncologist is capable.

In conclusion, this study showed that while a question prompt sheet addressed by the physician significantly increased question-asking, the addition of one-to-one intensive coaching with a psychologist before an initial oncology consultation did not further enhance question-asking. A prompt sheet that the physician endorses is an effective and inexpensive means of encouraging patient involvement in the cancer consultation.

References

Bertakis, K.D., Roter, D. and Putnam, S.M. (1991) 'The relationship of physician medical interview style to patient satisfaction', *Journal of Family Practice*, 32: 175–81.

Butow, P.N., Dunn, S.M., Tattersall, M.H.N. and Jones, Q.J. (1994) 'Patient participation in the cancer consultation: evaluation of a question prompt sheet', *Annals of Oncology*, 5: 199–204.

Cassileth, B.R., Zupkis, R.V., Sutton-Smith, K. and March, V. (1980) 'Information and participation preferences among cancer patients', *Annals of Internal Medicine*, 92: 832–6.

Derogatis, L.R., Morrow, G.R. and Fetting, J. (1983) 'The prevalence of psychiatric disorders among cancer patients', *Journal of the American Medical Association*, 249: 751–7.

Girgis, A. and Sanson-Fisher, R.W. (1995) 'Breaking bad news: consensus guidelines for medical practitioners', *Journal of Clinical Oncology*, 13: 2449–56.

Green, L.W., Werlin, S.H. and Schauffler, H.H. (1977) 'Research and demonstration issues in self care: measuring the decline of medicocentrism', *Health Education Monographs*, 5: 161–89.

Kaplan, S.H., Greenfield, S., Gandek, B., Rogers, W.H. and Ware, J.E. (1996) 'Characteristics of physicians with participatory decision-making styles', *Annals of Internal Medicine*, 124: 497–504.

Korsch, B.M., Gozzi, E.K. and Francis, V. (1968) 'Gaps in doctor–patient communication: doctor patient interaction and patient satisfaction', *Pediatrics*, 42: 855–70.

Kupst, M., Dresser, K., Schulman, J.L. and Paul, M.H. (1975) 'Evaluation of methods to improve communication in the physician–patient relationship', *American Journal of Orthopsychiatry*, 45: 420–9.

Levin, L., Katz, A.H. and Holst, E. (1976) *Lay Initiatives in Health*, New York: Prodist.

Ley, P., Bradshaw, P.W., Eaves, D. and Walker, C.M. (1973) 'A method for increasing patients recall of information presented by doctors', *Psychological Medicine*, 3: 217–20.

Molleman, E., Krabbendam, P.J., Annyas, A.A., Koops, H.S., Sleijfer, D.T. and Vermey, A. (1984) 'The significance of the doctor–patient relationship in coping with cancer', *Social Science and Medicine*, 18: 475–80.

Mosconi, P., Meyerowitz, B.E., Liberati, M.C. and Liberati, A. (1991) 'Disclosure of breast cancer diagnosis: patients and physician reports', *Annals of Oncology*, 2: 273–80.

Oken, D. (1961) 'What to tell cancer patients: a study of medical attitudes', *Journal of the American Medical Association*, 175: 1120–8.

Reiser, S.J. (1980) 'Words as scalpels: transmitting evidence in the clinical dialogue', *Annals of Internal Medicine*, 92: 837–42.

Roter, D.L. (1977) 'Patient participation in the patient provider interaction: the effects of patient question asking on the quality of interaction, satisfaction and compliance', *Health Education Monographs*, 5: 281–315.

Spielberger, C.D. (1983) *Manual for the State Trait Anxiety Inventory (Form Y)*, Palo Alto, CA: Consulting Psychologists Press.

Tattersall, M.H.N., Butow, P.N., Griffin, A.M. and Dunn, S.M. (1994) 'The take home message: patients prefer consultation audiotapes to summary letters', *Journal of Clinical Oncology*, 12: 1305–11.

Thomasma, D.C. (1983) 'Beyond medical paternalism and patient autonomy: a model of physician conscience for the physician–patient relationship', *Annals of Internal Medicine*, 98: 243–8.

Watson, M., Greer, S., Young, J., Inayat, Q., Burgess, C. and Robertson, B. (1988) 'Development of a questionnaire measure of adjustment to cancer: the MAC scale', *Psychological Medicine*, 18: 203–9.

This article can be found complete, and unedited as Brown, R., Butow, P.N., Boyer, M.J. and Tattersall, M.H.N., 'Promoting patient participation in the cancer consultation: evaluation of a prompt sheet and coaching in question-asking', in the *British Journal of Cancer* (1999) Volume 80, pages 242–8.

Chapter 10

Health care rationing: the public's debate

Ann Bowling

Abstract

Objective: To elicit the views of a large nationally representative sample of adults on priorities for health services.

Design: An interview survey based on a random sample of people aged 16 and over in Great Britain.

Subjects: The response rate to the survey was 75%, and the total number of adults interviewed was 2005.

Main outcome measures: A priority ranking exercise of health services supplemented with attitude questions about priorities, who should set priorities, and budget allocation.

Results: The results of the main priority ranking exercise of 12 health services showed that the highest priority (rank 1) was accorded to 'treatments for children with life-threatening illness', the next highest priority (rank 2) was accorded to 'special care and pain relief for people who are dying'. The lowest priorities (11 and 12) were given to 'treatment for infertility' and 'treatment for people aged 75 and over with life-threatening illness'. Most respondents thought that surveys like this one should be used in the planning of health services.

Conclusions: The public prioritise treatments specifically for younger rather than older people. There is some public support for people with self-inflicted conditions (for example, through tobacco smoking) receiving lower priority for care, which raises ethical issues.

Source: *British Medical Journal*, 312, 1996, 670–4.

Introduction

Prioritisation or rationing of health services is on government agendas across the world; different countries have adopted different approaches, ranging from policies of rationing by exclusion of specified treatments to rationing by guidelines (Citizen's Committee on Biomedical Ethics (New Jersey) 1988; National Health and Medical Research Council (Australia) 1990; Oregon Health Services Commission 1991; Honigsbaum *et al.* 1995).

In Britain Nicholson (1995) called for a public debate on health priorities and for the establishment of a Royal Commission on Priorities, with the public represented along with politicians and the medical profession. A study of the five-year purchasing plans of 66 district health authorities in England shows a considerable increase in the number of purchasers adopting explicit policies on rationing health care. For example, 11 of the 66 plans specified treatments that will not be purchased, in contrast with four in the team's previous survey, and many others conceded that similar rationing may be unavoidable (Redmayne 1995). These developments highlight the need to measure public opinion on rationing.

Several local surveys of the priorities of the public and doctors have been conducted in the UK (Lutton and Garrol 1991; Richardson *et al.* 1992; Whitty and Jessop 1992; Bowling 1993). Apart from one survey based on a quota sample drawn by a market research company (Heginbotham 1993), however, there have been no published nationally representative surveys of health care priorities anywhere in the world. The studies in the UK have consistently shown that acute interventions that are perceived to be life-saving are prioritised very highly by the public compared with many preventive initiatives (such as family planning and health education and promotion) and care for people with chronic illnesses and disabilities (such as people with mental illnesses and older people). In the United States the public consultation exercises of the Oregon Health Commission also found that the highest ranking priorities were for treatments for life-threatening conditions (particularly acute conditions), maternity care, preventive care (but only for children) and palliative care (Oregon Health Services Commission 1991).

Obtaining a representative response from the public can be difficult (Bowling 1993). Rapid appraisal techniques that may be useful at neighbourhood level (Murray *et al.* 1994) are relatively resource intensive across a whole population and are not a substitute for the need for representative information which deals with specific questions. This study aimed to obtain the views on priorities for health services of a random sample of the British population and used the Office of Population Censuses and Surveys omnibus survey as the vehicle.

Subjects and methods

The study design was an interview survey that was based on a random sample of people aged 16 and over in Great Britain. The sampling frame was stratified by region, housing tenure and socioeconomic group. The postal sectors were selected with probability proportionate to size and, within each sector, 30 addresses were selected randomly. If an address contained more than one household, the interviewer used a standard procedure to select just one household randomly. Within households with more than one adult member just one person aged 16 or over was selected with the use of random number tables. Because only one household member was interviewed, people in households that contained few adults had a better chance of selection than those in households with many. A weighting factor was applied to correct for this unequal probability, and the individual adult was the unit of analysis.

Questionnaire design

The questionnaire was based on an earlier version developed and tested for the City and Hackney survey (Bowling 1993) and on questions from surveys in the United States (Citizen's Committee on Biomedical Ethics (New Jersey) 1991). The original pilot survey tested respondents' understanding and acceptability of different forms of question wording and methods of prioritising on 326 members of community groups in Hackney. The number of services listed was reduced from 16 to 12, and services were listed without any examples in brackets because examples may have caused bias. The service items were deliberately biasing – for example, treatments for life-threatening illness were itemised separately for children, for people aged 75 and over, and with no age specification to assess age biases in relation to these treatments. Respondents were asked to look at a card displaying the 12 services and 'choose the four services that you consider the most essential', then they were asked to 'choose the four services that you consider the next most important', The bottom four services, by deduction, were the four remaining services, and respondents were asked to check the order.

Respondents were asked about the extent of their agreement or disagreement (strongly disagree to strongly agree) with six statements about priorities. They were asked who they thought should set priorities and asked to select their preference from a precoded list of doctors at local level, the public at local level, local NHS managers, local health authorities, and politicians or government at national level. Finally, they were asked about how they themselves would allocate £100,000. These further sets of questions on priorities were developed for use in the studies in Hackney and the United States, as with the main priority ranking exercise.

Results

Prioritisation exercises

Table 10.1 shows the frequency distributions and the mean priority rankings for the 12 services and treatments. The table shows that the highest priority (rank 1) was accorded to 'treatments for children with life-threatening illness', the next highest priority (rank 2) was accorded to 'special care and pain relief for people who are dying'. 'Preventive screening services and immunisations' were ranked next highest (3). 'Psychiatric services' was given a middle ranking (6) as was 'high technology surgery' (7); 'health promotion' was given a middle to low ranking (8). The lowest priorities were assigned to 'treatment for infertility' (11) and 'treatment for people aged 75 and over with life-threatening illness' (12).

A further question on attitudes was asked in which respondents were asked if they strongly disagreed to strongly agreed (on a five-point scale) with each of six statements. Table 10.2 shows the responses to these statements. Most respondents agreed or strongly agreed that high cost technology should be available to all, regardless of age, which somewhat contradicts their bottom ranking of treatments for people aged 75 and over with life-threatening illness (Table 10.1), illustrating the complexity of prioritisation by age group. However, in agreement with earlier research (Bowling 1993), most respondents agreed or strongly agreed that the patient's quality of life should be considered. More consistent with the priority ranking exercise of the 12 services, half (979) of respondents agreed or strongly agreed that if resources are to be rationed then higher priority should be given to treating the young rather than elderly people.

Table 10.2 also shows that respondents were more evenly divided on whether people who contribute to their own illness (for example, through smoking, obesity or drinking) should have lower priority for health care, although 42 per cent (842) agreed or strongly agreed with this. Most respondents agreed or strongly agreed that the responsibility for rationing spending on health care should rest with doctors rather than managers, health authorities or the government, echoing a similar direct question asked (see below). Consistent with this again most people disagreed or strongly disagreed with the statement that the government should issue guidelines to doctors about rationing life-saving treatments.

Priority setting

Respondents were asked who should set priorities and shown a precoded list: 56 per cent (1104) said 'doctors at local level', 19 per cent (377) said 'local health authorities', 17 per cent (336) said 'the public at local level', 5 per cent (89) said 'local NHS managers' and 3 per cent (61) said 'politicians and the government at national level'. In reply to a separate question 88 per cent (1739) said that they thought that 'surveys of the general public's opinions, like this one, should be used in the planning of health services', 7 per cent (149) disagreed with this, and 5 per cent (91) said that they did not know.

They were also asked how they themselves would allocate £100,000. Seventy-one per cent (1393) of respondents selected 'a health screening and education programme which could prevent a large number of people needing life-saving operations in the future (for example, screening for cancers)' and 26 per cent (521) selected '12 extra immediate life-saving operations this year (for example, heart bypass)'; 3 per cent (65) said they did not know.

There were few associations between health service priorities and sociodemographic characteristics, although those that were found did make theoretical sense. For example, 44 per cent (426) of people aged between 16 and 45 prioritised as their first choice 'treatments for children with life-threatening illness', in comparison with 26 per cent (218) of people aged between 45 and 75 and 21 per cent (30) of people aged 75 and over ($\chi^2 = 79.29$; df $= 2$; $P < 0.001$); and whereas just 1 per cent (15) of people aged under 75 years prioritised as first 'treatments for people aged 75 and over with life-threatening illness', 10 per cent (14) of people aged 75 and over prioritised this as first ($\chi^2 = 75.13$; df $= 1$; $P < 0.001$).

Discussion

The study presented here is the first prioritisation exercise based on a random sample of a total (national) population. The methodology of ranking lists of treatments and services may be criticised as superficial in relation to the complexity of the decisions to be made about health service priorities, which necessitate consideration of the costs and effectiveness of treatments and care programmes rather than sole reliance on values that may include prejudices. The prioritisation exercise presented here mostly entailed the ranking of broader treatments and services for specific groups of people rather than ranking individual procedures and diagnostic groups as in the Oregon experiment (Oregon Health Services Commission 1991). This focus was deliberate to measure the public's values in relation to specific groups of patients and age groups. In the context of a lack of adequate knowledge about the costs and effectiveness of much medical care it is important to be democratic and involve everyone in an open debate about rationing. One first step must be to measure baseline public opinions and values. If the public's values seem to conflict with firm medical evidence on effectiveness or to be prejudiced against certain groups, then open debate and the provision of sound, unbiased information for public consumption and education is even more essential.

Table 10.1 Priority rating of health services: figures are percentages (numbers)

Priority	Priority rank												Mean	Mean P rank
	1	2	3	4	5	6	7	8	9	10	11	12		
Treatments for children with life-threatening illnesses	34 (674)	21 (409)	9 (185)	7 (143)	10 (196)	6 (119)	3 (64)	3 (59)	2 (36)	3 (63)	1 (14)	1 (3)	3.2	1
Special care and pain relief for people who are dying	23 (442)	6 (127)	7 (129)	9 (183)	19 (337)	6 (104)	6 (124)	8 (153)	12 (241)	1 (26)	1 (26)	1 (25)	4.8	2
Preventive screening services and immunisations	9 (174)	15 (301)	15 (302)	10 (198)	7 (140)	10 (195)	9 (181)	5 (92)	2 (39)	7 (127)	7 (135)	3 (67)	5.3	3
Surgery, such as hip replacement, to help people carry out everyday tasks	4 (82)	12 (232)	11 (213)	8 (164)	8 (160)	13 (259)	12 (223)	7 (135)	2 (49)	11 (207)	10 (195)	2 (31)	6	4
District nursing and community services/ care at home	4 (72)	7 (141)	12 (235)	17 (337)	8 (152)	10 (196)	11 (219)	12 (237)	1 (21)	2 (30)	4 (74)	12 (240)	6.1	5
Psychiatric services for people with mental illness	3 (68)	10 (201)	9 (183)	6 (109)	11 (222)	16 (311)	11 (219)	8 (153)	4 (79)	13 (247)	5 (106)	3 (51)	6.2	6

Service													Mean	
High technology surgery, organ transplants and procedures which treat life-threatening conditions	7 (145)	7 (140)	9 (190)	18 (345)	7 (124)	6 (114)	9 (175)	14 (73)	2 (39)	2 (48)	2 (44)	17 (326)	6.3	7
Health promotion/education services to help people lead healthy lives	8 (164)	8 (157)	6 (115)	6 (106)	11 (206)	9 (167)	6 (108)	6 (118)	11 (223)	22 (430)	6 (108)	3 (51)	6.7	8
Intensive care for premature babies who weigh less than 680 g with only a slight chance of survival	3 (56)	6 (111)	9 (167)	7 (133)	5 (87)	7 (144)	8 (156)	8 (154)	4 (70)	16 (309)	20 (392)	8 (169)	7.7	9
Long-stay hospital care for elderly people	2 (44)	4 (70)	7 (144)	7 (146)	5 (98)	7 (135)	12 (223)	15 (287)	3 (52)	4 (77)	10 (205)	24 (469)	7.9	10
Treatment for infertility	1 (24)	1 (14)	1 (13)	1 (22)	6 (117)	4 (83)	4 (69)	5 (104)	53 (1028)	11 (221)	5 (90)	8 (162)	8.4	11
Treatment for people aged 75 and over with life-threatening illness	2 (30)	3 (69)	5 (96)	4 (83)	3 (65)	6 (113)	9 (179)	9 (175)	4 (71)	8 (162)	29 (346)	18 (346)	8.7	12
No. of respondents*	1975	1974	1972	1969	1944	1941	1939	1939	1949	1945	1944	1940		

*Number of respondents varied.

Table 10.2 Attitudes about health priorities*: figures are percentages (numbers)

Possible answers	Strongly disagree	Disagree	Neither disagree nor agree	Agree	Strongly agree	No. of respondents
High cost technology (for example, transplantation and kidney machines) should be available to all regardless of age	2 (32)	11 (216)	7 (133)	55 (1092)	25 (505)	1978
People who contribute to their own illness – for example, through smoking, obesity or excessive drinking – should have lower priority for their health care than others	10 (188)	33 (656)	15 (289)	33 (656)	9 (186)	1975
The responsibility to ration health care spending should rest with the doctor rather than a hospital manager, health authority, politician or government minister	1 (30)	14 (271)	10 (196)	48 (946)	27 (524)	1966
The government should issue guidelines to doctors about when not to use life-saving medical treatment/technology	28 (548)	49 (962)	8 (165)	12 (245)	2 (47)	1968
If resources must be rationed, higher priority should be given to treating the young than the elderly	5 (94)	24 (476)	21 (422)	40 (776)	10 (203)	1971
The patient's quality of life should be considered in determining whether or not to use life-saving treatment/technology	2 (52)	12 (237)	12 (227)	51 (1004)	23 (451)	1971

*'I am now going to read out a series of statements about health priorities, please tell me whether you agree or disagree. Choose your answer from this card.'

Probably the most important shortcoming of the setting of public priorities is that priorities chosen by the public do not necessarily offer the most equitable solutions in relation to the original aspiration of the NHS of equal treatment for equal need. Overall, this research confirms the results of earlier surveys which showed that the public's priorities are not value-free – they are most likely to prioritise treatments specifically for younger rather than older people and particularly life-saving treatments (Richardson *et al.* 1992; Bowling 1993; Heginbotham 1993); it also shows some public support (42 per cent) for people with self-inflicted conditions receiving lower priority for care, which raises ethical issues. It clearly shows that different groups of people – for example, age groups – hold different values that need to be reconciled in policies on rationing. The debate about how to weight different value systems in every decision on the allocation of resources is in its infancy, as is the education of the public when prejudices are detected in their priority setting. These issues were not satisfactorily resolved in the largest exercise on rationing health care in Oregon (Oregon Health Services Commission 1991).

Finally, most people wanted to be involved in the planning of health services. Three quarters thought that the responsibility for rationing spending on health care should rest with doctors rather than managers, health authorities or the government. Health authorities should listen to the public's views on health priorities to add legitimacy to their decision making, given their own position as democratically unaccountable bodies. They also need to be seen by the public to be working with and not against their clinical colleagues in prioritisation or rationing exercises to retain the trust of the public.

References

Bowling, A. (1993) *What People Say about Prioritising Health Services*, London: King's Fund Centre.

Citizen's Committee on Biomedical Ethics (1988) *Your Health, Your Choices, Whose Decisions*, New Jersey: Citizen's Committee on Biomedical Ethics.

Heginbotham, C. (1993) 'Health care priority setting: a survey of doctors, managers, and the general public', in *Rationing in Action*, London: British Medical Journal Publishing.

Honigsbaum, F., Calltorp, J., Ham, C. and Holmstrom, S. (1995) *Priority Setting for Health Care*. Oxford: Radcliffe Medical Press.

Lutton, G. and Carroll, G. (1991) *Fourth Public Health Forum; 25th April, 1991*. Witham: Mid-Essex Health Authority.

Murray, J., Tapson, J., Turnbull, L., McCallum, J. and Little, A. (1994) 'Listening to local voices: adapting rapid appraisal to assess health and social needs in general practice', *British Medical Journal*, 308: 698–700.

National Health and Medical Research Council (1990) *Discussion Paper on Ethics and Resource Allocation in Health Care*, Canberra, Australia: National Health and Medical Research Council.

Nicholson, R. (1995) *The World Tonight*, BBC Radio 4, 24 May 1995.

Oregon Health Services Commission (1991) *Health Care in Common*, Salem, Oregon: Oregon Health Decisions.

Redmayne, S. (1995) *Reshaping the NHS: Strategies, Priorities and Resource Allocation*, Birmingham: National Association of Health Authorities and Trusts.

Richardson, A., Charny, M. and Hanmer-Lloyd, S. (1992) 'Public opinion and purchasing', *British Medical Journal*, 304: 680–4.

Whitty, P. and Jessop, E. (1992) *Priorities for Health Care: A Population Survey in Colchester*, Colchester: Department of Public Health, North East Essex Health Authority.

This article can be found complete, and unedited as Bowling, B., 'Health care rationing: the public's debate', in the *British Medical Journal* (1996) Volume 312, pages 670–4.

Part 3

Workforce issues

Part 3

Workforce issues

Introduction

The past decade has witnessed increasing concern about the health care workforce. These concerns extend from the recruitment and training of staff to their retention and regulation. The sustainability of health services in all countries, both developed and developing, is under threat as policy-makers and managers struggle to maintain sufficient staff and to ensure the quality of their work. This section includes five papers that illustrate some of the ways in which research can contribute to resolving these problems. They focus on three key issues: the recruitment and retention of staff; the reassignment of tasks between professions; and the impact of workforce on quality of care.

While recognition of workforce issues has increased in recent times, it is salutary to realise that these concerns are not new. Carol Helmstadter demonstrates this in her historical research on London teaching hospitals in the nineteenth century. The reasons she identifies for difficulties in recruiting and retaining nurses 150 years ago will be familiar to a modern reader – poor pay, understaffing, menial tasks and lack of affordable accommodation. Then, as now, the key solution was perceived to be the need to raise the esteem and status of nurses through education. This would, it was perceived, also help raise the quality of hospital care. Historical research of this type teaches us that some apparently new problems are in fact long-standing and it may be worthwhile to explore and understand how they have been addressed in the past. In this particular case, one successful solution was to introduce externally managed nursing services (an approach that returned to consideration in modern times), although this in turn created problems of conflicting authority within hospitals and cost inflation.

A contrasting approach to the difficulties of recruiting and retaining staff is provided by Alastair Gray and Victoria Phillips. Using economic analysis they assessed the extent to which the turnover of three key groups – nurses, midwives, clerical staff – was related to the characteristics of the local labour markets. Studying English health districts in the 1980s, they show how the turnover of registered nurses in the National Health Service was dependent on their age, the pay levels and the size of the local private hospital sector. In contrast, other features of the local labour market, such as the level of unemployment, had little influence. This paper also serves to illustrate the shortcomings of routinely available data on workforce. It's possible that with more sophisticated data other determinants of recruitment and retention would have been detected. Despite this, they demonstrated how private or 'independent' hospitals contribute to the difficulties faced by public sector managers – an issue of contemporary importance with the encouragement of private providers alongside public providers.

Another example of the need to consider factors outwith the health sector is provided by an occupational psychology study. Vivien Swanson and her colleagues' concern was an issue assuming increasing importance for all working people, that of the balance between work and home life, prompted by changing social mores and expectations. They looked at the vulnerability of male and female doctors in Scotland to work stress on home life and home stress on work life. In a mailed survey to around 1000 doctors (half general practitioners, half hospital specialists), they found that although traditional gender patterns of domestic responsibilities had been maintained, increasing domestic demands were related to stress for both sexes. They concluded that it was 'important for employers to recognise the need of individuals to fit the demands of work into a normal working day'. While pay remains a key issue for recruitment and retention, other rewards and terms of employment are taking on greater importance. Health care managers need to ensure that doctors, and indeed all health care workers, have the opportunity to achieve an optimal balance.

The impact of professional esteem on the quality of care recognised in nineteenth-century hospitals is demonstrated in contemporary times by Linda Aiken and colleagues. They conducted an epidemiological study to see if there was an association between good nursing care and patient outcomes in US hospitals. In-hospital mortality in 'magnet hospitals', designated on the basis of their reputation for attracting and retaining nurses, was shown to be about 5 per cent lower among elderly patients than in other hospitals. They attributed this advantage to 'the greater status, autonomy and control afforded nurses in magnet hospitals and their resulting impact on nurses' behaviours on behalf of patients'. The study illustrates the challenges of conducting and interpreting non-randomised comparisons. Recognising that the result could be due to insufficient adjustment for confounding factors, the authors rightly stop short of claiming a causal relationship and recognise the need for further confirmatory studies. If confirmed, such findings are of considerable importance for the planning and management of hospital services.

Finally, there has been a considerable amount of research on staff substitution, seen as a potential solution to the lack of sufficient staff in certain professions. An example is the comparison of general practitioners and nurse practitioners conducted by Pamela Venning and colleagues. Despite limited research evidence as to the cost-effectiveness of nurse practitioners, they have increasingly been introduced in many health care systems. In the NHS in England and Wales, nurse practitioners are the mainstay of initiatives such as the telephone advice service (NHS Direct) and primary care walk-in centres. In general practices they function autonomously, being permitted to make clinical decisions and instigate treatment decisions. In a randomised trial in 20 practices, patients wanting an appointment the same day were invited to be randomly allocated to a doctor or a nurse practitioner. The latter were found to spend longer with the patient, order more tests, and more likely to ask the patient to return. There was, however, no difference in costs and patients who saw a nurse practitioner were more satisfied (even after allowing for the longer consultation period). These and other similar findings question basic assumptions and perceptions of the roles of different health care professions which go to the heart of how we organise and deliver care. It suggests that part of the solution to some of the workforce challenges facing managers lies in greater flexibility in staff deployment and the potential to redesign the way services are delivered.

Nurse recruitment and retention in nineteenth-century London teaching hospitals

Carol Helmstadter

Abstract

Difficulty in recruiting sufficient nurses of the right calibre is nothing new. This historical paper explores the situation in the London teaching hospitals during the nineteenth century. It uses contemporary archives and published accounts to explore the organisation of nursing services. Different models were tried at different times, involving the identification of new pools of potential recruits, the need to provide accommodation, and a focus on improving working conditions. By the end of the century a standard model had emerged.

Introduction

One of the greatest difficulties which occurs in completing the arrangements of a hospital is the procuring of proper persons to act as nurses; since as much perhaps depends on the humane endeavours of a kind and attentive female as upon the ability of the medical attendant.

So wrote Benjamin Golding, the founder of Charing Cross Hospital, in 1819. He had just qualified as a doctor at St Thomas' and was impressed by the way a skilful nurse could often secure a patient's recovery when the doctor had given up all hope (Golding 1819).

There were 12 hospitals with medical schools in London by the middle of the nineteenth century. St Bartholomew's and St Thomas' were medieval foundations; the Westminster, Guy's, St George's, the London and the Middlesex were eighteenth century foundations; while the Royal Free, Charing Cross, University College, King's College and St Mary's Hospitals were established in the nineteenth century. All were charitable

Source: *International History of Nursing Journal*, 2.1, 1996, 58–69.

institutions depending on endowments, gifts and subscriptions for their funding. Most ran at a deficit, and some were on the brink of financial disaster most of the time (HMSO 1892).

In efforts to attract and keep better nurses during the second half of the century, each of these hospitals reorganised its nursing service at different times and in different ways. Nevertheless, by the end of the century a standard model, severely compromised by the hospitals' financial difficulties, had emerged.

A shortage of nurses

In 1834, Golding opened his new hospital at Charing Cross. The new institution set out over 100 pages of rules and regulations for officers and servants of the institution, but did not include nurses as a separate category. Nurses were mentioned, however, in the five pages devoted to the duties of the Sisters or Dames of the Wards. They were responsible for orderly discipline, regularity and comfort in their wards, and for the sobriety and good behaviour of patients, nurses and visitors. The Sisters were to employ the nurses for the heavier domestic duties and see that they were performed with system and regularity (Charing Cross Archives 1845). These nurses worked a 17-hour day if they were day nurses, and a minimum of 11 hours if they were night nurses. These working hours were not unusual in England in the first part of the nineteenth century, when the working day was longer than at any other time (Kucyzynski 1936).

Job opportunities for women were few, narrow and overcrowded. Apart from domestic service, street selling, prostitution and the various forms of the needle trade were the main options for unskilled women. The term 'women's work' generally meant unskilled and low-paid work, frequently involving, as did nursing, heavy physical labour. Many women broke down under the severe physical strain (Alexander 1983). One of the major objections to the new-style lady nurses later in the century was that they were young women who did not have the physical strength of the older nurses, and could not shift and change the patients as easily and quickly (GLRO 1880).

Where heavy physical work was not involved, as with unskilled needlewomen, the pay was lower. They made as little as £9 to £12 per year. A woman could earn more by the day washing and charring but she could rarely count on more than three to five days' work a week. Women's work in London was usually casual and irregular. Nurses' work, however, was entirely regular: they had to work seven days a week (London Hospital Archives 1850).

Not only was nursing regular work but it was well compensated, comparatively speaking. While the value of money remained essentially unchanged, nurses' wages climbed steadily from the eighteenth century until the introduction of the new training schools in the latter part of the nineteenth century. Nurses were paid £18 a year at St Thomas' in 1741, £25 in 1819, and by 1858 some were making as much as £33 (GLRO 1864).

At Charing Cross nurses started at £24 a year in 1834. Their wages were raised to £27 in 1849, a year when unemployment reached unprecedented heights and women's and children's wages dropped to unprecedented depths. In 1862, the hospital raised the nurses' wages to £30 a year (Charing Cross Archives 1865). In addition, the hospital generally provided some kind of sleeping accommodation which was usually wretched, plus beer and often some food (Abel-Smith 1960). But despite the relatively good pay, the shortage of nurses was acute.

Solutions to recruitment and retention problems

In December 1818 the House Committee of the London Hospital met to discuss the nursing situation. Sir William Blizard, the senior surgeon, was present with two of his juniors, Drs Buxton and Robertson. The committee felt the matron was unequal to the duties which had devolved to her. She needed to keep better accounts and she needed the power to suspend the nurses and servants. The committee found it very discouraging: the problems were not so much due to faulty regulations as to the regulations not being enforced.

They concluded that the key to the problem was to find a more respectable class of woman to provide the nursing and to induce them to stay for longer periods. In an effort to attract this better class of woman and to achieve a lower rate of turnover, they raised the nurses' wages and set aside £50 for gratuities for those nurses who remained for a whole year.

The committee also tightened up and elaborated hospital regulations. Strict adherence to a time schedule was to be enforced: the nurses were to be in the wards from 6 am to 10 pm and in bed by 11 pm. They were to wear a distinctive dress or at least a medal, and were to do their washing in the wash-house, not in the wards. The strictest attention should be paid to the personal cleanliness of the patients, who should be served their meals at a stated time. Nurses were never to accept money from patients. The custom of taking turns going out on Sunday was to be stopped: nurses were never to leave the hospital without the express permission of the matron (London Hospital Archives 1818).

Sixty years later, in 1879, Margaret Burt arrived at Guy's Hospital as the new matron. Dr Steele, the administrator, had made major efforts at improving the nursing service over the previous 25 years, but things were not very different from the situation which Sir William Blizard found so unsatisfactory in 1818. The nurses accepted tips from the patients, there was no difference between the nurses' indoor dress and that of the ward maids, and the nurses' outdoor dresses were dirty.

The nurses had regular working hours but they were not enforced. The sisters had no regular hours of work but came and went as they pleased. Some were sleeping with the medical students in their rooms adjoining the ward. The hospital did not provide food for the night nurses, so they appropriated the patients' food. Patients with broken legs and others who should not have been moved were taken out of bed so that their beds could be made more easily. No medicines were given on Sunday afternoons because it spoiled the pleasure of the day. No reports were exchanged between day and night nurses. The patients were not clean: some were in the hospital for weeks with only their hands and faces washed. Worse still, the nurses were allowed to leave without giving notice (Counsell 1943).

This 'lack of order and regularity' was not confined to hospital nursing services but existed throughout the early nineteenth century workforce. How to secure adherence to a structured time schedule and workday was something which was only beginning to be worked out. In the first three quarters of the century the basic problem for managers was getting the work done. The labour supply was extremely unpredictable and rates of turnover very high. Nurses were not the only workers who came and went as they pleased. Regular attendance at work was the central problem in the new industries (Booth 1902).

The nursing reforms of St John's House

These problems were intimately associated with those of social discipline, and it was Dr Robert Bentley Todd of King's College Hospital who first realised this. He saw that the conventional method of addressing the problem, by raising wages and writing stricter rules which hospital administrators were not able to enforce, was ineffective.

Rather than trying to attract a better class of woman, Todd and a group of men who were deeply committed to education for women proposed creating a new type of nurse by educating young women systematically in hospital nursing (Cartwright 1968). The training institution which they founded in 1848 took the form of a lay Anglican community, the Sisterhood of St John the Evangelist, better known as St John's House.

The sisterhood consisted of three groups: the sisters (who were ladies working for no pay), experienced nurses and probationers (GLRO 1908). The aim of the institution was threefold: to train the probationers systematically in a regular course to nurse in a trustworthy and professional manner; to offer nurses a better social position; and to open a legitimate field of labour to middle and upper class ladies, who traditionally were not allowed to work (GLRO 1848).

Three obvious obstacles to recruitment which the sisters faced were the heavy menial duties of the nurses, their wretched living conditions and the degraded social status of nursing. The sisters met these problems by hiring domestic staff to do the charring, cooking and laundry so that the nurses could spend all their time attending the sick, and they provided comfortable living arrangements both in the community home and in the hospitals where they later nursed (Kamm 1965).

The problem of social status was overcome by making the training institution a religious sisterhood. The religious organisation offered working class women an improved social standing and it enabled middle class women to remain ladies, for they did not receive a salary. Most women had, of course, always worked, but they were lower or working class women. The Victorians believed that when a lady accepted a salary she not only gave up her status as a lady but also deprived a needy woman of a living. Even though their nursing work was considered religious charity, it was a radical departure for upper class ladies to hold regular jobs.

Perhaps the three most revolutionary changes were that the sisters had to be trained nurses themselves; that the sisterhood allowed its nurses and sisters time off when they became too tired; and that the sisters treated the working class nurses with respect. 'Every nurse is an object of personal solicitude to the superior, who endeavours to allot to each the work for which she is best fitted', Sister Caroline Lloyd, the Lady Superior, wrote in 1874. She deplored the way nurses were worked for the convenience of others until they were worn out, at which point they were cast aside as useless. At St John's House, she said, the sisters treated the nurses with sympathy and consideration and as members of the community (GLRO 1852).

In 1856 St John's House took over the nursing at King's College Hospital. Subsequently, parties came from all over the world to study the sisters' nursing arrangements, and within a year other hospitals were emulating their reforms. When Florence Nightingale began planning her school at St Thomas' she constantly consulted Sister Mary Jones, the Lady Superior of St John's House. Nightingale greatly admired her, and she was one of her closest friends. She believed Jones had the 'firmest, clearest mind'.

The cost of nursing reform

In the 1860s and 1870s the nursing shortage reached crisis proportions. In 1872 the Westminster Hospital found itself unable to staff its nursing department. It therefore set up a Sub-Committee on Nursing to investigate how best to obtain and keep a well trained and efficient staff of nurses. After looking at the nursing systems in nine other London teaching hospitals and the Liverpool Royal Infirmary the committee concluded that the old system was not capable of providing a constant supply of good nurses. They thought that outside associations such as the sisterhoods were highly efficient and satisfactory, but expensive. There could also be conflicts of authority because the sisterhoods maintained a high degree of control over the nursing.

The sisterhoods' new nursing systems were indeed more expensive than the old. When St John's House took over the nursing at Charing Cross in 1866, Sister Mary Jones insisted on a larger support staff, a higher nurse to patient ratio and an even higher ratio of nurses for children. There were only three night nurses in the hospital, one for each floor. There were four wards on each floor with a total of 48 women on the first floor, 47 men on the second, and 20 children on the third. Jones felt that no night nurse should have to look after more than 30 patients, and even then, only if all the beds were in one room. She suggested an additional two night nurses.

After careful consideration, the Westminster Sub-Committee decided to adopt the training school system which the Liverpool Royal Infirmary used. The nursing service was completely under the control of the hospital administration. Furthermore, it was the cheapest of the 11 nursing services surveyed, costing £5 per bed to nurse as compared with the most expensive nursing service, St John's House at King's College Hospital, which cost £13 per bed. The training institution in Liverpool not only provided the nurses for the hospital but made a profit sending nurses out to private families (GLRO 1874).

The committee identified four major stumbling blocks to the recruitment and retention of a superior and qualified class of women: inadequate pay, understaffing, menial work such as cleaning and scrubbing, and want of proper accommodation for eating and sleeping. In their analysis inadequate pay and understaffing created much less of a barrier than menial work and proper accommodation. So the new training schools improved the sleeping quarters for the nurses and provided them with better meals. There was less of the heavy cleaning work, but there were fewer staff than those of the sisterhoods, and salaries were lower.

This training school model was to become the standard paradigm by the end of the century. Its introduction was facilitated by a major shift in the labour market. By the 1890s nursing had become a recognised option for women and, in the London teaching hospitals, was attracting more applicants than the training schools could accept. This was partly because many middle class women were working in other occupations making it more socially acceptable to work for a salary, and partly due to the excellent publicity which Nightingale and her Fund Council were obtaining. The reversal of the supply and demand ratio proved temporary but it enabled hospitals to phase out the sisterhoods which, in the 1850s and 1860s, were often the only reliable and educated nursing services. By the end of the 1890s the new era of the training school had begun (Morten 1895).

Conclusion

In 1891 William Rathbone appeared as a witness before a Select Committee of the House of Lords. The committee was investigating the operation of the London hospitals. Rathbone was a well known nursing reformer and a member of the Nightingale Fund Council. 'We have been told over and over again' Lord Thring explained to Mr Rathbone 'that it is a law of necessity that nurses should be worked so hard and for such long hours, but on analysing the situation, it was simply a matter of the hospitals not wishing to spend the money on the nurses'. Mr Rathbone replied:

> *The patients are our first objects in hospitals, and if hospital work is such work that a woman of ordinary health and strength can do it and remain in health, at least as well as she could in other work by which women have to earn their livelihood, I think that you have done all that you are bound to do until the public gives you money to do more.*
>
> (HMSO 1892)

The committee was not certain that Rathbone was right. They pointed out in their final summary that even those witnesses who considered the nursing staffs adequate hoped that nurses could have shorter hours, longer holidays and better pay in the near future.

Charles Booth objected to using the nurses until their health broke on the grounds of the cost to society. 'Hospitals', he said, require the services of nurses for a few years only and the supply of probationers is abundant. But the long hours and excessively hard work during the period of training damaged the nurses' strength physically and mentally. And thus the hospitals themselves may be well and economically served', he concluded, 'but the nurses, and ultimately the community as a whole, pay the penalty' (Booth 1902).

In 1904 Sidney Holland, the Chairman of the Board at the London Hospital, explained that there was a shortage of the right class of women applying to nursing school. 'We sometimes despair a great deal of the class of women that are applying', he explained. 'There just weren't that many people who wanted to be nurses. The Florence Nightingales of the world had been exhausted', he said. 'There was a great rush at one time and a very few places to go to. Now it is increasingly difficult to get these people to come in' (HMSO 1892).

The supply and demand relationship had returned to its secular norm. Perhaps in the long run the hospitals' strategy for supplying nurses served them less well than they thought.

References

Abel-Smith, B. (1960) *A History of the Nursing Profession*, London: Heinemann.

Alexander, S. (1983) *Women's Work in Nineteenth Century London: A Study of the Years 1820–50*, London: Routledge.

Booth, C. (1902) *Life and Labour of the People of London*, London, 1st Series, IV: 321–6.

Cartwright, F. (1968) *The Story of the Community of the Nursing Sisters of St. John the Divine*, London: Greater London Record Office.

Charing Cross Archives (1845) *Minutes of the Board of Governors*, London: Charing Cross Hospital.

Charing Cross Archives (1865) *Minutes of the Board of Governors*, London: Charing Cross Hospital.

Counsell, H. (1943) *The Broad: The Memoirs of an Oxford Doctor*, London: Scientific Press.

Golding, B. (1819) *Historical Account of the Origin and Progress of St Thomas's Hospital, Southwark*, London: Longman, Hurst, Rees, Orme and Brown.

GLRO (1848) *Training Institutions for Nurses for Hospitals, Families and the Poor*, London: Greater London Record Office, GLRO/H1/ST/SJ/A34/1.

GLRO (1852) *Lady Superintendent's Reports 1849–52*, London: Greater London Record Office, GLRO/H1/ST/SJ/A19/2.

GLRO (1864) *St. Thomas's Hospital Report to the Charity Commissioners*, London: Greater London Record Office.

GLRO (1874) *Report of the Westminster Hospital Sub-committee on Nursing 1871–74*, London: Greater London Record Office, GLRO/H2/WH/AI/44.

GLRO (1880) *Minutes of the General Court*, London: Greater London Record Office, H9/GY/A225/2. 176–80.

GLRO (1908) *St John's House: A Brief Record of Sixty Year's Work*, London: Greater London Record Office, GLRO/H1/ST/SJ/YA10. 3–4.

HMSO (1892) *Parliamentary Papers* 1892. XIII; viii–xxviii; 1904. VI; 747, 765. London.

Kamm, J. (1965) *Hope Deferred: Girls' Education in English History*, London: Methuen.

Kucyzynski, J. (1936) *Labour Conditions in Western Europe 1820–1935*, New York: Harper.

London Hospital Archives (1818) *Minutes of the House Committee*, 28 November and 19 December, 1818. London: London Hospital, LH/A5/16.

London Hospital Archives (1850) *Standing Orders*, London: London Hospital, 7–14.

Morten, H. (1895) *How to Become a Nurse and How to Succeed*, London: Scientific Press.

A complete, unedited version of this article can be found as Helmstadter, C.S. 'Nursing recruitment and retention in the 19th century London teaching hospitals' in the *International History of Nursing Journal* (1996) Volume 2, pages 58–69.

Chapter 12

Labour turnover in the British National Health Service: a local labour market analysis

Alastair M. Gray and V.L. Phillips

Abstract

This study uses regression analyses to examine the relationship between staff turnover in the British National Health Service (NHS) and a range of labour market, job and worker characteristics. Two variables consistently emerge as significantly related to turnover across a range of staff groups: the size of the private health care sector, as measured by the number of beds in private hospitals and in private nursing homes, and the pay of the staff group relative to the local average for comparable workers. The results suggest that staff groups of different skill levels each have distinct labour markets.

Introduction

For most of its existence, the National Health Service (NHS), Britain's largest employer, has managed its human resources centrally with pay and conditions of employment determined at a national level. Under this system periodic concern has arisen in relation to the rate of staff turnover and to sustained recruitment and retention difficulties relative to particular skill groups or in specific geographical areas. Discussions have focused on factors likely to influence turnover, such as pay, management practices, age and gender of the workforce, and aspects of the wider labour market (King's Fund Institute 1990; National Audit Office 1991; Review Body 1992). Although the absence of empirical information in this area is striking, recent reforms to the NHS have clearly underlined the Government's belief that local labour market conditions affect staff behaviour.

Initially set out in *Working for Patients* (Department of Health 1989), the NHS reforms devolve many aspects of labour management to the local

Source: *Health Policy*, 36, 1996, 273–89.

level. NHS Trusts are now free to adjust pay and conditions of employment in response to individual supply and demand needs and to local labour market conditions.

These reforms have major implications for the management of the NHS's human resources – for example, pay rises can now be used to attract nurses to an area experiencing a shortage – and they have given rise to heated debate in the medical and nursing press (Smith and Simpson 1994; Fox 1995). In an effort to inform this discussion, this paper assesses the extent to which labour turnover is systematically related to the characteristics of the local labour markets.

An economic approach to turnover

In explaining quits or voluntary turnover, economists tend to emphasise wages as the central factor affecting worker behaviour. Workers are assumed to maximise lifetime income, and as part of this process, workers join firms which provide the best employment package on offer at a particular point in time. When considering job changes, workers take account of their wage in the firm in which they are employed, that on offer in alternative employment, and the value of their time out of the formal labour market. Quits arise as they re-evaluate their initial employment decision in light of changes in market conditions or in their own circumstances and decide not to continue existing employment.

Firms, on the other hand, recognise that wages affect quits and set remuneration rates with an expected level of quits in mind. Information is revealed to firms through worker quits and an employer may modify the employment package on offer to induce a change in the level of turnover.

The economic literature on labour turnover, both theoretical and empirical, is extensive (Parsons 1977; Jovanovic 1979). Empirical studies of the job-quit relationship generally fall into two categories: those that use longitudinal data to analyse the quit behaviour of individuals, and those that use cross-sectional industry data to systematically link quit behaviour and labour market characteristics. Both types produce consistent results: that quits are negatively related to wage rates in the current job, to the costs of search, to the skill level of the workers in question, and to their time on-the-job, and that quit rates are affected by labour market conditions and characteristics of the workforce.

Despite the general interest in the subject, however, and the specific interest in relation to the NHS, there have been few attempts to measure turnover rates in the health service or to establish any empirical relationship between local labour market conditions and a provider's ability to recruit or retain staff. Similarly, apart from anecdotal evidence, little documentation exists on the characteristics of the local labour markets which providers face or even how they should be defined.

Hypotheses

As described above, turnover results from an individual reassessing his or her current employment situation in light of new information related to their characteristics, their job, or the wider labour market. Although desirable, longitudinal data on individuals are not available from the NHS and the unit of observation under study here is the District Health Authority (DHA). Specifically, the dependent variables are the average annual turnover rates across all providers within the geographical area of a DHA for various staff groups by sex and contract status. Individual behaviour is thus aggregated across providers within a district's area.

Workforce variables

A number of factors may influence an individual's propensity to quit. These include: her or his qualifications, which determine the relevant job market; time spent on the job in which firm-specific capital could have been acquired; age; contract status; family obligations; and gender. Many such data on the NHS workforce are not available. Turnover rates are disaggregated by skill level, contract status and gender, and age is included in the regression as an important workforce characteristic. Its relationship to turnover, however, is difficult to predict.

Generally, age and quits are held to be inversely related as age correlates with length of service and the acquisition of firm-specific capital leading to higher pay. In the NHS it is unclear if this generalisation holds true across staff groups. Younger workers, on the whole, are more likely to be mobile as they have lower investments in their job and community. Older workers may have lower quit rates as they settle into a job or a community, but they may continue to have relatively high quit rates if they move for promotion or for family reasons. Data suggest that quit rates for nurses rise initially, fall and plateau, then rise again as workers approach retirement age (Gray and Phillips 1994). An average turnover rate for a staff group aggregated across a DHA is likely be a reflection of the average age of its workforce, although the direction will depend on the career structure of the staff group in question.

Job characteristics

Features of employment in provider units are also likely to affect turnover rates. For example, providers serving large *populations* may be able to offer greater opportunities for promotion and employee-job matching, thus reducing quit rates.

The workload may also be important: providers with particularly high *throughput* rates may be operating more efficiently, but also increasing pressure on their workforce and raising quit rates.

Labour market variables

The opportunities for alternative employment can be captured through a number of variables. The assumption here is that each DHA's boundaries represent not just an administrative boundary, but also a *functional* space, the labour market within which providers recruit labour. The district *unemployment/vacancy ratio* is an indicator of the volume of employment available generally in the local labour market. A high ratio is likely to be associated with lower turnover rates, as it signals job scarcity. Alternatively, poor local employment conditions could increase female turnover rates if women migrate from the area with their spouses or partners who are in search of work.

A large *service sector* offering part-time employment in a local labour market will potentially be associated with higher turnover rates, especially among administrative, clerical, professional and technical staff. Local *pay levels* are also likely to play a key role in a provider's ability to retain staff. Prior to the reforms, providers were constrained by national pay agreements. In this situation, if the remuneration levels in the local labour market are high relative to the national average, a provider will not be able to offer a competitive salary compared with the local going rate because the provider has to adhere to a nationally determined pay rate. As a result, they may have difficulty retaining staff and experience higher turnover rates.

While conditions in the local labour market generally are likely to be influential, the availability of employment in the *private health care sector* may be of greater importance in influencing turnover rates. Many groups, particularly nurses, have occupation-specific skills and are not portable to other industrial sectors but could be transferred between the public and private health care sectors. Therefore a large private/registered nursing home and hospital sector are likely to be associated with high turnover rates. Similarly, high numbers of *nurse vacancies* may signal the availability of alternative nursing employment and thus be linked to a high turnover rate.

Data

The dependent variable

Data on leavers and staff-in-post for 19 staff groups by age, sex, length of service, and full-time and part-time status were requested from all English Regional Health Authorities. In total, the sample number of DHAs was 103, and an aggregate number of 311,000 employees were covered.

Turnover rates

The mean turnover rate for all staff groups was 13.8 per cent, while the turnover rate for all full-time staff was 15.2 per cent, compared to 11.6 per cent among all part-time staff. Nurses do not have the highest turnover rates: clerical and higher clerical officers are more subject to staff turnover than are nursing staff in the NHS.

Regression analysis and empirical results

A series of regression analyses were performed for each staff group. The independent variables consisted of the variables from each sub-group of explanatory variables: labour market, job and worker characteristics. The list of variables included in the equations are given in Table 12.1.

Table 12.2 contains a summary of the regression equations for the staff

Table 12.1 Definitions of explanatory variables

Variable name	Definition
INHOSBED	(Log of) number of beds in independent hospital sector in DHA in 1990
PRIVNHBD	(Log of) number of beds in private nursing home sector in DHA in 1990
REGRPFT	(Log of) full-time registered nurse pay as a percentage of average earnings of all non-manual full-time female employees in relevant NES region in 1990
REGRPPT	(Log of) part-time registered nurse pay as a percentage of average earnings of all non-manual full-time female employees in relevant NES region in 1990
ENRRPFT	(Log of) full-time enrolled nurse pay as a percentage of average earnings of all full-time female employees in relevant NES region in 1990
ENRRPPT	(Log of) part-time enrolled nurse pay as a percentage of average earnings of all part-time female employees in relevant NES region in 1990
UNQRPFT	(Log of) full-time unqualified nurse pay as a percentage of average earnings of all full-time female employees in relevant NES region in 1990
UNQRPPT	(Log of) part-time unqualified nurse pay as a percentage of average earnings of all part-time female employees in relevant NES region in 1990
NURSEVAC	Nurse vacancies reported in DHA, as a percentage of DHA population in 1990
UNVACRAT	Ratio of unemployed persons in DHA to number of vacancies in DHA in 1990
THRUGM	Throughput in general medicine wards in 1990
AGE	Age in years

Variables were entered in logged form to enable the coefficients to be interpreted as elasticities.

Table 12.2 Regressions: dependent variable = turnover rate

Variable	Registered nurses and HVs		Enrolled nurses		Other nursing staff		Midwives	Clerical workers	
	F-T	P-T	F-T	P-T	F-T	P-T	F-T	F-T	P-T
INHOSBED	0.027 (3.43)***	0.018 (0.27)	0.054 (1.64)*	0.022 (0.48)	0.023 (1.98)**	0.018 (0.89)	0.059 (2.07)**	0.017 (1.61)	0.065 (1.29)
PRIVNHBD	6.383×10^{-5} (0.002)	0.223 (2.72)*	−0.087 (−0.54)	0.280 (1.27)	0.078 (1.39)	0.368 (3.65)***	−0.051 (−0.35)	0.051 (1.09)	0.117 (0.53)
Relative pay	−1.147 (−2.83)***	−2.398 (−2.88)***	−1.515 (−1.02)	−6.108 (−2.75)**	−1.536 (−2.69)***	−3.519 (−3.50)***	−2.379 (−1.75)*	−0.957 (−1.81)*	−3.06 (−1.31)
NURSEVAC	0.004 (2.54)	0.006 (1.91)**	0.002 (0.35)	0.007 (0.86)	1.631×10^{-4} (−0.07)	0.003 (0.84)	0.004 −0.74		
UNVACRAT	0.002 (2.54)	0.015 (2.14)**	−0.031 (−2.21)**	−0.014 (−0.73)	-9.978×10^{-4} (−0.19)	0.011 (1.22)	−0.022 (−1.71)*	0.007 (−1.48)	0.006 (0.27)
Age	0.044 (5.33)***	-4.890×10^{-4} (−0.04)	0.092 (3.19)***	−0.054 (−1.51)	0.013 (1.58)	−0.020 (−1.51)	−0.018 (−0.79)	−0.015 (−1.94)**	−0.006 (−0.21)
THRUGM	0.002 (0.98)	1.749×10^{-4} (0.03)	−0.001 (−0.13)	0.002 (0.16)	0.009 (2.56)***	2.219×10^{-4} (0.03)	−0.017 (−1.87)*	0.002 (0.72)	−0.007 (−0.49)
Adjusted R^2	0.452	0.167	0.239	0.069	0.239	0.174	0.131	0.143	0.001
F-statistic significance	0.000	0.001	0.000	0.099	0.000	0.001	0.007	0.021	0.426

B coefficient (T-statistic), significance: * = <10%; ** = <5%; *** = <1%.
HV, health visitor; F-T, full-time; P-T, part-time.

groups covered by this study: registered, enrolled and unqualified nurses, midwives and clerical workers.

The largest staff group in the analysis were registered nurses. Among full-timers, the regression equation explained 45 per cent of the variation in turnover between DHAs in the sample, a higher level of explanation than for any other staff group. Relative pay, age and the number of beds in the private hospital sector were highly significant.

For part-time registered nurses, the adjusted R^2 was much lower at around 17 per cent (Table 12.2). However, the relative pay variable was again highly significant, while the nurse vacancy ratio, unemployment rate and private sector nursing home beds were also significant variables.

For full-time enrolled nurses, the regression equation explained around 24 per cent of the variation in turnovers between DHAs. The main significant variables were age, the unemployment to vacancies ratio (the more the unemployed in relation to vacancies, the lower the turnover rate among full-time enrolled nurses), and to a lesser extent the number of beds in private hospitals in the district. For part-time enrolled nurses, the overall explanatory power of the equation was lower than for full-time unqualified nurses.

The regression results for full-time midwives attained an adjusted R^2 of just 0.13, with no variables achieving a significance level better than the 5 per cent level. The skills of midwives are probably less transferable to other employers than any other group in this study: even the private health care sector only offers potential employment opportunities for this group as nurses rather than midwives. Viewed from this perspective, the results of the regression analyses for this group are not surprising: midwives would not necessarily be expected to be responsive to most of the labour market variables included here.

Finally, in the regression equations for full-time clerical officers, the only variables in any way significant were age and relative pay. Unlike other staff groups, the sign on the age variable was negative, suggesting that turnover is lower among these staff in DHAs with a higher than average age. This result may be related to the unusual age and length of service structure of the clerical staff group. There are relatively small numbers in the youngest age categories, but in these categories turnover rates are particularly high: for full-time clerical workers the turnover rate among those aged 25 or less is 25 per cent. The regression results for part-time clerical workers produced no significant results.

Elasticity of turnover with respect to relative pay and to the private sector

From the analyses reported above, two variables were repeatedly and significantly related to turnover across several NHS staff groups: the private health care sector and relative pay. Two main measures of the private health care sector were used in the regression equations: the number of beds in nursing homes in each local labour market, and the number of beds in independent hospitals in each local labour market.

Private sector hospital beds appear to be directly related with the turnover rate of full-time staff, while private sector nursing home beds in the case of registered nurses are directly related with part-time staff. Only in the case of registered nurses did the results for full-time staff attain a 1 per cent level of significance, whereas both results for part-time staff were highly significant. Turnover rates are relatively unresponsive to small changes in the size of the private sector and the elasticities are much smaller for the private hospital sector than for the nursing home sector. A 10 per cent increase in the number of private nursing home beds would be associated with approximately a 2.5 per cent increase in the turnover rate.

In relation to relative pay, the elasticity of turnover with respect to pay is uniformly lower among full-time compared with part-time staff. A 5 per cent increase in the relative pay of full-time registered or unqualified nurses would be associated with reductions in the turnover rate of 6 per cent and 8 per cent respectively. However, among part-time staff the elasticities are significantly larger. For example, a 5 per cent increase in the relative pay of part-time unqualified nurses would be associated with reductions in the turnover rate of 17.6 per cent.

Conclusions

Several features of the results merit discussion. It is noteworthy that relative pay, despite the fairly crude way in which it was measured due to data limitations, achieved striking and consistent significance across staff groups. This suggests that the reforms have placed an extremely powerful tool in the hands of local managers to influence worker behaviour.

The results indicate that alternative employment opportunities in the private health care sector affect the behaviour of most staff groups. A large private hospital sector was associated with higher turnover rates among full-time staff, and a large nursing home sector with higher turnover rates among part-time staff. This finding suggests that labour demands differ by facility type. Private hospitals prefer full-time qualified staff, while nursing homes demand part-time, less qualified staff. Thus, both the size and the composition of the local private health care sector will affect employment patterns within NHS providers.

Conditions in the general labour market, measured by the unemployment/vacancy ratio, suggest that local labour market tightness has little impact on most NHS staff groups. The turnover of part-time nurses rises with the unemployment/vacancy ratio, while that of full-time enrolled nurses and midwives falls. The latter two groups may be opting for job security, while the migration effect (i.e. with spouse or partner) may be influencing the former group.

Both worker and job characteristics sporadically influenced the behaviour of staff groups. Age was a significant factor affecting turnover for full-time registered and enrolled nurses and for full-time clerical workers. For the nursing groups the relationship between turnover and age was negative, which suggests that both groups accumulate human capital and quit for promotion or family obligations. Clerical workers, on the other hand, appear to settle into employment as they get older. This group of workers is relatively unusual among those included in the study in that the skills they acquire on the job are less specific to the NHS than are the skills of most other staff groups. They are more easily transferable to a wide range of other employers and in consequence their labour market may be very different to the geographic area of the DHA. This may go some way towards explaining why no significant results could be produced for part-time clerical workers.

The reforms to the NHS have been introduced and their consequences are now unfolding. The analysis presented here indicates that these reforms have given local managers some potentially powerful levers to alter the behaviour of NHS employees. These may help to redress some local problems of staff recruitment and retention, but will also have wider implications for the structure and remuneration of the NHS labour force.

References

Department of Health (1989) *Working for Patients: The Health Service, Caring for the 1990s*, CM555, London: HMSO.

Fox, J. (1995) 'Should nurses have to negotiate local pay awards?', *British Journal of Nursing*, 4: 126–7.

Gray, A.M. and Phillips, V. (1994) 'Turnover, age and length of service: a comparison of nurses and other staff in the NHS', *Journal of Advanced Nursing*, 19: 819–27.

Jovanovic, B. (1979) 'Job matching and the theory of turnover', *Journal of Political Economy*, 87: 972–90.

King's Fund Institute (1990) *New for Old? – Prospects for Nursing in the 1990s*, London: King's Fund Institute Research Report No. 8.

National Audit Office (1991) *NHS Administrative and Clerical Manpower. Session 1990–91*, HC276, London: HMSO.

Parsons, D.O. (1977) 'Models of labour turnover: a theoretical and empirical survey', in R. Ehrnbeg (ed.) *Research in Labour Economics*, Vol. 1, Greenwich, CT: JAI Press, 185–223.

Review Body for Nursing Staff, Midwives, Health Visitors and Professions Allied to Medicine (1992) *Report on Nursing Staff, Midwives and Health Visitors*, London: HMSO.

Smith, J. and Simpson, J. (1994) 'Locally determined performance related pay', *British Medical Journal*, 309: 495–6.

A complete, unedited version of this article can be found as Gray, A.M. and Phillips, V.L., 'Labour turnover in the British NHS: a local labour analysis', in *Health Policy* (1996) Volume 36, pages 273–89.

Chapter 13

Occupational stress and family life: a comparison of male and female doctors

V. Swanson, K.G. Power and R.J. Simpson

Abstract

Characteristics of medical work suggest that doctors are especially vulnerable to stress between work and home. The present study adopted a theoretical approach towards the study of the relationship between occupational stress and home life in doctors in Scotland, comparing male and female general practitioners (GPs) and specialist consultants. First, the relationship between role complexity and occupational stress, workload, job satisfaction and domestic stress and satisfaction was examined. Second, the theory of asymmetric permeability of occupational and domestic roles was used to compare the impact of work-to-home (WH) and home-to-work (HW) stress. Gender and medical speciality differences were considered as intervening variables.

Increased role complexity was related to stress for both male and female doctors in the study, suggesting an increasing convergence in the occupational and domestic roles of male and female doctors. Higher levels of occupational stress were also recorded for WH variables than HW variables for both male and female doctors, confirming the asymmetric permeability of such roles, and failing to identify significant gender differences in this asymmetry. Role complexity was related to reduced occupational workload for females only, and to increased domestic workload for male and female doctors. Aspects of occupational and domestic stress were significantly related to increased role complexity, although role complexity was not significantly related to job satisfaction. When medical specialities were compared, GPs were found to record greater stress in the home/work interface than consultants.

Source: *Journal of Occupational and Organisational Psychology*, 71, 1998, 237–60.

Introduction

Although stresses in the domains of work and home life are often studied in isolation, it is acknowledged that the relationship between the demands of work and home is an important source of occupational stress. This relationship is conceived as being bidirectional, with satisfactions and stressors experienced at work having an impact on satisfactions and stress in home life, and vice versa.

There have been two main approaches to the study of the interface between work and home life, and within these approaches the home/work interface can be seen as contributing positively or negatively to well-being. The first approach suggests that multiple role demands of work and home domains are additive, with combined overload leading to increased stress, strain and illness (Goode 1974; Sekaran 1983). The positive aspect of role additivity theory is that multiple occupational and domestic roles complement one another, resulting in enhanced well-being (Verbrugge 1986). Linked to the concept of additivity is the idea of transfer or 'spillover', where attitudes or behaviour employed in one domain are carried over into and influence the other (Greenhaus and Beutell 1985).

The relationship between home and work can alternatively be seen as 'compensatory', or negatively associated, where problems or deficiencies in one domain are compensated for in the other (Haw 1982). This approach has been adopted in many studies of the relationship between home and work, carried out in mainly female participants, with the weight of evidence suggesting that involvement in occupational roles offers opportunities for self-growth or fulfilment not found in non-work roles and is therefore associated with greater mental well-being (Haw 1982; Nelson *et al.* 1990; Kopp and Ruzicka 1993; Campbell *et al.* 1994).

There are, however, many factors that might affect the relationship between occupation of multiple roles and the experience of stress or strain. Individual factors may include personality, positive/negative affectivity, and mental or physical health status. Social structural factors include status level of the occupation, socioeconomic and financial status, degree of work and family responsibility, and family variables such as number and age of children and degree of support from spouse or others.

Pleck developed the concept of the 'asymmetric permeability' of domestic and work roles, whereby work roles are seen as having a greater influence on home life than vice versa (Pleck 1977). Subsequent studies have developed models of work–family conflict suggesting that work interferes with family life to a greater degree than family life interferes with work (Hall and Richter 1988; Frone *et al.* 1994). With responsibilities as the main breadwinner, males have traditionally been required to allow work to take precedence over family demands, whereas females have had primary domestic responsibility with family demands requiring precedence over work (Haw 1982; Pleck 1985).

The present study aimed to investigate stress in the interface between home and work, comparing male and female doctors working in general practice and in consultant specialities. First, it was hypothesised that females, but not males, with greater 'role complexity' would be more likely to adapt working hours, time on call and domestic work hours to family demands. The nature of general practice compared with consultant medical specialities may also affect this relationship. Second, increased complexity of domestic roles may be significantly associated with increased occupational stress or decreased job satisfaction, and the nature of this relationship would be expected to be more significant for females rather than male doctors and because of their differing work roles, more significant for general practitioners (GPs) than consultants. Third, with reference to the theory of asymmetric permeability of home and work roles, it was hypothesised that levels of home-to-work (HW) stress, but not work-to-home (WH) stress would increase with increasing role complexity. It was also expected that female doctors, particularly GPs, would have greater HW stress, but not greater WH stress than males.

Method

A survey compared levels and sources of occupational stress and job satisfaction for male and female GPs and consultants. The sampling frame of 1668 doctors was selected to represent all Scottish Health Boards. Replies were returned anonymously to maintain confidentiality.

Measures

1 *Demographic information:* A variable was constructed to reflect increasing domestic 'role complexity': group 1, single without children; group 2, married/cohabiting, without children; group 3, married/cohabiting with children, youngest child 5–18 years; group 4, married/cohabiting, youngest child under 5 years.
2 *Workload:* Average number of hours worked per week, including time spent on call during the day; hours per day spent on housework and/or childcare.
3 *Occupational stress:* Sources of Pressure Scale, comprises 61 items and 6 subscales (Cooper *et al.* 1988).
4 *Home/work stress:* 'Home/work Interface Scale', divided into two components: WH items are *(a)* taking my work home; *(b)* not being able to 'switch off' at home; *(c)* demands work makes on my relationship with my spouse/children; *(d)* demands work makes on my

private/social life; (e) pursuing a career at the expense of home life. HW items are (f) my spouse's attitude towards my job and career; (g) absence of emotional support from others outside work; (h) lack of practical support from others outside work; (i) home life with a partner who is also pursuing a career; (j) absence of stability or dependability in home life.

5 *Job satisfaction:* 22-item Job Satisfaction Scale with five subscales.
6 *Home stress:* 'How stressful is your home life?'.
7 *Domestic conflict:* Dichotomous item 'does your job cause conflict with your spouse/partner?'.
8 *Domestic satisfaction:* Two-item scale, assessing satisfaction with spouse's contribution to housework and childcare.

Analysis

For the whole sample, males and females were compared in terms of age, marital status and parental status using *t*-tests or chi-square analysis. To test the theories of additivity, or 'role complexity' and 'asymmetric permeability' of roles, analyses were carried out with a subsample of participants divided into four domestic role groupings representing increased complexity, as described above. Dependent variables were: hours worked, time on call and domestic workload; occupational stress subscales, total job satisfaction, factors representing WH, and HW stress, and overall home stress. Since age was found to be significantly correlated with each of the dependent variables apart from job satisfaction, factorial analysis of covariance (ANCOVA) was carried out with age as the covariate, and 'role complexity', gender and speciality as independent variables. Interaction effects of role complexity, gender and speciality were also calculated. Interactions that were statistically significant are reported. Hierarchical regression analyses were carried out separately for males and females in the 'role complexity sample' with the total home/work interface scale score as the dependent variable.

Results

A total of 986 responses was received, the response rate being slightly higher in female (62 per cent) than male participants (57 per cent). The final sample comprised 283 female GPs, 224 female consultants, 264 male GPs and 215 male consultants. Approximately a quarter (26 per cent) of GPs in the sample worked in rural and 49 per cent in urban practices, the rest being classified as suburban. Mean individual GP list size was 1544, compared with 1569 for Scotland overall. Male doctors in the sample were significantly older, more likely to be married/cohabiting, to have children and to have more children than female doctors (Table 13.1).

Table 13.1 Characteristics of the study sample (n = 986)

	Females (n = 507)	Males (n = <479)	Comparisons
Mean age (years)	41.6	44.9	$t\,(979) = 5.90^{*}$
Marital status: no. (%)			
Single/separated/widowed/divorced	128 (25.2)	33 (6.8)	$\chi^{2}(1) = 60.75^{*}$
Married/cohabiting	379 (74.8)	446 (93.2)	
Children: no. (%)			
Yes	326 (64.3)	419 (87.8)	$\chi^{2}(1) = 74.06^{*}$
No	181 (35.7)	58 (12.2)	
Mean no. of children (SD)	2.18 (0.9)	2.58 (0.9)	$t\,(742) = 5.90^{*}$

$^{*}P < 0.001$.

Workload

After adjusting for age, each of the dependent variables was shown to vary significantly by degree of role complexity, gender and speciality (Table 13.2). Post hoc examination of means revealed that female GPs with children spent significantly fewer hours at work than those with no children, whereas this comparison was not significant for female consultants or for male doctors. A similar pattern emerged in terms of time on call, with the

Table 13.2 Change in hours worked, time on call and domestic work with increasing role complexity in four groups

(a) Means (SD)	→ Increasing role complexity			
	1. (n = 109)	2. (n = 120)	3. (n = 310)	4. (n = 205)
Hours worked				
GP				
Female	42.21 (7.6)	39.98 (16.5)	34.46 (10.8)	31.58 (10.9)[a]
Male	47.54 (11.7)	44.87 (7.2)	46.46 (7.9)	46.31 (8.9)
Consultant				
Female	47.84 (9.1)	47.54 (10.7)	43.33 (10.7)	43.56 (8.8)
Male	51.57 (5.6)	50.0 (11.2)	52.25 (11.0)	53.06 (10.6)
On call				
GP				
Female	7.19 (2.3)	6.59 (3.4)	5.33 (3.5)	5.06 (3.2)[b]
Male	7.23 (3.4)	8.17 (1.6)	8.05 (2.1)	8.00 (1.9)
Consultant				
Female	7.24 (3.4)	7.46 (2.9)	6.50 (3.1)	7.49 (2.9)
Male	8.14 (1.9)	6.93 (3.2)	8.42 (2.2)	8.33 (2.5)

Table 13.2 continued

(a) Means (SD)	→ Increasing role complexity			
	1. (n = 109)	2. (n = 120)	3. (n = 310)	4. (n = 205)
Domestic work				
GP				
Female	1.54 (1.5)	1.52 (0.6)	3.70 (1.8)	5.78 (2.9)[c]
Male	1.18 (0.6)	0.74 (0.8)	1.19 (1.1)	1.79 (0.9)[d]
Consultant				
Female	1.60 (0.8)	1.47 (0.8)	2.96 (1.4)	4.15 (1.8)[e]
Male	1.25 (0.9)	1.14 (0.5)	1.30 (1.0)	1.85 (0.9)[f]

(b) Analysis of variance	Source	d.f.	MS	F
Hours worked				
	Error	727	106.41	
Covariate	Age	1	678.58	6.4*
Main effects	Roles	3	301.08	2.83*
	Gender	1	6308.24	59.28*
	Speciality	1	3705.33	34.82*
Interactions	Roles × gender	3	511.47	4.81*
On call				
	Error	728	7.6	
Covariate	Age	1	40.05	5.27*
Main effects	Roles	3	9.59	1.26
	Gender	1	176.76	23.26***
	Speciality	1	13.24	1.74
Interactions	Roles × gender	3	27.6	3.63*
	Gender × speciality	1	35.1	4.62*
Domestic work				
	Error	712	1.9	
Covariate	Age	1	6.66	3.50
Main effects	Roles	3	114.63	60.23**
	Gender	1	257.61	135.36***
	Speciality	1	1.49	0.78
Interactions	Roles × gender	3	49.73	26.13***
	Roles × speciality	3	6.66	3.50*
	Gender × speciality	1	16.45	8.64**

Groups: 1. Single (SWD), no children; 2. married/cohabiting, no children; 3. married/cohabiting, youngest child 5–18; 4. married/cohabiting, youngest child under 5. Post hoc Scheffé: all comparisons non-significant apart from [a]1–3, 1–4, 2–4; [b]1–3, 1–4; [c]1–3, 1–4, 2–3, 2–4, 3–4; [d]2–4, 3–4; [e]1–3, 1–4, 2–3, 2–4, 3–4; [f]1–4 (groups separated by a dash differ significantly from each other, $P < 0.05$).
* $P < 0.05$.
** $P < 0.01$.
*** $P < 0.001$.

effect of gender being highly significant: female GPs with children spent significantly less time on call than other groups. Time spent on domestic work was shown to increase for both male and female parents in both speciality types with youngest child under 5 in comparison with those with youngest child aged 5–18, and those without children.

Occupational stress

Role complexity was significantly related to occupational stress in two scales, 'factors intrinsic to the job' and the 'home/work interface'. Although no occupational stress scale revealed a significant main effect for gender, the 'factors intrinsic to the job' scale revealed significant interaction effects of roles and gender, and speciality and gender, suggesting that gender may moderate the relationship between parental roles, speciality and this aspect of occupational stress. Similarly, the 'organizational structure and climate' scale showed a significant interaction effect of gender and speciality.

Job satisfaction

Age, role complexity and speciality were not significantly related to job satisfaction (Table 13.3). However, there was a highly significant main effect of gender on this scale, with female GPs and consultants recording significantly higher job satisfaction scores than male GPs and consultants.

Stress between home and work

Examination of means indicates consistently higher scores for WH stress in comparison with HW stress for all participants. Analysis of variance revealed that age was not significantly related to WH or to HW stress. However, the main effect of roles was shown to be significantly related to WH stress: doctors with youngest child under 5 recorded significantly greater scores than those without children. There was no significant effect of role complexity for HW stress. For both WH and HW stress, GPs tended to record higher stress than consultants.

A highly significant effect of role complexity was also observed in terms of the global rating of stressfulness of home life. Post hoc comparisons showed that females with children recorded significantly more 'home stress' than those without children, whereas this was not the case for males.

There was no significant effect of role complexity or speciality in terms of satisfaction with spouse's contribution to housework and to childcare for parents. However, male doctors expressed greater satisfaction with their spouse's contribution to domestic work than females.

Table 13.3 Association between job satisfaction and increasing role complexity in four groups

(a) Means (SD)	→ Increasing role complexity			
	1. (n = 114)	2. (n = 112)	3. (n = 305)	4. (n = 192)
Job satisfaction total				
GP				
Female	82.98 (18.1)	83.64 (14.7)	83.88 (16.3)	85.56 (14.9)
Male	81.18 (14.3)	74.17 (18.1)	79.77 (13.7)	76.97 (15.1)
Consultant				
Female	77.69 (20.1)	82.95 (17.0)	87.15 (13.7)	81.87 (15.5)[a]
Male	73.12 (27.8)	78.14 (15.8)	84.40 (17.3)	82.39 (10.8)

(b) Analysis of variance	Source	d.f.	MS	F
Job satisfaction	Error	748	265.15	
	Age	1	5.51	0.02
Main effects	Roles	3	640.31	2.5
	Gender	1	2261.54	8.83*
	Speciality	1	1.81	0.01

Groups: 1. Single (SWD), no children; 2. married/cohabiting, no children; 3. married/cohabiting, youngest child 5–18; 4. married/cohabiting, youngest child under 5. Post hoc Scheffé: all comparisons non-significant apart from [a]1–3 (groups separated by a dash differ significantly from each other, $P < 0.05$).
**$P < 0.01$.

Predictors of stress in the home/work interface

Overall, 57 per cent of the variance in stress due to the home/work interface was predicted for both female and male doctors (Table 13.4). Demographic variables accounted for a slightly larger amount of variance in female (13 per cent) than in male doctors (6 per cent). The combined workload variables predicted less than 1 per cent of variance in home/work stress. Hours worked was a significant predictor of home/work stress for females but not for male doctors, and time on call was a significant predictor of home/work stress for male but not for female doctors.

The remaining five Occupational Stress Scales jointly predicted an additional 34 per cent of variance for female and an additional 41 per cent for male doctors. Job satisfaction made no significant contribution. Indicators of domestic stress predicted a further 9 per cent of variance.

Discussion

Increasing domestic role demands were related to stress not only for female doctors, but also for male doctors. This could be taken as evidence

Table 13.4 Hierarchical regression analysis of stress in the home/work interface for female and male doctors

Step	1. Females			2. Males		
	β	Multiple R	Adjusted R^2	β	Multiple R	Adjusted R^2
1 Demographic variables		0.3611	0.1304		0.2676	0.0634
Age	−0.0765			−0.1351*		
Speciality	−0.0873			−0.0675		
Roles	0.3093***			0.1826***		
	Overall F (3,423) = 21.15***			Overall F (3,348) = 8.95***		
2 Workload variables		0.3822	0.1339		0.2989	0.0735
Hours worked	0.1381*			0.0764		
Time on call	0.0228			0.1080*		
Domestic work	0.0375			0.028		
	Overall F (6,420) = 11.98***			Overall F (6,345) = 5.64***		
3 Occupational stress		0.698	0.4737		0.7037	0.4788
Factors intrinsic to the job	0.2689***			0.3577***		
Managerial role	0.1078			0.2175**		
Relationships with others	0.2574***			0.1527*		
Career achievement	0.1155*			0.1297*		
Organisational structure and climate	−0.0749			−0.1071		
	Overall F (11,415) = 35.85***			Overall F (11,340) = 30.32***		
4 Job satisfaction	−0.0608	0.7001	0.4755	−0.0439	0.7048	0.479
	Overall F (12, 414) = 33.2***			Overall F (12,339) = 27.88***		
5 Domestic stress		0.7644	0.5691		0.766	0.5686
Home stress	0.2178***			0.2417***		
Conflict	0.1365***			0.1112***		
Spouse satisfaction	−0.1511***			−0.0764*		
	Final F (15,411) = 38.51***			Final F (15,336) = 31.85***		

* $P < 0.05$.
** $P < 0.01$.
*** $P < 0.001$.

of an increasing convergence in the occupational and domestic roles of male and female doctors, and therefore has implications for health service planners in ensuring that doctors of both sexes have the opportunity to achieve an optimal balance between home and work roles.

Increased domestic role complexity, and parenthood in particular, were related to reduced occupational working hours, and reduced hours on call, but increased time spent on domestic work for female doctors. However, for male doctors with young children, in comparison with non-parents in this study, working hours and time on call are maintained or even increased, and time spent on housework or childcare increased, albeit to a lesser extent than for females. Nevertheless, for both male and female doctors, combined occupational and domestic workload variables added little to the prediction of 'home/work stress' in this study. One explanation for the differential impact of domestic role complexity on the occupational and domestic *work hours* of male and female doctors may be the unequal weighting given to home and work roles, whereby home exerts greater demands on female doctors, and work exerts a greater demand on males. An alternative explanation may lie in male and female doctors' differing family circumstances: male doctors in the sample were older, more likely to be married/cohabiting, and had more children than female doctors. Opportunities for working less than full-time hours, job sharing, or taking career breaks are generally more available to females than males, and also more common in general practice than in hospital medicine, where career paths are more rigid (Allen 1988). It may also be the case that professional females are generally more satisfied with their work hours and their achieved balance between work and family time than are males (Bartoleme and Evans 1979; Grant *et al.* 1990).

Male doctors recorded significantly greater satisfaction with their spouse's contribution to domestic work than did females, suggesting that traditional patterns of domestic responsibilities were maintained, similar findings being reported in Lewis and Cooper's (1987) study of two-earner couples in a wider range of occupations.

Male doctors recorded lower job satisfaction than females overall. It has been suggested that job satisfaction for both GPs and consultants has reduced in recent years (Myerson 1991; Sutherland and Cooper 1992; British Medical Association 1996). The existence of high levels of dissatisfaction in medical practitioners is obviously a cause for concern, as it has implications for the well-being of individuals themselves, for the future manpower resources of the NHS, and for the quality of medical care offered to patients.

In terms of domestic stress, this study found a positive association between role complexity and increased WH stress, but not HW stress. This suggests that the demands of work on home life but not the demands of home life on work, are at their most stressful at a life stage when family life is also likely to be at its most demanding. It is therefore possible to conclude that the theory of asymmetric permeability of home and work roles is supported by this study. Interestingly, there was no significant gender difference in the relationship.

For parents, impact of work on home life was perceived as more stressful overall than the impact of home on work. Parents of children under 5 recorded highest WH stress scores. Since responsibility for very young children is both physically and mentally demanding, the fact that work demands have the strongest impact on home life for this group must give cause for concern.

There are obviously many potential contributors to 'role complexity', reflecting a wide range of domestic arrangements and demands, including single parenthood and caring for dependent adults, which it was not possible to accommodate in the sample for the present study. Also, although the role of some potential moderators of the stressor–strain relationship were considered, other potential intervening variables were not investigated. Similarly, some reservations exist as to the comprehensiveness of the measures of home/work stress adopted and the possibility of common method variance arising from the use of intercorrelated measures of occupational stress and home/work stress taken from the OSI questionnaire. Similarly the limitations of the self-report, cross-sectional questionnaire methodology adopted for this study are acknowledged.

Since greater well-being is derived from individuals' ability to be able to function effectively in both domains, and it is clear from this rather exploratory study that the relationship between home and work is a definite source of stress, it is important for employers to recognise the need for individuals to fit the demands of work into a normal working day.

References

Allen, I. (1988) *Any Room at the Top? A Study of Doctors and Their Careers*, London: Policy Studies Institute.

Bartoleme, F. and Evans, P. (1979) 'Professional lives versus private lives – shifting patterns of managerial commitment', *Organisational Dynamics*, 8: 3–29.

British Medical Association (BMA) (1996) 'Doctors under stress', *BMA News Review*, April, 32–4.

Campbell, D.J., Campbell, C.M. and Kennard, D. (1994) 'The effects of family responsibilities on the work commitment and job performance of non-professional women', *Journal of Occupational and Organisational Psychology*, 67: 283–96.

Cooper, C.L., Sloan, S.J. and Williams, S. (1988) *Occupational Stress Indicator Management Guide*, Windsor: ASE Division, NFER-Nelson.

Frone, M.R., Russell, M. and Cooper, M.L. (1994) 'Relationship between job and family satisfaction: causal or noncausal variation?', *Journal of Management*, 20: 565–79.

Goode, W.J. (1974) 'A theory of strain', *American Sociological Review*, 25: 483–96.

Grant, L., Simpson, L.A., Rong, X.L. and Peters-Golden, H. (1990) 'Gender, parenthood and work hours of physicians', *Journal of Marriage and the Family*, 52: 39–49.

Greenhaus, J.H. and Beutell, N.J. (1985) 'Sources of conflict between work and family roles', *Academy of Management Review*, 10: 76–88.

Hall, D.T. and Richter, J. (1988) 'Balancing work life and home life: what can organisations do to help?', *Academy of Management Executive*, 2: 213–23.

Haw, M.A. (1982) 'Women, work and stress: a review and agenda for the future', *Journal of Health and Social Behaviour*, 23: 132–44.

Kopp, R.G. and Ruzicka, M.F. (1993) 'Women's multiple roles and psychological wellbeing', *Psychological Reports*, 72: 1351–4.

Lewis, S.N. and Cooper, C.L. (1987) 'Stress in two-earner couples and stage in the lifecycle', *Journal of Occupational Psychology*, 60: 289–303.

Myerson, S. (1991) 'Doctors' methods of dealing with 'ongoing' stress in general practice', *Medical Science Research*, 19: 267–9.

Nelson, D.L., Quick, J.C., Hitt, M. and Moesel, D. (1990) 'Politics, lack of career progress and work/home conflict: stress and strain for working women', *Sex Roles*, 23: 169–85.

Pleck, H. (1977) 'The work-family role system', *American Journal of Sociology*, 50: 417–25.

Pleck, H. (1985) *Working Wives/Working Husbands*, Beverly Hills, CA: Sage.

Sekaran, U. (1983) 'Factors influencing the quality of life in dual career families', *Journal of Occupational Psychology*, 56: 161–74.

Sutherland, V.J. and Cooper, C.L. (1992) 'Job stress, satisfaction and mental health among general practitioners before and after the introduction of the new contract', *British Medical Journal*, 304: 1545–8.

Verbrugge, L.M. (1986) 'Role burdens and physical health in women and men', *Women and Health*, 11: 47–77.

A complete, unedited version of this article can be found as Swanson, V., Power, K. and Simpson, R., 'Occupational stress and family life: a comparison of male and female doctors' in the *Journal of Occupational and Organisational Psychology* (1998) Volume 71, pages 237–60.

Chapter 14

Lower Medicare mortality among a set of hospitals known for good nursing care

Linda H. Aiken, Herbert L. Smith and Eileen T. Lake

Abstract

Objective: To investigate whether hospitals known to be good places to practice nursing have lower Medicare mortality than hospitals that are otherwise similar with respect to a variety of non-nursing organisational characteristics.

Methods: We capitalise on the existence of a set of studies of 39 hospitals that, for reasons other than patient outcomes, have been singled out as hospitals known for good nursing care. We match these 'magnet' hospitals with 195 control hospitals, selected from all nonmagnet US hospitals with over 100 Medicare discharges, using a multivariate matched sampling procedure that controls for hospital characteristics. Medicare mortality rates of magnet versus control hospitals are compared using variance components models, which pool information on the five matches per magnet hospital, and adjust for differences in patient composition as measured by predicted mortality.

Results: The magnet hospitals' observed mortality rates are 7.7 per cent lower (nine fewer deaths per 1000 Medicare discharges) than the matched control hospitals ($P = 0.011$). After adjusting for differences in predicted mortality, the magnet hospitals have a 4.6 per cent lower mortality rate ($P = 0.026$ [95% confidence interval 0.9 to 9.4 fewer deaths per 1000]).

Conclusions: The same factors that lead hospitals to be identified as effective from the standpoint of the organisation of nursing care are associated with lower mortality among Medicare patients.

Source: *Medical Care*, 38.8, 1994, 771–87.

Introduction

Those familiar with the inner workings of hospitals will not be surprised that there is a relationship between the practice of nursing and the mortality experience of hospital patients (Sunshine and Wright 1988; Koska 1989; Findlay *et al.* 1990). The connection between nursing and mortality rates dates as far back as the reforms in British hospitals made under Florence Nightingale during the Crimean War (Cohen 1984). Nurses are the only professional caregivers in hospitals who are at the bedside of hospital patients around the clock. What nurses do or do not do (or in some circumstances are not allowed to do) is directly related to a variety of patient outcomes, including in-hospital deaths (Benner 1984). Nurses often must act in the absence of the physician when timely intervention is required (Mechanic and Aiken 1982; Stein *et al.* 1990)

Six American Academy of Nursing (AAN) hospital nursing experts in each of eight regions of the country were selected to nominate 6–10 hospitals that met the following three criteria: 1) nurses consider the hospital a good place to practise nursing; 2) the hospital has the ability to recruit and retain professional nurses, as evidenced by a relatively low turnover rate; and 3) the hospital is located in an area where it will have competition for staff from other institutions and agencies. A total of 165 hospitals was nominated; 155 agreed to participate. Each participating hospital provided information on a range of nursing-related issues including nurse vacancy, turnover and absentee rates; the ratio of inexperienced to experienced nurses; use of supplemental staffing agencies; nursing staffing policies; educational preparation of nurses in leadership positions; and the predominant mode of nurse organisation on the units (i.e. primary, team, functional or other). Hospitals were then ranked according to evidence of being able to attract and retain professional nurses and to create an environment conducive to nursing care. The top-ranked 41 institutions were subjected to a subsequent round of data collection interviews with staff nurses and directors of nursing. These were the hospitals that ultimately came to be designated 'magnet' hospitals.

The nurses practising in the designated magnet hospitals cited the following organisational attributes as important in making their hospitals good places to work: 1) the importance and status of nurses in the organisation as reflected in the formal organisational structure and its relationship to the organisation of the hospital; 2) nurse autonomy to make clinical decisions; 3) control over the practice environment; 4) organisation of nurses' clinical responsibilities at the unit level to promote accountability and continuity of care and 5) an established culture signifying nursing's importance in the overall mission of the institution (McClure *et al.* 1983; Kramer and Schmalenberg 1988, 1991; Kramer and Hafner 1989; Kramer 1990).

The original study of these hospitals was conducted in 1982 (McClure *et al*. 1983). A follow-up study was conducted in a geographical stratified subsample of the magnet hospitals in 1986 (Kramer and Schmalenberg 1988, Kramer and Hafner 1989) and again in 1989 (Kramer 1990; Kramer and Schmalenberg 1991). At each point, the magnet hospitals were found to have maintained their ability to attract and recruit nurses, and to have retained the organisational features found in the initial study. With this as backdrop, we turn to the question of whether magnet hospitals have lower mortality than hospitals with similar structural features, except for the organisational facilitation of professional nursing practice.

Methods

Our analysis of the mortality experience of Medicare patients at the magnet hospitals is based on a comparison of these hospitals with a set of hospitals not known for good nursing care, but comparable with respect to other factors thought to be correlated with hospital mortality. The 195 control hospitals, 5 for each magnet hospital, were selected by a multivariate matching procedure.

Our response variable is the 1988 mortality rate (death within 30 days of admission) among hospitalised Medicare beneficiaries, as reported in the Health Care Financing Administration (HCFA) Medicare hospital mortality rate file (Health Care Financing Administration 1989). Thirty-nine of the original 41 magnet hospitals could be found in this file.

Potential control hospitals were sought among the 5053 'non-magnet' hospitals that had at least 100 Medicare discharges and could be linked to the 1988 American Hospital Association (AHA) annual survey of hospitals (American Hospital Association 1989). The AHA annual survey of hospitals provides the most comprehensive data available on hospital organisational structure, facilities and services, beds and utilisation, finance, personnel by occupational category, medical staff and other hospital characteristics. We compared magnet hospitals with other hospitals along a variety of dimensions, and then used these organisational characteristics to construct a matched sample of control hospitals.

The matching procedure worked as described below.

Propensity scores

For the entire sample, a dichotomous variable (coded 1 if the hospital was a magnet hospital and 0 otherwise) was (logistically) regressed on the 12 organisational characteristics in the first column of Table 14.1 (Rosenbaum and Rubin 1985). The resultant discriminant function was used to obtain, for each hospital in the sample, a predicted logit (log-odds on being a magnet hospital). This predicted logit is the propensity score.

Table 14.1 Characteristics of the study hospitals

Characteristics	Magnet hospitals (n = 39)	Potential control hospitals (n = 5053)	Matched control hospitals				
			1st (n = 39)	2nd (n = 39)	3rd (n = 39)	4th (n = 39)	5th (n = 39)
1 Ownership (%)							
Public	7.7	28.2[a]	2.6	12.8	0.0	5.1	10.3
Private for-profit	7.7	14.2	18.0	5.1	12.8	12.8	2.6
Private not-for-profit	84.6	57.7[a]	79.5	82.1	87.2	82.1	87.2
2 Member – Council of Teaching Hospitals (%)	28.2	5.8[a]	23.1	33.3	30.8	30.8	28.2
Hospital size							
3 Average daily census (ADC)	305.5 ± 148.9	112.0 ± 137.6[a]	326.2	323.5	294.1	274.6	302.9
4 Hospital beds	412.6 ± 180.4	160.6 ± 167.4[a]	444.9	452.4	399.9	372.9	407.7
5 Medicare discharges	5006 ± 2229	1873 ± 1927[a]	5357	5227	4877	4915	5306
Financial status							
6 Payroll ($million)	46.7 ± 29.5	13.3 ± 20.4[a]	45.1	49.6	42.3	45.6	45.1
7 Occupancy rate	0.722 ± 0.115	0.556 ± 0.190[a]	0.72	0.679	0.707	0.712	0.737
8 Board-certified physicians/all physicians	0.756 ± 0.086	0.661 ± 0.194[a]	0.759	0.749	0.741	0.774	0.743
9 Payroll expense/hospital bed ($1000)	109 ± 35	64 ± 35[a]	95[b]	105	100	110	108
10 High-technology index score[c]	2.57 ± 1.68	0.59 ± 1.12[a]	2.68	2.75	2.74	2.68	2.36
11 No. of emergency visits/ADC	117.7 ± 69.6	181.6 ± 144.4[a]	121.9	127	96.4	127.2	129.8
12 Metropolitan statistical area size[d]	4.49 ± 1.254	2.14 ± 2.296[a]	4.26	4.44	4.54	4.33	4.51
13 Propensity score	3.530 ± 1.142	6.589 ± 1.956[a]	3.531	3.532	3.533	3.525	3.523
14 RNs/ADC	1.569 ± 0.556	1.216 ± 0.704[a]	1.471	1.503	1.329[b]	1.454	1.424
15 RNs/total nursing personnel	0.760 ± 0.130	0.581 ± 0.149[a]	0.692[b]	0.690[b]	0.682[a]	0.708[b]	0.671[a]
16 Predicted mortality	0.113 ± 0.016	0.123 ± 0.024[a]	0.117	0.114	0.117	0.115	0.119
17 Mortality rate	0.105 ± 0.021	0.126 ± 0.035[a]	0.117[b]	0.109	0.117[b]	0.111	0.116[b]

Plus-minus values are means ± standard deviation. [a]$P < 0.01$. [b]$P < 0.05$.
[c]The high-technology index score ranges from 0 to 5 based on the presence or absence of the following items: a cardiac catheterisation laboratory, an extracorporeal lithotriptor, a facility for magnetic resonance imaging, a facility for open-heart surgery and organ transport capability.
[d]Metropolitan statistical area size is an ordinal variable with values ranging from 0 to 6 corresponding to the following Census Bureau MSA population size categories: 0 = non-metropolitan area – areas with no city with a population of 50,000 or more nor a total population of 100,000 or more; 1 = under 100,000; 2 = 100,000 to 250,000; 3 = 250,00 to 500,000; 4 = 500,000 to 1,000,000; 5 = 1,000,000 to 2,500,000; 6 = over 2,500,000.

Random order, nearest available pair-matching

A set of random numbers was generated, one for each of the 39 magnet hospitals (Rubin 1973). Beginning with the lowest random number, and proceeding in random number size order, each magnet hospital was matched with the non-magnet hospital in the sample with the nearest propensity score. That control hospital, or 'match,' was then removed from the sample, so that no hospital served as the control for more than one magnet hospital. Random order, nearest available pair-matching was repeated four more times, until each magnet hospital was matched with five unique control hospitals.

Even after matching on numerous organisational characteristics, magnet hospitals clearly employ more registered nurses as a percentage of total nursing personnel (variable no. 15; this was *not* a predictor in the discriminant function) than do their matched controls. Matching on organisational characteristics does, however, reduce differences between hospitals in patient characteristics affecting mortality.

Results

The matching procedures previously described resulted in five comparison hospitals for each of our 39 magnet hospitals. In concept, our analysis is simple. We compare the average mortality of the 39 magnet hospitals with those of the 195 ($= 5 \times 39$) comparison (control) hospitals. In practice, the analysis is somewhat more complex, because having multiple controls (matches) for each magnet hospital allows us to examine whether the mortality differences between magnet and non-magnet hospitals varies across the set of magnet hospitals. Thus, we have embedded familiar *t*-tests for paired comparisons in the framework of the random effects analysis of variance (ANOVA). We do this by conceptualising each difference between a magnet hospital and a matched control hospital as attributable to 1) the 'general' effect of magnet hospitals on mortality; 2) an effect that is specific to a particular magnet hospital; and 3) chance error. An advantage of this general model is that it is easily extended to include control variables, such as predicted mortality (as a function of patient composition).

The first row of Table 14.2 gives the basic ANOVA estimates (model I). The estimate of -0.0087 corresponds to a reduction of approximately nine deaths per 1000 Medicare admissions. With hospital death rate averages in the order of 113 per 1000 in the study sample, this is equivalent to an estimated 7.7 per cent diminution in mortality.

Table 14.2 also contains estimates of the variation in mortality differences between magnet hospitals and matched control hospitals in its final two columns. There are significant differences between magnet hospitals

Table 14.2 Estimated parameters for three models of hospital mortality

Model	Control for predicted mortality?	Response variable	Mean difference between magnet hospitals and matched controls γ_{00}	Between-block progression of predicted mortality difference on observed mortality differences γ_{01}	Within-block regression of predicted mortality differences on observed mortality differences γ_{10}	Between blocks of matched hospitals τ_{00}	Within blocks of matched hospitals σ_2
I	No	Mortality difference between magnet hospital and matched control hospital	−0.0087 −0.0032 $P = 0.011$			0.00029 ($\chi^2 = 154$) $P < 0.001$	0.00048
II	Yes	Mortality difference between magnet hospital and matched control hospital	−0.0052 −0.0022 $P = 0.026$	0.93 −0.133 $P < 0.001$	1.01 −0.074 $P < 0.001$	0.00013 ($\chi^2 = 145$) $P < 0.001$	0.00022
III	Yes	Natural logarithm of the ratio of excess (observed over predicted) mortality in magnet versus control hospitals	−0.048 −0.021 $P = 0.034$			0.0139 ($\chi^2 = 154$) $P < 0.001$	0.0167

'Blocks' are a magnet hospital and its five matched control hospitals. There are 39 blocks in the analysis. For fixed effects, estimated standard errors are in parentheses. For variance components, estimated χ^2 statistics are in parentheses.

regarding their effects on mortality, as indicated by the high level of variance between blocks of matched hospitals. This means that the average mortality reduction, of nine deaths per 1000 Medicare admissions, blends substantial differences in effects, across magnet hospitals. Having multiple matches per magnet hospital allows us to estimate these hospital-specific effects with moderately good precision. The reliability of the estimated mortality reduction effect for specific hospitals is 0.75.

Hospitals appear well matched with respect to a variety of organisational characteristics, such as size and ownership, found by some previous studies to be related to mortality. However, as revealed in Table 14.1, the predicted mortality of magnet hospitals is somewhat lower than that of matched controls. The estimated mortality difference under model I might reflect differences in patient composition, as measured by their functional composite, predicted mortality. Thus, in model II of Table 14.2, we control for differences between magnet hospitals and matched control hospitals in predicted mortality. Some, but not all, of the observed mortality difference is attributable to differences in patient characteristics, as the estimate of the general magnet hospital effect on mortality shrinks from -0.0087 to -0.0052. The 95 per cent confidence interval for the effect of magnet hospitals on mortality, with adjustment for hospital-specific predicted mortality, is from 0.9 to 9.4 fewer deaths per 1000.

Controlling for differences in patient composition (i.e. predicted mortality) also substantially attenuates differences between magnet hospitals in their effect on observed mortality. A comparison, between models I and II, of the estimated variance in effects between blocks of matched hospitals reveals that over half the original variability in estimates of mortality reduction across magnet hospitals is attributable to not having controlled for differences between hospitals in patient characteristics.

Similar results are obtained when we adjust for predicted mortality not as a covariate, but as the denominator in a measure of excess mortality (i.e. the ratio of observed to expected mortality). This is model III, the final line of Table 14.2. In this formulation, the estimated effect of -0.048 corresponds to 4.8 per cent less excess mortality in the magnet hospitals. There is still significant variance across magnet hospitals in the extent to which their mortality differs from that of their matched controls. Excess mortality across magnet hospitals is well measured. The reliability of estimates of hospital-specific excess mortality, under model III, is 0.81.

Discussion

The magnet hospitals were selected on the basis of their reputations, not on objective evidence of the presence of a unique set of organisational attributes. Their common organisational dimensions were only identified subsequently. The estimated effects on mortality might not be the same as would be found were we to: 1) enumerate the important organisational characteristics; 2) seek to identify hospitals on the basis of objective measures of those characteristics; and 3) compare them to hospitals without such characteristics. We do not know the extent to which our matched comparison hospitals share those organisational features of nursing that we have deemed conducive to lower mortality, because the only information available on the matched comparison hospitals is macro-level hospital characteristics from the AHA annual survey. However, to the extent that the control hospitals do share these characteristics, our estimates are conservative with respect to their effects on mortality.

One thing we can do to clarify these issues is to examine nursing skill mix (RNs as a percentage of total nursing personnel) in magnet and matched non-magnet hospitals. The mix of nursing personnel is one of the distinguishing characteristics of magnet hospitals and a variable on which information is available on matched hospitals from the AHA annual survey of hospitals. Additionally, higher ratios of registered nurses to other nursing personnel have been associated with lower hospital mortality in other studies, raising the possibility that this is the major explanation for lower mortality in magnet hospitals. As noted in Table 14.1, magnet hospitals do have significantly higher ratios of RNs to total nursing personnel and slightly higher nurse to patient ratios. This provides some evidence that non-magnet hospitals do indeed differ from magnet hospitals in nursing organisational features that comprise the 'intervention' in our quasi-experimental study design.

To test whether this particular variable provides the full explanation for the mortality effect, we extended model II to include terms for both within-block and compositional differences in the ratio of RNs to total nursing personnel. We found no evidence that average differences between magnet hospitals and matched controls, with respect to either skill mix or nurse to patient ratios, significantly affect mortality nor do they explain any of the variability in effects across magnet hospitals.

On the basis of this analysis, we conclude that the matched comparison hospitals are not identical in nursing organisation to the magnet hospitals. At the same time, we have also demonstrated that one of the attributes of magnet hospitals – a greater proportion of nursing service personnel being registered nurses – is not the sole explanation for their lower mortality. This finding reinforces our belief that the mortality effect derives from the greater status, autonomy and control afforded nurses in the magnet hospitals, and their resulting impact on nurses' behaviours on behalf of patients.

As with any observational comparison, our results are potentially subject to biases for unobserved covariates (Rosenbaum and Rubin 1985). We cannot rule out the possibility that variables omitted from the analysis explain the lower mortality in magnet hospitals. If this is the case, such omitted variables will be correlated with the set of nursing variables operationalised by the magnet hospital construct. Although there may be other variables that we have not measured that affect mortality on their own accord, we believe they are as likely to be functions of the within-hospital organisation of nursing as determinants of it.

We have utilised Medicare mortality data because of their availability for the hospitals of interest even though data on patients of all ages would have been preferable. It is uncertain how expanding the age range of patients on which mortality is observed would affect our findings. Mortality rates are lower among younger patients, which argues for a diminution in the size of the effect. However, within the aged Medicare population there are limits to the proportion of mortality that can be expected to be prevented by any intervention.

The practical importance of our findings is influenced by the extent to which the organisational characteristics of magnet hospitals can be replicated elsewhere. In another paper, we have demonstrated that hospital unit level reforms, such as enabling nurses to specialise, also stimulate greater autonomy, control and intra-organisational status towards nursing. However, institution-wide professional nursing practice models (as in the magnet hospitals) stimulate them further.

Conclusion

Our narrowest conclusion is that the hospitals in the magnet hospital study have mortality rates that are lower than those among matched control hospitals, by a factor of approximately 5 per 1000 Medicare discharges. This corresponds to a reduction in 'excess mortality' of 5 per cent. The magnet hospitals do differ from their matched controls in their nursing 'skill mix', but this is not the explanation for the mortality differential. Based on adjunct studies of the magnet hospitals, we are inclined to attribute this differential to hospital-level differences in the organisation of nursing care. Our broader conclusion is that such organisational factors are important in understanding why some hospitals achieve better patient outcomes than others. We point to the 39 magnet hospitals, that appear to be in many respects like other hospitals except in the organisation of nursing, as evidence that further reductions in excess hospital mortality may well be within our reach.

References

American Hospital Association (1989) *Hospital Statistics*, Chicago: American Hospital Association.
Benner, P. (1984) *From Novice to Expert*, Menlo Park, CA: Addison-Wesley Publishing.
Cohen, I.B. (1984) 'Florence Nightingale', *Scientific American*, 250: 128–37.

Findlay, S., Roberts, M. and Silberner, J. (1990) 'The best hospitals, from AIDS to urology', *U.S. News & World Report*, 108: 68.

Health Care Financing Administration (1989) *Medicare Hospital Mortality Information 1986, 1987, 1988*, Washington, DC: US Government Printing Office.

Koska, M.T. (1989) 'Quality – thy name is nursing care, CEOs say', *Hospitals*, 32: 32.

Kramer, M. (1990) 'The magnet hospitals: excellence revisited', *Journal of Nursing Administration*, 20: 35–44.

Kramer, M. and Hafner, L.P. (1989) 'Shared values: impact on staff nurse job satisfaction and perceived productivity', *Nursing Research*, 138: 172.

Kramer, M. and Schmalenberg, C. (1988) 'Magnet hospitals: institutions of excellence, Parts I & II', *Journal of Nursing Administration*, 18: 11–19.

Kramer, M. and Schmalenberg, C. (1991) 'Job satisfaction and retention. Insights for the '90s, Parts I & II', *Nursing*, 21: 50–5.

McClure, M., Poulin, M., Sovie, M.D. and Wandelt, M.A. (1983) *Magnet Hospitals: Attraction and Retention of Professional Nurses*, Kansas City, MO: American Academy of Nursing.

Mechanic, D. and Aiken, L.H. (1982) 'A cooperative agenda for medicine and nursing', *New England Journal of Medicine*, 307: 747–50.

Rosenbaum, P.R. and Rubin, D.B. (1985) 'Constructing a control group using multivariate matched sampling methods that incorporate the propensity score', *American Statistician*, 39: 33.

Rubin, D.B. (1973) 'Matching to remove bias in observational studies', *Biometrics*, 29: 159.

Stein, L.I., Watts, D.T. and Howell, T. (1990) 'The doctor-nurse game revisited', *New England Journal of Medicine*, 322: 546–9.

Sunshine, L. and Wright, J.W. (1988) *The Best Hospitals in America*, New York: Henry Holt and Co.

US Department of Health and Human Services (1988) *Secretary's Commission on Nursing, Final Report*, Washington, DC.

A complete, unedited version of this article can be found as Aiken, L.H., Smith, H.L. and Lake, E.T., 'Lower Medicare mortality among a set of hospitals known for good nursing care' in *Medical Care* (1994) Volume 32, pages 771–87.

Chapter 15

Randomised controlled trial comparing cost-effectiveness of general practitioners and nurse practitioners in primary care

P. Venning, A. Durie, M. Roland, C. Roberts and B. Leese

Abstract

Objective: To compare the cost-effectiveness of general practitioners and nurse practitioners as first point of contact in primary care.

Design: Multicentre randomised controlled trial of patients requesting an appointment the same day.

Setting: 20 general practices in England and Wales.

Participants: 1716 patients were eligible for randomisation, of whom 1316 agreed to randomisation and 1303 subsequently attended the clinic. Data were available for analysis on 1292 patients (651 general practitioner consultations and 641 nurse practitioner consultations).

Main outcome measures: Consultation process (length of consultation, examinations, prescriptions, referrals), patient satisfaction, health status, return clinic visits over two weeks, and costs.

Results: Nurse practitioner consultations were significantly longer than those of the general practitioners (11.57 *vs* 7.28 min; adjusted difference 4.20, 95% confidence interval 2.98 to 5.41), and nurses carried out more tests (8.7% *vs* 5.6% of patients; odds ratio 1.66, 95% confidence interval 1.04 to 2.66) and asked patients to return more often (37.2% *vs* 24.8%; 1.93, 1.36 to 2.73). There was no significant difference in patterns of prescribing or health status outcome for the two groups. Patients were more satisfied with nurse practitioner consultations (mean score 4.40 *vs* 4.24 for general practitioners; adjusted difference 0.18, 0.092 to 0.257). This difference remained after consultation length was controlled for. There was no significant difference in health service costs (nurse

Source: *British Medical Journal*, 320, 2000, 1048–53.

practitioner £18.11 vs general practitioner £20.70; adjusted difference £2.33, −£1.62 to £6.28).

Conclusions: The clinical care and health service costs of nurse practitioners and general practitioners were similar. If nurse practitioners were able to maintain the benefits while reducing their return consultation rate or shortening consultation times, they could be more cost effective than general practitioners.

Introduction

Although use of nurse practitioners is well developed in the USA, it is only in the past 10 years that they have become established in the UK. A nurse practitioner has been defined as 'an advanced level clinical nurse who through extra education and training is able to practice autonomously, making clinical decisions and instigating treatment decisions based on those decisions, and is fully accountable for her own practice' (Royal College of Nursing 1989). Models of nurse practitioner care have, however, developed in several different ways. In Britain, nurse practitioners working in general practice most commonly work as part of a team alongside general practitioners (GPs), and it is this model we have evaluated.

Nurse practitioners are increasingly used as points of first contact in primary care. The number of trained nurse practitioners is increasing as dedicated training programmes become more accessible. New government initiatives include nurses as front-line providers for a national telephone advice service (Department of Health 1999a) and for proposed new walk-in primary care clinics (Department of Health 1999b). Despite this, there have been few rigorous comparisons between doctors and nurses. Observational studies generally suggest that patients give positive reports of nurses in such roles (South Thames Regional Health Authority 1994; University of Newcastle upon Tyne 1998). However, the only two randomised controlled trials comparing the cost-effectiveness of nurses and doctors in first contact roles in primary care in the United States and Canada provide conflicting results (Spitzer et al. 1974; Diers et al. 1986). These studies were conducted on single sites with a small number of nurses. A recent meta-analysis commented on the limited evidence available to compare the cost-effectiveness of doctors and nurses in primary care (Brown and Grimes 1995).

The aim of this study was to compare the process, outcome and costs of care given by GPs and nurse practitioners for patients requesting a same-day appointment in 20 general practices. This group of patients was chosen because a high proportion would be likely to agree to randomisation, as they would not have a strong preference for one practitioner who was already involved in their ongoing care.

Participants and methods

The study took place in 20 geographically dispersed practices in England and Wales. Each practice employed a nurse who had completed a one- or two-year nurse practitioner training programme at diploma, BSc or MSc level. The median length of time the nurses had been qualified as nurse practitioners was 3 (range 1–5) years and the median time as registered nurses was 22 (9–35) years. Each nurse practitioner had been seeing patients as first point of contact for at least two years.

Randomisation

In each practice, experimental sessions were booked when both the nurse practitioner and a GP had appointments available for patients who asked to be seen on the same day. Patients were eligible for entry to the study if they requested an appointment the same day and were able to come to the experimental session. A method of coded block randomisation was developed which meant that neither the receptionist nor the patient could determine the group to which a patient had been allocated at the time of booking.

Data collection

The GPs and nurse practitioners booked appointments at their normal intervals. For each consultation they recorded details of history, diagnosis, examination, tests carried out, prescriptions and referrals. The time of each consultation, including interruptions, was recorded with an electronic time stamp. This included time taken by the nurse practitioners to get a prescription signed by a general practitioner. We extracted details of consultations in the following two weeks from the medical records.

Patients completed health status measures before the initial consultation and by post two weeks later (SF-36 for adults or the child health questionnaire for parents of children aged 5–16). For children under 5 years, parents completed a brief health status questionnaire which had been developed for a previous study in general practice (McKinley *et al.* 1997). After the consultation, patients completed the medical interview satisfaction scale (Wolf *et al.* 1978) or the paediatric version of this scale (Lewis *et al.* 1986) and the patient enablement instrument (Howie *et al.* 1998).

We coded patients' diagnoses and prescriptions using Read codes. Data were double-coded, double-entered and verified. For health status and satisfaction scales, scores were reported if 50 per cent or more of items had been completed, and we used the method advised for the SF-36 scale to impute missing values. Costs of GPs' and nurse practitioners' time were taken from Netten *et al.* (1998) using the actual grades on which the study nurses were employed. Costs of prescriptions were derived from the *British National Formulary*, and costs for investigations and referrals were supplied by the individual provider units associated with the practices.

Analysis

Because of potential correlation between the outcomes of patients treated by the same health professional, estimates of variation between health professionals may be over precise unless intra-cluster correlation is adjusted for. We adjusted outcome for the age and sex of the patients, as these characteristics may also influence outcome. The statistical modelling used generalised estimating equations (Zeger and Liang 1986). A logistic regression model was used for binary outcomes. As some of the cost data were highly skewed, estimates for costs were compared with estimates based on non-parametric clustered bootstrap to check the robustness of the analysis (Barber and Thompson 1998). Both estimates gave similar results and so only the direct estimates are presented.

Results

A total of 1316 (76.7 per cent) eligible patients were randomised (Figure 15.1). Fifteen patients subsequently did not attend the appointment that they had booked. Table 15.1 shows the demographic characteristics of the patients and the main diagnoses.

The nurse practitioners spent a mean of 11.57 minutes face-to-face with patients compared with 7.28 minutes for GPs (Table 15.2). In addition, the nurses spent a mean of 1.33 minutes per patient in getting prescriptions signed. Table 15.3 shows that there was no significant difference in the percentage of patients who had a physical examination (nurse practitioners 88.1 per cent vs GPs 85.7 per cent). Nurse practitioners issued fewer prescriptions than GPs, but the difference was not significant (391 (61.0 per cent) vs 421 (64.6 per cent); odds ratio 0.88, 95 per cent confidence interval 0.66 to 1.17). Nurses ordered more tests and investigations than GPs (56 (8.7 per cent) vs 37 (5.6 per cent); 1.66, 1.04 to 2.66). In particular, the nurse practitioners carried out more tests associated with opportunistic screening such as urine testing and cervical screening. Nurse practitioners were also significantly more likely to ask patients to return (37.2 per cent vs 24.8 per cent; 1.93, 1.36 to 2.73). In 81 (12.6 per cent) consultations the nurse discussed the patient with a doctor, and in 26 (4.1 per cent) consultations the patient was seen by the doctor.

Table 15.1 Demographic information and the five most common diagnoses: values are numbers (%) of patients

	Total (n = 1292)	Nurse practitioners (n = 641)	General practitioners (n = 651)
Age (years)			
>16	866 (67.0)	414 (64.6)	452 (69.4)
5–15	200 (15.5)	114 (17.8)	86 (13.2)
<5	224 (17.3)	112 (17.5)	112 (17.2)
Sex			
Male	547 (42)	269 (42)	278 (43)
Female	743 (58)	371 (58)	372 (57)
Diagnosis*			
Upper respiratory tract infection	475 (36.8)	236 (36.8)	239 (36.7)
Viral illness	147 (11.4)	81 (12.6)	66 (10.1)
No specific diagnosis	142 (11.0)	76 (11.9)	66 (10.1)
Minor injuries	119 (9.2)	70 (11.0)	49 (7.5)
Eye and ear conditions	98 (7.6)	45 (7.0)	53 (8.1)

*362 (28 per cent) of patients had more than one diagnosis.

The satisfaction questionnaires (Table 15.4) showed that patients were more satisfied after consultations with nurses. Scores were significantly higher for the adult medical interview satisfaction scale scores and all its subscales and for the paediatric medical interview satisfaction scale scores in children and two of its subscales. There were no significant differences in enablement scores between the groups. The differences in satisfaction scores were still significant when the scores were additionally controlled for the length of face-to-face contact (mean difference 0.16, 95 per cent confidence interval 0.08 to 0.24).

In the two weeks after the initial consultation, patients who had seen a nurse practitioner were more likely to make a return visit to the clinic (mean number of returns 0.49 vs 0.36). These return visits were mainly to GPs because there were more GPs than nurses in the practices and many of the nurses worked part-time. There were no differences in health status at the end of two weeks.

Table 15.5 shows health service costs. These include the basic salary costs of each health professional plus the costs of prescriptions, tests, referrals, and the cost of return consultations in the following two weeks. Since return consultations were not timed, we estimated that they lasted an average of 7 minutes for GP consultations and 11.5 minutes for nurse practitioner consultations. There was no significant difference in the cost of care given by the nurse practitioners and the GPs. Further details of costings are available from us on request.

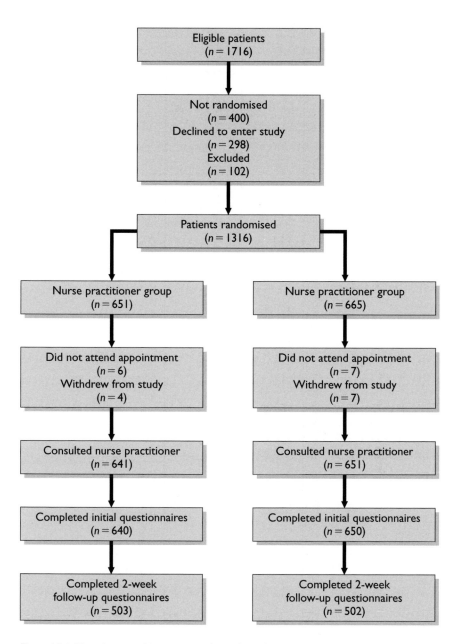

Figure 15.1 Flowchart tracking patients through study.

Table 15.2 Differences in care given at initial consultation (values adjusted for age, sex and intra-cluster correlation)

	Nurse practitioners		General practitioners		Adjusted mean difference (95% CI)	P value	Intra-cluster correlation
	No. of patients	Mean (SD)	No. of patients	Mean (SD)			
Total consultation time (min)	639	12.9 (6.28)	639	7.49 (4.75)	5.46 (4.16 to 6.78)	<0.001	0.19
Face-to-face consultation time* (min)	639	11.57 (5.79)	651	7.28 (4.80)	4.20 (2.98 to 5.41)	<0.001	0.17
Mean number of physical examinations per patient	612	2.28 (1.55)	635	1.95 (1.57)	0.19 (−0.03 to 0.71)	0.072	0.19
Mean number of return visits	638	0.49 (0.79)	651	0.36 (0.66)	0.14 (0.05 to 0.22)	0.002	0.00[†]

*Face-to-face consultation time = total consultation time minus time to have prescription signed or time to sign a prescription.
[†]Negative estimate of intra-cluster correlation coefficients.

Table 15.3 Differences in actions taken during consultation with nurse and general practitioners (values adjusted for age, sex and intra-cluster correlation)

Action	Nurse practitioners		General practitioners		Odds ratio (95% CI)	P value	Intra-cluster correlation
	No. of patients	%	No. of patients	%			
Physical examination	590/640	88.1	572/649	92.2	1.76 (0.90 to 3.42)	0.097	0.10
Prescription given	391/641	61.0	421/651	64.7	0.88 (0.66 to 1.17)	0.375	0.03
Antibiotic prescribed	195/641	30.4	207/651	31.7	0.94 (0.76 to 1.17)	0.576	0.00*
Investigation carried out	56/641	8.7	37/651	5.6	1.66 (1.04 to 2.66)	0.033	0.01
Hospital referral	11/641	1.7	25/651	3.8	0.50 (0.16 to 1.63)	0.25	0.08
Asked to return	236/634	37.2	161/648	24.8	1.93 (1.36 to 2.73)	<0.001	0.05
Actually returned	224/634	35.3	184/647	28.4	1.42 (1.18 to 1.71)	<0.001	0.00*

*Negative estimate of intra-cluster correlation coefficient.

Table 15.4 Differences in satisfaction after consultation (adjusted for age, sex, time and intra-cluster correlation)

	Nurse practitioners		General practitioners		Adjusted mean difference (95% CI)	P value	Intra-cluster correlation
	Mean (SD) score	No. of patients	Mean (SD) score	No. of patients			
Adults							
Medical interview satisfaction scale	4.40 (0.46)	388	4.24 (0.52)	390	0.18 (0.09 to 0.26)	<0.001	0.04
Communication	4.35 (0.54)	370	4.21 (0.60)	384	0.13 (0.06 to 0.21)	0.001	0.0*
Distress relief	4.43 (0.47)	390	4.26 (0.57)	400	0.19 (0.08 to 0.29)	0.001	0.01
Clinician behaviour	4.44 (0.49)	375	4.22 (0.57)	369	0.23 (0.15 to 0.32)	<0.001	0.2
Enablement score	4.92 (3.62)	335	4.43 (3.65)	361	0.65 (−1.50 to 0.19)	0.13	0.14
Children							
Medical interview satisfaction scale[†]	4.39 (0.46)	220	4.17 (0.57)	181	0.23 (0.12 to 0.34)	<0.001	0.3
Communication with parent	4.58 (0.51)	223	4.48 (0.65)	190	0.07 (−0.26 to 0.16)	0.159	0.0
Communication with child	4.16 (0.63)	176	3.67 (0.77)	147	0.47 (0.29 to 0.67)	<0.001	0.11
Distress relief	4.41 (0.53)	222	4.21 (0.64)	186	0.21 (0.08 to 0.34)	0.002	0.04
Adherence intent	4.47 (0.53)	218	4.44 (0.53)	185	−0.01 (−0.10 to 0.08)	0.817	0.0*

*Negative estimate of intra-cluster correlation coefficient.
[†]Paediatric version.

Table 15.5 Difference in cost of consultation with nurse and general practitioners based on salary costs (adjusted for age, sex and intra-cluster correlation)

	Nurse practitioners		General practitioners		Adjusted mean difference (95% CI)	P value	Intra-cluster correlation
	Mean (SD) cost (£)	Range	Mean (SD) cost (£)	Range			
Initial consultation							
Total time	11.71 (25.23)	0.66–297.1	14.14 (29.62)	0.78–246.5	2.17 (−1.18 to 5.51)	0.204	0.009
Face-to-face time*	11.29 (25.18)	0.66–297.1	14.11 (29.63)	0.79–246.5	2.58 (−0.73 to 5.89)	0.127	0.009
Return consultation	6.40 (21.20)	0.0–219.3	6.56 (22.85)	0.0–217.3	−0.03 (−2.25 to 2.20)	0.98	0.008
Total costs							
Total time	18.11 (33.43)	0.66–297.1	20.70 (33.43)	0.78-300.6	2.33 (−1.62 to 6.28)	0.247	0.0†
Face-to-face time*	17.69 (33.41)	0.66–297.1	20.68 (33.41)	0.78–300.6	2.73 (−1.20 to 6.66)	0.173	0.0†

*Face-to-face time = total consultation time minus time to get a prescription signed or time to sign a prescription.
†Negative estimate of intra-cluster correlation coefficient.

Discussion

We have evaluated care given by nurse practitioners working as part of primary care teams alongside GPs. Our results do not therefore relate to nurse practitioners who are working independently. It is often assumed that when nurses substitute for doctors, the same service is provided (Richardson and Maynard 1995). However, the British literature suggests that the combination of nursing and medical skills provides a more comprehensive and flexible service for patients than that provided by doctors (NHS Executive 1996). Our study provides limited support for this theory.

In many respects the behaviour of the nurses was similar to that of general practitioners, but some important differences existed. Nurse practitioners spent more time with patients and were more likely to ask patients to return. There were no differences in health outcome, although the study did not have sufficient power to detect a difference in rare serious events.

The differences in working styles between nurse practitioners and GPs are shown by the number and types of tests ordered and the numbers of patients who were asked to return to surgery. Nurse practitioners carried out more opportunistic screening. This was also found in a comparative study in the USA (Diers *et al.* 1986).

In Britain only two groups of nurses (district nurses and health visitors) are able to prescribe drugs, and then from a limited list of items. During training nurse practitioners do an extensive pharmacology module with supporting modules in pathophysiology and disease management, and they argue that they are able to use the same range of drugs as doctors (Mayes 1996). We found that the nurse practitioners had similar prescribing behaviour to the general practitioners. As they had been qualified for some time, unlike nurse practitioners in other British studies (South Thames Regional Health Authority 1994; NHS Executive 1996; Reveley 1998) and were experienced nurses, this finding is not unexpected. These nurses were working in teams alongside GPs and consistent prescribing behaviour should, in theory, be adopted by all practice staff. Indeed, some practices had developed specific prescribing protocols for both GPs and nurse practitioners.

Patient satisfaction is an important component of nearly all studies looking at the role of nurse practitioners, and patients generally report high levels of satisfaction with nurse practitioner care (Office of Technology Assessment 1986; South Thames Regional Health Authority 1994; NHS Executive 1996; Reveley 1998; University of Newcastle upon Tyne 1998). Increased satisfaction has been linked with longer consultations, and nurse practitioners have been shown to spend longer with patients than GPs. However, the differences in satisfaction remained in our study after we had controlled for differences in consultation time.

The health service costs of consultation with nurse practitioners were 12.5 per cent lower than those for GPs, but this difference was not significant. However, a larger study with greater power to detect cost differences is needed. We were unable to do power calculations for cost before the study because none of the British studies of nurse practitioners have compared cost of consultations for GPs and nurse practitioners (South Thames Regional Health Authority 1994; NHS Executive 1996; Reveley 1998; University of Newcastle upon Tyne 1998). In the USA studies have shown conflicting results (Office of Technology Assessment 1986). Nurses were paid less than the GPs, but they took longer to see patients and more of their patients returned for further consultations. This reduced the overall difference in consultation costs. If lifetime training costs were included the GP costs would be higher.

Conclusion

Our results relate to patients requesting a same-day appointment in general practice and cannot necessarily be generalised to other situations. Overall, the clinical care and outcome were similar for nurse practitioners and GPs. Patients who requested a same-day appointment were satisfied with nurse practitioner consultations. If nurse practitioners were able to work in different ways, for example, to shorten their consultation times (which our results suggest will not alter higher patient satisfaction with nurse practitioners) or reduce their return consultation rate, they could be more cost-effective than GPs for this group of patients.

References

Barber, J.A. and Thompson, S.G. (1998) 'Analysis and interpretation of cost data in randomised controlled trials: review of published studies', *British Medical Journal*, 317: 1195–200.

Brown, S.A. and Grimes, D. (1995) 'A meta-analysis of nurse practitioners and nurse midwives in primary care', *Nursing Research*, 44: 332–8.

Department of Health (1999a) *New Opportunities for NHS Direct*, London: DoH (press release 1999/0227).

Department of Health (1999b) *Up to £30 Million to Develop 20 NHS Fast Access Walk-in Centres*, London: DoH (press release 1999/0226).

Diers, D., Hamman, A. and Molde, S. (1986) 'Complexity of ambulatory care: nurse practitioner and physician caseloads', *Nursing Research*, 35: 310–14.

Howie, J.G.R., Heaney, D., Maxwell, M. and Walker, J.J. (1998) 'A comparison of the patient enablement instrument (PEI) against two established satisfaction scales as an outcome measure of primary care consultations', *Family Practice*, 15: 165–71.

Lewis, C., Scott, D., Pantell, R. and Wolf, M. (1986) 'Patient satisfaction with children's medical care: development, field test and validation of a questionnaire', *Medical Care*, 24: 209–15.

McKinley, R.K., Cragg, D.K., Hastings, A.M., French, D.P., Manku-Scott, T.K., Campbell, S.M., Van, F., Roland, M.O. and Roberts, C. (1997) 'Comparison of out of hours care provided by patients' own general practitioners and commercial deputising services: a randomised controlled trial. 2. Outcome of care', *British Medical Journal*, 314: 190–3.

Mayes, M. (1996) 'A study of prescribing patterns in the community', *Nursing Standard*, 10: 34–7.

Netten, A., Knight, J., Dennett, J., Cooley, R. and Slight, A. (1998) *A Ready Reckoner for Staff Costs in the NHS. Volume 1. Estimated Unit Costs*, Canterbury: Personal Social Services Research Unit, University of Kent.

NHS Executive (1996) *Nurse Practitioner Evaluation Project: Final Report*, Uxbridge: Coopers and Lybrand.

Office of Technology Assessment (1986) *Nurse Practitioners, Physician Assistants and Certified Midwives: A Policy Analysis*, Washington, DC: US Government Printing Office (Health technology case study 37, OTA-HCS-37).

Reveley, S. (1998) 'The role of the triage nurse practitioner in general medical practice: an analysis of the role', *Journal of Advanced Nursing*, 28: 584–91.

Richardson, G. and Maynard, A. (1995) *Fewer Doctors? More Nurses? A Review of the Knowledge Base of Doctor-Nurse Substitution*, York: Centre for Health Economics, University of York.

Royal College of Nursing (1989) *Nurse Practitioners in Primary Health Care Role Definition*, London: RCN.

South Thames Regional Health Authority (1994) *Evaluation of Nurse Practitioner Pilot Projects: Summary Report*, London: Touche Roche Management Consultants, STRATA.

Spitzer, W.O., Sackett, D.L., Sibley, J.C., Roberts, R.S., Gent, M., Kergin, D.J., Hackett, B.C. and Olyrich, A. (1974) 'The Burlington randomised controlled trial of the nurse practitioner', *New England Journal of Medicine*, 290: 251–6.

University of Newcastle upon Tyne, Centre for Health Services Research (1998) *Evaluation of Nurse Practitioners in General Practice in Northumberland: The EROS Projects 1 and 2*, Newcastle upon Tyne: CHSR.

Wolf, M.H., Putnam, S.M., James, S.A. and Stiles, W.B. (1978) 'The medical interview satisfaction scale: development of a scale to measure patient perceptions of physician behaviour', *Journal of Behavioural Medicine*, 1: 391–401.

Zeger, S.L. and Liang, K.Y. (1986) 'Longitudinal data analysis for discrete and continuous outcomes', *Biometrics*, 42: 121–30.

A complete, unedited version of this article can be found as Venning, P., Durie, A., Roland, M., Roberts, C. and Leese, B., 'Randomised controlled trial comparing cost effectiveness of general practitioners and nurse practitioners in primary care' in the *British Medical Journal* (2000) Volume 320, pages 1048–53.

Part 4

Evaluating models of service delivery

Introduction

Evaluation has been described as: '... a comparative assessment of the value of ... [an] ... intervention using systematically collected and analysed data, in order to decide how to act'. (Ovretveit J., *Evaluating Health Interventions*, Open University Press, 1998.)

In this section of the Reader there are five articles each describing different methods of evaluation and of systematically collecting and analysing data. Methods range from meta-analysis of randomised controlled trials through observational studies to qualitative enquiries. The models of service delivery also vary and include stroke care, both within and outside stroke units, the use of an emergency helicopter, clinical policies in intensive care and the effects on the outcome of the volume of procedures or interventions undertaken.

This section inevitably invites the reader to ask questions about how best to evaluate models of service delivery – using randomised trials, qualitative studies or a mixture of methods? Should comparisons be made against standard practice or best practice? Should evaluation ever be undertaken without an economic component? Is it possible to generalise from randomised trials of complex interventions?

One of the most problematic issues in evaluation of models of service delivery is in the precise definition of the model or intervention to be evaluated. This is often much more difficult than it might seem, for example, in interventions such as stroke units. Even a helicopter (the intervention in the first article) presents a challenge, as any benefits of the helicopter are almost certainly dependent on who or what is inside it and the details of how care is delivered!

The conundrum of how to define the intervention is often matched only by how to define the relevant outcome. Death is frequently used in evaluations, but is a poor proxy for the intended outcomes of most health care, as Amanda Sowden and Trevor Sheldon point out in their article on volume and outcome. Lastly, even with the intervention and outcomes well defined, there is still a problem of identifying and adequately accounting for other factors which might affect observed differences. This is a theme in four of the papers, where case-mix factors (age, severity and co-morbidity) are important determinants of outcome.

In the first study John Brazier and colleagues evaluate the London Helicopter Emergency Medical Service (HEMS). In a prospective comparison of the costs and effectiveness of the use of the HEMS, compared to the London Ambulance Service, they found no difference in case-mix adjusted disability among the survivors for an extra incremental cost of the helicopter of £1.97 million per year at 1996 prices. Nonetheless, the authors report that there is continuing diffusion of helicopter emergency medical services – despite a similar finding by the US Department of Transport.

The second paper asks, 'How do stroke units improve patient outcomes?' Langhorne and colleagues undertook a secondary analysis of a collaborative systematic review of all randomised trials which compared stroke unit care with conventional care. The problem is that while stroke units have been found to be beneficial, the exact mechanism by which this benefit is brought about is not understood. They suggest that the net effect of stroke units is a more favourable outcome for all stroke patients. It is clear, however, that further research will be needed in defining the intervention more precisely. The 'black box' to discover what is included in a stroke unit still needs further exploration!

The third paper asks whether volume really affects outcome. Sowden and Sheldon describe the effects of inadequate adjustment for case-mix that may result in apparently higher mortality for patients treated in smaller volume hospitals and conclude that volume-quality effects found previously may well partly be an artefact. They question the validity of previous research and suggest that 'most research in this area is insufficiently reliable to inform policy'.

In the fourth paper the effects of discharging patients from intensive care units (ICUs) at night are investigated. Caroline Goldfrad and Kathy Rowan found that after careful adjustment for case-mix outcomes appeared to be poorer for patients discharged prematurely at night. Many evaluations are set up to evaluate a new service. But this is no innovation. It is a model of care driven by the necessity to deal with increased bed pressures in ICUs in the UK and this study is important in pointing out that this practice is not without risks.

The fifth paper is refreshingly different in its approach to evaluation of a Pilot Community Stroke Service. Analysis of in-depth interviews describes a range of 'system-induced setbacks' which Elizabeth Hart suggests reflect 'the enduring impact of fragmentation and poor co-ordination on service provision'. An important theme is that of the uniqueness of the health care experience for individuals. Evaluation of models of service delivery often relies on aggregated, quantitative data from large numbers of people but it is important to remember that health care is delivered to individuals one at a time. The aim of many evaluations should be to improve that individual experience of health care. And Ovretveit, in his definition of evaluation says that evaluation is undertaken 'in order to decide how to act'. Evaluation can be expensive and is not a frivolous undertaking. It is a useful exercise to ask which of these evaluations have affected decisions – and how?

Chapter 16

The cost and effectiveness of the London Helicopter Emergency Medical Service

John Brazier, Jon Nicholl and Helen Snooks

Abstract

Objectives: To assess the incremental consequences of the London Helicopter Emergency Medical Service for the outcomes of survivors in terms of disability and health status, and cost.

Methods: Prospective comparison of outcomes in cohorts of seriously injured patients attended either by the HEMS or by paramedically crewed land ambulances. In survivors, disability was assessed using an 11-point disability scale, and general health status was measured by the six dimensions of the 100-point Nottingham Health Profile (NHP) assessed six months after the injury. Costs were estimated for the HEMS and associated facilities at the Royal London Hospital, and the extra admissions attributable to the HEMS.

Results: There was no evidence of reduced disability in HEMS survivors (estimate: +0.8 disability grades worse; 95% CI: 0, 1.6), and no evidence of improvement in the six NHP dimension scores or in the mean number of problems with seven aspects of daily living (estimated difference: +0.5; 95% CI: −0–2, 1.2). The incremental costs of HEMS were estimated to be £2.0 million a year.

Conclusion: As there is no evidence of any improvement in outcomes overall for the extra cost, the HEMS has not been found to be a cost-effective service.

Source: *Journal of Health Services Research and Policy*, 1.4, 1996, 232–7.

Introduction

The US Department of Transport concluded that the use of the helicopter as an emergency ambulance could provide only limited benefits and was likely to be too costly (US Department of Transportation 1972). However, the diffusion of this technology has taken place with little conclusive evidence concerning its effectiveness and cost-effectiveness (Nicholl *et al.* 1994a, 1995; Snooks *et al.* 1996).

The London helicopter operates from the Royal London Hospital (RLH) during daylight hours. The helicopter is called out via the ambulance service control centre. A paramedic tries to establish the condition of the patient before activating the helicopter so as to minimise abortive missions. Typical signs indicating that HEMS is required are: falls of greater than 2 m; road traffic accidents (RTAs) where a patient is trapped; patients reported as unconscious or not breathing; limb survival threatened in trauma patients; burns; patient under a train; a confirmed gunshot or stabbing.

Compared to patients attended by the Land Ambulance Service (LAS), HEMS patients receive medical attention (on the scene from HEMS doctors) 25 minutes earlier, on average, but arrive in hospital 10–20 minutes later (Nicholl *et al.* 1994b). They are more intensively managed on scene and spend an average of 6 minutes longer at the scene. HEMS triage their patients to hospitals with appropriate facilities on site. Despite these differences in the process of pre-hospital care and after taking into account age and the nature and severity of the injuries, the survival rates in HEMS and LAS patients have been found to be the same (Nicholl *et al.* 1995).

In this paper the authors assessed the overall cost-effectiveness of this service compared with other health care interventions.

Methods

Inclusion criteria

All the activity of HEMS during a two-year period (1 August 1991 to 31 July 1993) was identified from records completed by ambulance control and the HEMS staff.

Patients meeting operational and clinical inclusion criteria (Box 16.1) and who were taken to any one of a group of 20 primary receiving hospitals in the operational area during the first 21 months were eligible to be included in the follow-up. Information was collected from all available sources including pre-hospital records, accident and emergency department records, inpatient notes, coroners' records and, for a sample of survivors, an outcome assessment by interview or postal questionnaire.

Box 16.1 London HEMS review inclusion data

1. OPERATIONAL	a)	Helicopter case: patient attended by HEMS crew from 'primary missions' resulting in 'helicopter transfer' 'ground escort' and ground assist' Land case: patient attended by an LAS paramedic-crewed land ambulance and HEMS was not in attendance
and	b)	Patient who was taken to any one of 20 study hospital casualty departments, or died on scene but would have been taken to a study hospital if attended by the LAS, between 8 am and 9 pm
2. CLINICAL	a)	Externally caused ('trauma') incident including drownings, but excluding medical complications following surgery and falls within the home of less than 1 m
and	b)	Any patient attended by air or ground ambulance on whom resuscitation is attempted, and for land ambulance cases on whom paramedic skills were used
and	c)	1) who died on scene or at hospital (during first admission episode)
	or	2) who stayed in hospital for 72 hours or more
	or	3) who had an initial TRTS of 10 or less
	or	4) who had an initial GCS of 12 or less with a head injury
	or	5) who had an ISS greater than 10

The sample consisted of one in three HEMS patients flown to the RLH and all other HEMS patients taken to the 20 study hospitals.

Missions undertaken by land ambulances included during the same 21 months were all trauma patients attended by ambulance service paramedics, who were trained in the extended skills of intubation and infusion, for whom extended skills were used and who arrived at hospital between 08:00 and 21:00 hours. Children and all patients with single system head injuries attended during the daytime who met the other inclusion criteria were also included (Nicholl *et al.* 1994b). All patients were followed-up in the same way as HEMS patients.

Outcome measures in survivors

All survivors in the outcome evaluation were followed-up by postal questionnaire or interview at two months and six months after their injury, unless they were under five years old, were involved in an assault or other crime, or had attempted suicide. Patients were offered an interview if they were accessible to a team of ten interviewers resident in the London area; otherwise, they were sent questionnaires by mail. When possible, the interview was done with the patient themselves, whether at home or in hospital. The mailed questionnaire was similar to the interview schedule but excluded the disability assessment.

Disability was assessed using the Office of Population Censuses and Surveys survey instruments (Martin et al. 1988). It covers locomotion, dexterity, sensory and mental functioning, incontinence and disfigurement. Despite being multidimensional, it can generate a single score from 0 to 10 (with zero indicating no disability). These 11 severity grades, which indicate qualitatively different levels of disability, have been used in this analysis. The instrument was adapted for use with trauma patients by asking them during the interview whether any disability had arisen as a result of the accident or was worse since the accident. Only those disabilities so identified have been included in the analysis of residual disability.

General health status was measured using the Nottingham Health Profile (NHP) (Hunt et al. 1986), which has been used in a wide range of conditions, although not trauma. It covers a wide range of health concepts, generating scores for six dimensions: physical mobility, pain, emotional reaction, energy, sleep and social isolation. The second part of the NHP asks dichotomous questions about difficulties in different areas of life, including job, hobbies and holidays.

Costing

The aim was to estimate the incremental (i.e. extra) costs of the HEMS both pre-hospital, and for six months following the injury. The pre-hospital costs of the helicopter include the aircraft, its pilots, associated medical personnel, maintenance, landing facilities and the ambulance control staff involved in deploying it. These were supplied by local providers and funders, and were mostly directly attributable to the London HEMS. Information on subsequent use of health and other services was collected for HEMS and LAS cases, including length of stay, readmission, outpatient attendance and major investigations. Data were obtained from medical records and the patient follow-up questionnaires (at two and six months). The number of contacts with general practitioners, district nurses, social workers and other health care providers was obtained from patients, as well as time off work and other main activities.

Use of resources has been costed using the same method for both HEMS and LAS patients in order to avoid differences arising due to accounting practice. A national set of average speciality costs per diem and per attendance have been used for hospital episodes (NHS Executive 1993). Stay in intensive therapy has been costed using data from a UK study of general intensive care unit cases (Shiell 1991). Unfortunately, cost data relating specifically to trauma cases were not available at the time of the study. All costs are presented at 1991–1992 price levels, and all capital items have been converted into an annual equivalent using a 6 per cent discount rate.

Injury and severity measures

Injury descriptions were taken from hospital notes and coded using the Abbreviated Injury Scale (AIS) dictionary (AAAM 1990). For multiply injured patients, AIS scores were combined to produce an Injury Severity Score (ISS) (Wisner 1992; Copes *et al.* 1996).

Glasgow Coma Scores (GCS), respiratory rate and systolic blood pressure assessed before arrival at hospital were obtained from LAS and HEMS records. Revised Trauma Scores (RTS, the weighted sum of coded values of these three components) and Triage Revised Trauma Scores (TRTS, the unweighted sum) (Champion *et al.* 1989) were calculated.

Data analysis

The analysis involved comparing outcomes and resource costs of HEMS and LAS calls after adjusting for possible confounding factors. The confounding factors considered were age, sex, ISS, GCS, RTS, AIS body region scores and type of incident. Only those possible confounders found to be associated with each of the outcomes considered have been included in each of the multivariate models used to compare the HEMS and LAS cohorts. For comparing the HEMS and LAS in terms of the semiquantitative validity outcomes (disability grades and other scores) and (log-transformed) lengths of stay and costs, multivariate models have been estimated by least squares but tested using permutation tests. For the proportions of patients admitted to intensive care units, standard logistic regression models were used.

Results

Study numbers

During the study period, 337 HEMS patients met the inclusion criteria for the mortality assessment, as did 466 patients attended by LAS paramedics.

Morbidity

Six months after their injury, 116 HEMS patients were interviewed or returned a questionnaire (73 per cent of those approached) and 157 LAS patients (63 per cent) (Table 16.1). There was no evidence that response rates varied with injury severity, although age and sex were associated with response. Both the NHP scores and the disability grade detected a marked improvement in both cohorts between two and six months (Table 16.2).

The factors found to be strongly associated with the six-month residual disability grades were age, sex, ISS score, GCS score, and an AIS score for

Table 16.1 Results of six-month follow-up

	HEMS	LAS
Not approached		
Dead	92	77
Ineligible for other reasons*	86	140
Approached		
Not responded	43	92
Responded	116	157
All	337	466

*Cases involving attempted suicide, crime or children under five years old.

Table 16.2 Unadjusted disability scores* at two months and six months after injury

Outcome	Measure	Two months		Six months	
		HEMS	LAS	HEMS	LAS
Total disability grade	Mean	5.5	4.4	4.5	3.4
(for problems worse	(SD)	(3.0)	(3.2)	(3.3)	(3.1)
since the accident)	Median	5.0	5.0	4.0	3.0
Nottingham Health Profile					
Energy	Mean	43.8	29.0	29.5	23.7
Pain		32.0	29.2	24.6	23.6
Emotion		24.5	20.0	21.0	19.3
Sleep		39.0	34.4	28.7	22.2
Social isolation		15.6	12.2	12.7	12.2
Mobility		36.5	34.7	24.9	21.1
No. of problems	Mean	4.5	3.7	2.9	2.4
	(SD)	(2.1)	(2.4)	(2.1)	(2.3)
	Median	(5.0)	4.0	3.0	2.0

*Higher scores indicate more disability.

the lower extremities (Table 16.3). These factors together explained 38 per cent of the variance in the six-month residual disability scores. At most levels of these factors, the mean disability grade was higher in the HEMS cohort than in the LAS cohort, indicating a greater degree of residual disability. The exception to this general rule was for patients with the most severe injuries (ISS 25–74, or TRTS score 0–9). In these cases the HEMS cohort appeared to have the better outcomes, although the numbers were small (ISS 25–74: HEMS, $n = 16$; LAS, $n = 9$; TRTS 0–9; HEMS, $n = 15$; LAS, $n = 2$). After adjusting for the factors associated with disability grades at six months, the estimate of the difference in mean grade in the

Table 16.3 Mean six-month residual grades[a] by patient characteristics

Characteristic	Values	Cohort			
		HEMS		LAS	
		Mean	(SE)	Mean	(SE)
Age (years)	5–49	4.4	(0.4)	3.0	(0.3)
	50–75	3.8	(0.7)	3.6	(0.5)
	75+	7.3	(1.0)	5.0	(0.2)
ISS score	0–8	3.1	(0.5)	3.1	(0.4)
	9–15	4.0	(0.5)	2.9	(0.4)
	16–24	4.6	(0.7)	3.3	(0.7)
	25–76	6.6	(0.8)	7.1	(1.4)
(not scored: HEMS 2, LAS 1)	–	(4.5)	–	(10.0)	–
GCS score	3–9	6.1	(0.8)	5.4	(1.1)
	10–14	4.0	(0.8)	3.8	(0.7)
	15	3.7	(0.4)	2.8	(0.3)
(not scored: HEMS 1, LAS 7)	–	(2.0)	–	(6.3)	(1.4)
TRTS score	0–9	5.9	(1.0)	8.5	(1.5)
	10–11	5.1	(0.8)	4.2	(0.8)
	12	3.6	(0.4)	3.0	(0.4)
(not scored HEMS: 10, LAS 40)	–	(3.9)	(1.0)	(3.6)	(0.5)
Head injury score	1	3.7	(0.4)	3.2	(0.3)
	2	4.4	(0.8)	3.0	(1.0)
	3	6.1	(0.9)	4.8	(1.1)
(not scored: HEMS 3, LAS 2)	–	(3.3)	(2.3)	(7.5)	(2.5)
Lower extremities score	1	4.1	(0.5)	3.0	(0.5)
	2	3.8	(0.5)	3.3	(0.3)
	3	6.0	(0.7)	4.6	(1.0)
(not scored: HEMS 3, LAS 2)	–	(3.3)	(2.3)	(7.5)	(2.5)
Sex	Male	4.3	(0.4)	2.9	(0.3)
	Female	5.0	(0.6)	4.3	(0.5)

[a]Higher scores indicate more disability.

HEMS cohort relative to the LAS cohort was small: $+0.82$ (95% CI: 0.01, 1.63) on the scale 0–10 ($P = 0.04$).

The six NHP dimension scores had slightly different distributions in the two cohorts at both two months and six months, with worse health in the HEMS cohort on all dimensions (Table 16.4). Both age and AIS score in the lower extremities were associated with several of the NHP dimension scores six months after the injury. After adjusting for these and other associated confounding factors, there continued to be no evidence of any benefit from HEMS. Indeed, consistent with the results from the disability scores, there was some evidence of poorer physical mobility in the HEMS cohort than the LAS cohort even after adjusting for age and injury severity ($P = 0.03$) (Table 16.4). For all aspects of daily living, apart from participation in interests and hobbies, more HEMS patients reported problems at six months, although the differences were often small (Table 16.5). Adjusting for the ISS score and the AIS score in the lower extremities (accounting for 15 per cent of the variance in the number of problems at

Table 16.4 Difference in mean scores between HEMS and LAS six months after injury for each dimension of the NHP

NHP dimension	Unadjusted effect of HEMS*	Adjusted[†] effect on HEMS	(SE)	% variance explained	P value (permutation test)
Energy	+5.8	+1.2	(4.8)	7.0	0.81
Pain	+1.0	+4.6	(3.7)	20.5	0.27
Emotional reactions	+1.7	−3.0	(4.3)	12.9	0.53
Sleep	+6.5	+8.0	(4.2)	17.2	0.07
Social isolation	+0.5	+0.0	(3.9)	8.4	1.00
Physical mobility	+3.8	+6.7	(3.0)	32.5	0.03

*An increased score indicates worse health.
[†]Adjusted for age and injury severity.

Table 16.5 Problems with aspects of daily living at six-month follow-up

	Proportion (%) reporting problems	
	HEMS	LAS
Job of work (paid employment)	51.6	44.8
Looking after the home	54.3	41.9
Social life	35.6	33.1
Home life	21.3	20.3
Sex life	33.0	18.4
Interests and hobbies	52.8	55.6
Holidays	43.2	41.0

six months), the estimated difference in mean number of problems between the HEMS and LAS cohorts for all patients was not significant (estimated difference = +0.5 1, standard error = 0.34, $P = 0.1$).

Costs

The annual equivalent pre-hospital capital and running costs of the HEMS were estimated to be £1,146,861 (Table 16.6). The only major source of uncertainty is the appropriate residual value to assign to the helicopter in the annual equivalent cost calculation. Changing the central assumption from 50 per cent to 100 per cent or 0 per cent of the original purchase price results in a range in the total pre-hospital costs of £1,086,669 to £1,207,112.

Enhancements in the hospital accident and emergency department for the HEMS cases included building charges and equipment with an annual equivalent cost of £56,411 and four extra nursing posts (£97,492 per annum), resulting in an overall additional total annual cost of £153,903.

Table 16.6 Estimated annual costs of London HEMS

Pre-hospital	£ sterling*	
Capital costs (AEC)[†]		
Aircraft	365,334	
Landing deck	116,624	
Running costs		
Pilots and other staff	260,356	
Medical personnel (registrars)	125,200	
Maintenance	44,336	
Miscellaneous (e.g. insurance, fuel, fees, etc.)	137,377	
Ambulance service (e.g. paramedics, control and management support)	97,634	
	Subtotal	1,146,861
Hospital		
A&E department enhancements	56,411	
Capital (AEC)		
Staffing	97,492	
Difference in admission costs	672,400	
	Subtotal	826,303
		£1,973,164

*1991–1992 prices.
[†]Annual equivalent cost (see text).

After adjusting for age, ISS, TRTS and survival, it was estimated that the odds of HEMS patients being admitted to the intensive care unit were twice those of LAS patients (estimated odds ratio: 2.0; 95% CI: 1.4, 2.9), but there was little evidence that HEMS patients admitted to intensive care spent longer there (estimate: 11 per cent longer; 95% CI: −22 per cent, 58 per cent). In total, HEMS patients spent longer in hospital than LAS patients (estimate: 27 per cent; 95% CI: 4 per cent, 55 per cent). There were no significant differences in the use of other services.

Adjusting for age, ISS and TRTS, the extra admission cost per case attributable to HEMS was £1681 per HEMS case ($P < 0.05$). The confidence interval around this estimate was £57 to £3305 at the 95 per cent level, and £624 to £2743 at the 80 per cent level. The estimated extra admission costs for all HEMS patients would therefore be £672,400 per annum with an 80 per cent confidence interval of £283,300 to £1,245,000.

The incremental cost of HEMS is the sum of the costs of the helicopter, the accident and emergency department enhancements, and the difference in length of hospital stay and is estimated to be £1.97 million (Table 16.6).

Discussion

Despite an extensive analysis, we could find no evidence of an improved outcome among survivors associated with HEMS pre-hospital care. There was some evidence, in fact, that disabilities were comparatively worse in HEMS survivors, but little evidence of any difference in general health status. It is unlikely that this result is confounded by a survivor effect since the survival rates were similar in the two groups.

Of more concern than a possible survivor effect is the possibility of response biases among those who agreed to be interviewed. The response rate was better among HEMS patients than among LAS patients, but in both groups the numbers of patients not replying or refusing interview requests were large enough to introduce some uncertainty over their representativeness. Obviously, the comparison of the outcomes of HEMS and LAS survivors will only have been affected if the response rate of those with comparatively good outcomes and those with poor outcomes differed between the HEMS and LAS cohorts. There was no reason that this should have been the case and response rates did not vary with injury severity, but the size of the non-response does mean that the results would be susceptible to any such effect.

In addition, a large proportion of both HEMS (46 per cent) and LAS patients (39 per cent) were ineligible for interview, principally because they had died, but also because they had attempted suicide, were involved in crimes, or were children under five years of age and were thus not suitable for interview. This puts a further limitation on the disability results. Nevertheless, the lack of any evidence of benefit in those eligible for disability assessment makes it unlikely that there could have been any substantial benefit in the remainder.

In conclusion, the incremental costs of the HEMS have been estimated at £1.2 million per annum to run, and a further £0.8 million of cost consequences for health services, mainly as a result of increased use of intensive care facilities. Despite extensive analyses and review of 1145 HEMS patients and 700 patients attended by LAS, which identified for follow-up 337 HEMS patients and 466 LAS patients with non-minor injuries taken to any one of 20 study hospitals, there was no evidence of improvement in survival in the whole HEMS caseload and no benefit in terms of reduced disability for survivors.

Acknowledgements

The authors would like to thank the officers and staff of the London Ambulance Service (LAS), particularly those involved in the air ambulance and the LAS ground crews who provided information for this study about the patients they attended, and the air, ground and medical crew of HEMS based at the Royal London Hospital (RLH) for their wholehearted co-operation and assistance with this study. We would like to thank the LAS for allowing us to make a base in their headquarters, and the medical, nursing and administrative staff of the hospitals in London, particularly those at the RLU, for their help. The NHP was used with the agreement of Professor Jim McEwen. We would also like to thank our colleagues in London, Virginia Bergin, Jackie Neenan and Sharon Brereton, and at the MCRU, Janette Turner, and particularly Professor Brian Williams, who have helped us with this study.

References

AAAM (Association for the Advancement of Automotive Medicine) (1990) *The Abbreviated Injury scale, Revision*, Des Plaines AAAM.
Champion, H.R., Sacco, W.J., Copes, W.S., Gann, D.S., Generelli, T.A. and Flannagan, M.E. (1989) 'A revision of the Trauma Score', *Journal of Trauma*, 29: 623–30.
Copes, W.S., Champion, H.R., Sacco, W.J., Lawnick, M.M., Keast, S.L. and Bain, L.W. (1988) 'The Injury Severity Score revisited', *Journal of Trauma*, 28: 69–77.
Hunt, S.M., McEwan, J. and McKenna, S.P. (1986) *Measuring Health Status*, Beckenham, Kent: Croom Helm.
Martin, J., Meltzer, H. and Elliot, J. (1988) *The Prevalence of Disability Among Adults*, London: HMSO, OPCS Social Survey Division.
NHS Executive (1993) *NHS Financial Returns*, London: NHS Executive.
Nicholl, J.P., Beeby, N.R. and Brazier, J.E. (1994a) 'A comparison of the costs and performance of an emergency helicopter and land ambulances in a rural area', *Injury*, 25: 145–53.

Nicholl, J.P., Brazier, J.E., Snooks, H.A. and Lees-Mlanga, S. (1994b) *The Costs and Effectiveness of the London Helicopter Emergency Medical Service*, Sheffield: Medical Care Research Unit, University of Sheffield.

Nicholl, J.P., Brazier, J.E. and Snooks, H.A. (1995) 'Effects of London helicopter emergency medical services on survival after trauma', *British Medical Journal*, 311: 217–22.

Shiell, A.M. (1991) *Economics and Intensive Care: From General Principles to Practical Implications. Discussion Paper 80*, York: Centre for Health Economics, University of York.

Snooks, H.A., Nicholl, J.P., Brazier, J.E. and Lees-Mlanga, S. (1996) 'The costs and benefits of helicopter emergency ambulance services in England and Wales', *Journal of Public Health Medicine*, 18: 66–7.

US Department of Transportation (1972) *Helicopters in emergency medical service. NHSTA experience to date*, DOT HS 820231, Washington: NHSTA US Government Printing Office.

Wisner, D.H. (1992) 'History and current status of trauma scoring systems', *Archives of Surgery*, 127: 111–17.

A complete, unedited version of this article can be found as Brazier, J., Nicholl, J. and Snooks, H., 'The cost and effectiveness of the London Helicopter Emergency Medical Service' in the *Journal of Health Services Research and Policy* (1996) Volume 1, Number 4, pages 232–7.

Chapter 17

How do stroke units improve patient outcomes?

A collaborative systematic review of the randomised trials

Stroke Unit Trialists' Collaboration

Abstract

Background and Purpose: We sought to clarify the way in which organised inpatient (stroke unit) care can produce reductions in case fatality and in the need for institutional care after stroke.

Methods: We performed a secondary analysis of a collaborative systematic review of all randomised trials which compared organised inpatient (stroke unit) care with contemporary conventional care. Nineteen trials were included, of which 18 (3246 patients) provided outcome data. 12 trials (1611 patients) provided data analyses of timing and cause of death and outcomes at different levels of severity.

Results: The reduction in case fatality of patients managed in a stroke unit setting developed between 1 and 4 weeks after the index stroke. The reduction in the odds of death was evident across all causes and most marked for deaths considered secondary to immobility. However, data were insufficient to permit a firm conclusion. There was a relative increase in the number of patients discharged home from stroke units largely attributable to an increase in the number of patients returning home physically independent. Across the range of severity, stroke unit care was associated with non significant increases in the number of patients regaining independence.

Conclusions: Within the limitations of the available data, we conclude that organised inpatient stroke unit care benefits a wide range of stroke patients in a variety of different ways, i.e. reducing death from secondary complications of stroke and reducing the need for institutional care through a reduction in disability.

Source: *Stroke*, 28, 1997, 2139–44.

Introduction

Stroke patients who are managed in an organised (stroke unit) setting are less likely to die, remain physically dependent or require long-term institutional care (Stroke Unit Trialists' Collaboration 1997).

A number of mechanisms (Garraway 1986; Langhorne *et al.* 1995) have been proposed for the beneficial effects of stroke units, including the possibility of a more accurate diagnosis, more appropriate investigations, and more appropriate individualised patient care, improved assessment procedures, early active rehabilitation and earlier, more intense, and better coordinated rehabilitation procedures. However, there is a lack of direct evidence to support any of these proposals.

In this report we use data available from a collaborative systematic review of the available randomised trials (Stroke Unit Trialists' Collaboration 1997) to identify the aspects of recovery for which stroke unit care appeared to make the greatest impact. We wished to identify the following: (1) What causes of death were most likely to be prevented? (2) Did stroke unit care result in more patients surviving in a physically dependent state? (3) Did all groups of patients obtain similar benefit?

Methods

Systematic review

We identified randomised trials of organised inpatient (stroke unit) care for the period up to December 1995 using a variety of search strategies. We aimed to include all trials that compared management in an organised (stroke unit) setting with that of contemporary conventional care (usually provided within general medical wards). The co-ordinators of all relevant randomised trials were then contacted and invited to join a collaborative review group (Stroke Unit Trialists' Collaboration). The trial co-ordinators provided data in a standardised format concerning the trial characteristics, patient selection criteria and characteristics, and the numbers of patients in each outcome group (Stroke Unit Trialists' Collaboration 1997).

Subgroup data (either in the form of tabular or individual patient data) were also sought, in particular initial stroke severity, which was defined in terms of the functional status of the patient at the time of randomisation (Stroke Unit Trialists' Collaboration 1997). Mild stroke: equivalent functional status to a Barthel Index score of greater than 50/100 within the first week and greater than 65/100 within two weeks. Moderate stroke: Barthel Index score intermediate between the mild and severe subgroups. Severe stroke: Barthel Index score of less than 15/100 within the first week and less than 20/100 within two weeks after stroke.

Outcomes

The outcomes of interest in this analysis were (1) death, (2) the duration between the index stroke and death, (3) certified cause of death, (4) final functional status (Rankin score or equivalent measure of dependency), (5) requirement for long-term institutional care (i.e. within a residential home, nursing home or hospital setting).

The certified primary cause of death reported was allocated into the following categories (Bamford *et al.* 1991): (1) neurological – death attributable to the index stroke or recurrent stroke, (2) cardiovascular, (3) complications of immobility, e.g. sepsis (particularly chest or urinary tract), or venous thrombo-embolism, (4) other causes.

Statistical methods

A series of 'snapshots' of outcomes at various census times was used because insufficient individual patient data were available for more sophisticated survival curve analysis.

Proportions of patients were identified who were known to be dead at specific census times after the index stroke.

Differences in dichotomous outcomes were analysed by calculating the odds ratio (OR) (plus the 95% confidence interval [CI]) of an adverse outcome occurring in the stroke unit group relative to the control group (Der Simonion and Laird 1986; Peto 1987) and the risk difference was used to calculate absolute outcome rates.

If data from several trials were used to calculate a summary result, we calculated the heterogeneity between the individual trial data contributing to that summary result using standard techniques (Der Simonion and Laird 1986; Peto 1987). (Non-significant heterogeneity tests ($P > 0.05$) indicate that the results from the individual trials were all compatible with the summary result.) Fixed effects statistical models were used (Peto 1987) unless heterogeneity tests were significant when a 'random effects' model was used (Der Simonion and Laird 1986).

Results

Description of trials

Nineteen trials were identified up to December 1995; 17 were formally randomised with the use of random numbers or sealed envelopes (review papers 1–16, Table 17.1). An additional two trials used informal procedures (review papers 17 and 18, Table 17.1). Exclusion of these two quasi-randomised trials has no substantial effect on any of the conclusions reported here. One trial (review paper 4, Table 17.1) has not yet been completed; the remaining 18 have randomised 3249 patients.

Table 17.1 Review papers

1 Peacock PB, Riley CHP, Lampton TD, Raffel SS, Walker JS. Trends in epidemiology. In: Stewart GT, ed. *The Birmingham Stroke, Epidemiology and Rehabilitation Study.* Springfield, IL; Charles C Thomas Publishing; 1972: 231–345.
2 Stevens RS, Ambler NR, Warren MD. A randomised controlled trial of a stroke rehabilitation ward. *Age and Ageing* 1984;13: 65–75.
3 Garraway WM, Akhtar AJ, Hockey L, Prescott RJ. Management of acute stroke in elderly: follow-up of a controlled trial. *British Medical Jounal* 1980; 281: 827–9.
4 Fagerberg B, Blomstrand C. Do stroke units save lives? *Lancet* 1993; 342: 992.
5 Kaste M, Palomaki H, Sarna S. Where and how should elderly stroke patients be treated? A randomised trial. *Stroke* 1995; 26: 249–53.
6 Gordon EE, Kohn KH. Evaluation of rehabilitation methods in the hemiplegic patient. *Journal of Chronic Diseases* 1966; 19: 3–16.
7 Sivenius J, Pyorala K, Heinonen OP, Salonen JT, Riekkinen P. The significance of intensity of rehabilitation after stroke: a controlled trial. *Stroke* 1985; 16: 928–31.
8 Wood-Dauphinee S, Shapiro S, Bass E, Fletcher C, Georges P, Hensby V, Mendelsohn B. A randomized trial of team care following stroke. *Stroke* 1984; 5: 864–72.
9 Feldman DJ, Lee PR, Unterecker J, Lloyd K, Rusk HA, Toole A. A comparison of functionally orientated medical care and formal rehabilitation in the management of patients with hemi-plegia due to cerebrovascular disease. *Journal of Chronic Diseases* 1962; 15: 297–310.
10 Aitken PD, Rodgers H, French JM, Bates D, James OFW. General medical or geriatric unit care for acute stroke? A controlled trial. *Age and Ageing* 1993; 22 (Suppl 2): 4–5.
11 Juby LC, Lincoln NB, Berman P. The effect of a stroke-rehabilitation unit on functional and psychological outcome: a randomised controlled trial. *Cerebrovascular Disease* 1996; 6: 106–10.
12 Kalra L, Dale P, Crome P. Improving stroke rehabilitation: a controlled study. *Stroke* 1993; 24: 1462–7.
13 Kalra L, Eade J. Role of stroke rehabilitation units in managing severe disability after stroke. *Stroke* 1995; 26: 2031–4.
14 Hankey G, Deleo D, Stewart-Wynne EG. Acute hospital care for stroke patients: a randomised trial. *Cerebrovascular Disease* 1995; 5: 228.
15 Ilmavirta M, Frey H, Erila T, Fogelholm R. Does treatment in a non-intensive care stroke unit improve the outcome of ischaemic stroke? Presented at Nordiska Moter om Cerebrovasculara Sjukdomar, August 23–25, 1993, Jyvaskyla, Finland.
16 Indredavik B, Bakke R, Solberg R, Rokseth R, Haahein LL, Home I. Benefit of stroke unit: a randomised controlled trial. *Stroke* 1991; 22: 1026–31.
17 Strand T, Asplund K, Eriksson S, Hagg E, Lithner F, Wester PO. A nonintensive stroke unit reduced functional disability and the need for long-term hospitalization. *Stroke* 1985; 16: 29–34.
18 Hamrin E. Early activation after stroke: does it make a difference? *Scandinavian Journal of Rehabilitation Medicine* 1982; 14: 101–9.

Ten studies (2063 patients) evaluated units where admission was immediate; for the remaining eight (1186 patients) admission was usually delayed one to two weeks after stroke.

All patients allocated to a stroke unit received co-ordinated multidisciplinary rehabilitation by a team with a specialist interest in stroke disease and/or programmes of education and training in stroke (Stroke Unit Trialists' Collaboration 1997). Most of the control patients (1346 patients) received conventional care in a general medical ward. A small number (277) of control patients were exposed to multidisciplinary rehabilitation in a mixed rehabilitation setting (review papers 2, 11, 12, 15). For this analysis, they were analysed with the rest of the control group managed in general medical wards.

Case fatality

Data were available on the time of death for 14 trials (2463 patients), of which 10 trials could provide information on exact date of death and 4 gave information at census times. Figure 17.1 illustrates the proportion of patients known to be dead at intervals after the index stroke. In 13 of the

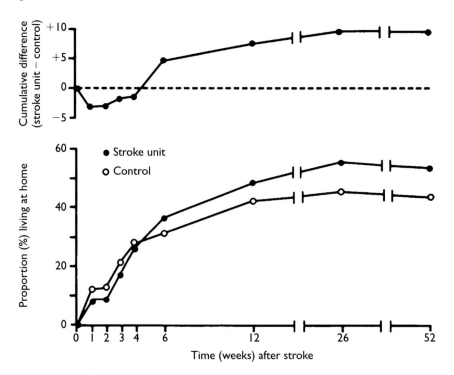

Figure 17.1 Percentage of patients living at home after stroke by treatment site (stroke unit or control) and by time after stroke.

14 trials the rise in case fatality among stroke unit patients was less than (or the same as) those in conventional care. The apparent number of lives saved is also shown. The observed differences largely developed during the period of one to four weeks after the index stroke.

Cause of death

Information on cause of death was available for 12 trials (1611 patients). Proportions of stroke unit and control group patients dying within particular categories of certified cause of death are shown in Table 17.2. There was no significant heterogeneity between trials within each of the outcome groups examined ($P > 0.2$).

The analysis lacks sufficient statistical power to draw unequivocal conclusions.

Other patient outcomes

We calculated the proportion of patients in four outcome categories at the end of scheduled follow-up (median, one year after stroke). These data were available for 14 trials (2770 patients) (Table 17.3). Stroke unit care was associated with:

- an increase in the number of patients residing at home in an 'independent' state (Rankin score 0–2)
- a marginal increase in the odds of a patient being at home in a 'dependent' state (Rankin score 3–5)
- reductions in the odds of death
- reductions in the requirement for institutional care.

In absolute terms the increase in independent survival appears to be the most striking consequence of organised inpatient (stroke unit) care.

Table 17.2 Proportions of stroke unit and control patients dying with particular categories of certified cause of death

	Stroke unit	Control
Neurological (%)	9.2	10.3
OR (95% CI)	0.92 (0.66–1.28)	
Cardiovascular (%)	5.2	7.0
OR (95% CI)	0.72 (0.47–1.09)	
Complications of immobility (%)	3.8	6.3
OR (95% CI)	0.62 (0.39–0.97)	
Other (%)	3.6	4.2
OR (95% CI)	0.9 (0.55–1.51)	

Table 17.3 Outcomes in stroke unit trials

Outcome	Stroke unit	Control	Odds ratio (95% CI)	Absolute difference in outcomes (95% CI)
Home (independent)	546 (39%)	463 (33%)	1.41[2] (1.19, 1.67)	+5 (+1, +8)
Home (dependent)	246 (18%)	226 (16%)	1.01 (0.72, 1.41)	0 (−4, +3)
Institutional care	270 (20%)	300 (22%)	0.83 (0.68, 1.03)	−1 (−4, +1)
Dead	320 (23%)	399 (28%)	0.80[1] (0.67, 0.95)	−4 (−7, 0)
Total	1382 (100%)	1388 (100%)		

CI, confidence interval. The table shows the number (%) of patients in the stroke unit and control groups who were in each outcome category at the end of scheduled follow-up (median, one year). Also shown is the odds ratio (95% CI) of a particular outcome occurring in the stroke unit vs control group and the absolute difference (95% CI in outcomes per 100 patients treated) calculated from the risk difference. The term 'independent' is equivalent to a Rankin score of 0–2 and 'dependent' is equivalent to a Rankin score of 3–5.
[1] $P < 0.05$.
[2] $P < 0.01$ based on z statistic of the odds ratio.

Figure 7.2 shows the proportion of subjects living at home and the cumulative difference between stroke unit patients and the control group.

The apparent impact of stroke unit care on patients with different degrees of initial stroke severity is shown in Table 17.4, which presents the numbers of patients surviving in either a physically dependent (Rankin score 3–5) or independent (Rankin score 0–2) state. Data were available for 13 trials (2091 patients) at the end of scheduled follow-up (median, one year).

Effects of stroke unit care

- Patients with mild stroke showed no net increase in survival but tended to be more likely to regain independence.
- Patients with moderate stroke showed a trend towards both increased survival and increased independent survival.
- Patients with severe stroke showed an apparent increase in both independent and dependent survival.

Overall, the trend is towards improvement in all outcome groups, but conclusions are limited by relatively small patient numbers.

Discussion

This article presents one part of a larger analysis of the randomised stroke unit trials. This analysis attempted to identify the way in which the apparent benefits of stroke units are achieved. This analysis is exploratory and is limited by two main problems. First, analyses were not always based on

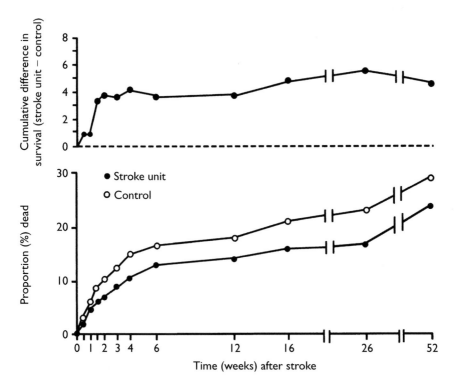

Figure 17.2 Percentage of patients dying after stroke by treatment site (stroke unit or control) and by time after stroke.

predefined a priori hypotheses. Second, analyses were frequently restricted to incomplete data sets.

Stroke unit care is thought to reduce the frequency of several common complications of stroke (e.g. cardiovascular complications, venous thrombo-embolism and infections) (Millikan 1979; Langhorne *et al.* 1995). The current analysis appears to support this view, as Figure 17.1 shows that most of the deaths prevented occurred between one and four weeks after the index stroke, which is the period of time in which many of the complications of immobility are believed to occur (Millikan 1979). However, there is insufficient statistical power to provide an unequivocal conclusion.

The reduction in the need for long-term hospital or institutional care, found as a result of stroke unit care, may result either from a more aggressive discharge policy or from a reduction in the number of patients who remained disabled. The current analysis (Table 17.3) indicates that the reduction is largely attributable to a reduction in patient dependency. Stroke unit care appeared to result in an increase in the numbers of survivors who were judged to be physically independent.

Table 17.4 Outcomes within stroke severity subgroups

Stroke subgroup	Outcome	Stroke unit	Control	Odds ratio (95% CI)	Absolute difference in outcomes (95% CI)
Mild	Independent	225 (78%)	186 (70%)	1.42 (0.95, 2.13)	+4 (−10, 18)
	Dependent	35 (12%)	52 (20%)	0.57[1] (0.35, 0.93)	−5 (−10, 0)
	Dead	30 (10%)	27 (10%)	1.04 (0.60, 1.91)	0 (−4, 5)
		290 (100%)	256 (100%)		
Moderate	Independent	208 (36%)	173 (31%)	1.26 (0.97, 1.62)	+6 (0, 11)
	Dependent	253 (44%)	237 (43%)	0.98 (0.76, 1.26)	−1 (−8, 6)
	Dead	120 (20%)	145 (25%)	0.76 (0.57, 1.01)	−3 (−6, 0)
		583 (100%)	555 (100%)		
Severe	Independent	20 (10%)	14 (7%)	1.30 (0.64, 2.65)	+1 (−3, 4)
	Dependent	86 (44%)	75 (37%)	1.27 (0.78, 2.07)	+3 (−9, 14)
	Dead	91 (46%)	112 (56%)	0.73 (0.47, 1.13)	−6 (−16, 4)
		197 (100%)	201 (100%)		

CI, confidence interval. The table shows the number (%) of patients in the stroke unit and control groups (subdivided by initial stroke severity) who were in each outcome category at the end of scheduled follow-up (median one year). Data are presented as in Table 17.3. Stroke severity subgroups are described in 'Methods'.
[1]$P < 0.05$ based on z statistic of the odds ratio.

The benefits of stroke unit care were apparent across a range of levels of stroke severity, although groups benefited in different ways (Table 17.4). Survivors of mild strokes were more likely to regain physical independence. Patients with moderate strokes were more likely to survive and to become independent. Those with severe stroke showed the largest absolute increase in survival with increases in both dependent and independent survivors. The increase in independent survivors is substantially greater than the increase in dependent survivors.

In summary, this secondary analysis of a systematic review of the randomised stroke unit trials has indicated that the observed benefits of stroke unit care probably resulted from a reduction in deaths caused by secondary complications of stroke (predominantly complications of immobility) and a reduced requirement for institutional care through a reduction in patient dependency. The net effect appears to be to shift the distribution of all observed outcomes in a favourable direction.

Acknowledgements

This study was supported by Chest, Heart, and Stroke, Scotland. Following is a list of collaborators (in alphabetical order): K. Asplund (Professor, Umea University Hospital, Umea, Sweden); P. Berman (Physician, City Hospital, Nottingham, England); C. Blomstrand (Neurologist, Sahlgrenska

University Hospital, Goteborg, Sweden); M. Dennis (Secretariat; Senior Lecturer, Western General Hospital, Edinburgh, UK); T. Erila (Neurologist, Tampere University Hospital, Tampere, Finland); M. Garraway (Professor, Public Health Sciences, University of Edinburgh, UK); E. Hamrin (Professor, Linkoping University, Linkoping, Sweden); G. Hankey (Neurologist, Royal Perth Hospital, Perth, Australia); M. Ilmavirta (Neurologist, Central Hospital, Jyvaskyla, Finland); B. Indredavik (Physician, University Hospital, Trondheim, Norway); L. Kalra (Professor, Orpington Hospital, Kent, UK); M. Kaste (Professor, University of Helsinki, Helsinki, Finland); P. Langhorne (Co-ordinator; Senior Lecturer, Royal Infirmary, Glasgow, UK); H. Rodgers (Physician, University of Newcastle, UK); J. Sivenius (Professor, University of Kuopio, Kuopio, Finland); J. Slattery (Secretariat; Statistician, University of Edinburgh, UK); R. Stevens (Retired Physician, formerly Dover, UK); A. Svensson (Professor, Ostra Hospital, Goteborg, Sweden); C. Warlow (Secretariat; Professor, Western General Hospital, Edinburgh, UK); B. Williams (Secretariat; Physician, Gartnavel General Hospital, Glasgow, UK); S. Wood-Dauphinee (Professor, McGill University, Montreal, Canada). In addition to the listed collaborators, important contributions were also made by D. Deleo (Perth), A. Drummond (Nottingham), R. Fogelholm (Jyvaskyla), N. Lincoln (Nottingham), H. Palomaki (Helsinki), T. Strand (Umea) and L. Wilhelmsen (Goteborg). Carl Counsell and Hazel Fraser (Cochrane Collaboration Stroke Group) provided invaluable assistance with literature searching.

References

Bamford, J., Sandercock, P., Dennis, M., Burn, J. and Warlow, C. (1991) 'Classification and natural history of clinically identifiable subtypes of cerebral infarction', *Lancet*, 337: 1521–6.

Der Simonion, R. and Laird, N. (1986) 'Meta-analysis in clinical trials', *Control Clinical Trials*, 7: 177–88.

Garraway, W.M. (1986) 'Stroke rehabilitation units: concepts, evaluation and unresolved issues', *Stroke*, 16: 178–81.

Langhorne, P., Dennis, M.S. and Williams, B.O. (1995) 'Stroke units: their role in acute stroke management', *Vascular Medicine Review*, 4: 33–44.

Millikan, C.H. (1979) 'Stroke intensive care units: objectives and results', *Stroke*, 10: 235–7.

Peto, R. (1987) 'Why do we need systematic overviews of randomised trials?', *Statistical Medicine*, 6: 233–40.

Stroke Unit Trialists' Collaboration (1997) 'Collaborative systematic review of the randomised trials of organised in-patient (stroke unit) care after stroke', *British Medical Journal*, 314: 1151–9.

A complete, unedited version of this article can be found as Langhorne, P. *et al.* (Stroke Unit Trialists' Collaboration), 'How do stroke units improve patient outcomes?' in *Stroke* (1997) Volume 28, pages 2139–44.

Chapter 18

Does volume really affect outcome? Lessons from the evidence

Amanda J. Sowden and Trevor A. Sheldon

Abstract

There is a prevailing consensus that the quality of health services can be improved by concentrating care in the hands of those providers who carry out larger volumes of activity. The substantial research literature indicates a positive volume-quality relationship. However, these conclusions are largely based on observational studies using administrative databases which are poorly adjusted for case-mix. Better control for confounding shows that volume-quality effects in several cases may be an artefact. The research is also difficult to interpret because of the limited measurement of outcomes, poor analysis of the relative contributions of the clinician and the hospital levels, and the lack of clarity about the direction of cause and effect. Most research is insufficiently reliable to inform policy on the use of volume for credentialing or for the reconfiguration of services.

Introduction

The concentration of hospital services into bigger units carrying out a higher volume of procedures has been proposed as a means of improving the quality of care. This is based on the assumption that an increase in the volume of activity – at the hospital and/or clinician level – will lead to better clinical outcomes. For example, the American College of Surgeons has recommended that open-heart surgery teams perform at least 150 operations per year so that the necessary skills can be maintained (American College of Surgeons 1984). Similarly, a number of service recommendations of the medical Royal Colleges in England are justified on this basis (Ferguson *et al.* 1997). Third-party payers and other organisations are

Source: *Journal of Health Services Research and Policy*, 3.3, 1998, 187–90.

increasingly using annual volume thresholds as the basis for credentialing hospitals, units or clinicians (Crawford *et al.* 1996). In some countries, legislation is used to impose minimum volume thresholds. In the Netherlands, for example, hospitals must obtain a licence to perform open-heart surgery, and the recommended number of procedures is 600 per year (Banta and Bos 1991).

The question raised is, to what extent is the assumption that quality improves as quantity increases supported by the research evidence? Over the past 15 years, publication of papers examining the relationship between volume and outcome has been prolific. In a recent systematic review of this research up to 1996, we identified approximately 220 separate analyses of volume and outcome after excluding those based on analyses of substantially the same data (NHS Centre for Reviews and Dissemination 1997). Studies have focused on groups of patients undergoing specific procedures or with particular diagnoses, and measured their outcome in relation to hospital and/or clinician volume. A number of reviews of this literature have also been published (Black and Johnston 1990; Luft *et al.* 1990). The overwhelming impression from this body of work is that, for many procedures and diagnoses, hospitals and clinicians that carry out larger numbers of a procedure have better patient outcomes.

It is argued here that, because of a number of methodological problems in the research which may affect the reliability and interpretation of the results, the scientific foundation of this consensus needs to be critically reexamined. Methodological issues such as the adequacy of adjustment for case-mix, data accuracy, level and type of analysis, and attribution of causality raise questions about whether improved patient outcomes can really be attributed to volume or whether other factors could account for the differences reported between high and low volume hospitals.

Case-mix adjustment

The majority of studies assessing the relationship between volume and outcome have used observational data such as hospital discharge abstracts. Variations in case-mix have a crucial influence on the interpretation of outcome data from observational studies. Differences in the patient populations between hospitals or clinicians with different volumes may produce misleading results if not adequately adjusted for differences in case-mix.

Our review of the international research suggests that data collected routinely are often not sufficient for this purpose. The importance of this is illustrated in a recent study examining the relationship between volume and outcome in over 20,000 patients undergoing coronary artery bypass grafting (CABG) (Shroyer *et al.* 1996). When no adjustment for case-mix or adjustment for age only was carried out, a relationship between hospital volume and 30-day mortality was found. However, with better adjustment for case-mix this relationship was no longer evident. The phenomenon of significant benefits associated with higher volume, or specialisation found with simple analysis, disappearing after better adjustment for case-mix has been reported in a number of other clinical areas such as cancer surgery (Sagar *et al.* 1996), stroke care (Davenport *et al.* 1996) and intensive care (Jones and Rowan 1995). The need for good case-mix adjustment is further illustrated by a recent meta-analysis of studies of the volume–outcome relationship for CABG, which showed that the greater the adjustment, the lower the estimate of benefit associated with increased volume (Sowden *et al.* 1995), a finding confirmed when the analysis was recently updated (see Figure 18.1) (NHS Centre for Reviews and Dissemination 1997).

Despite the clear centrality of case-mix adjustment, many publications in this area appear to have ignored this issue when interpreting the results, and studies with obviously inadequate adjustment continue to be published. For example, a recent study examining the relationship between surgeon volume and outcome in patients undergoing carotid endarterectomy did not include any risk adjustment when reporting a statistically

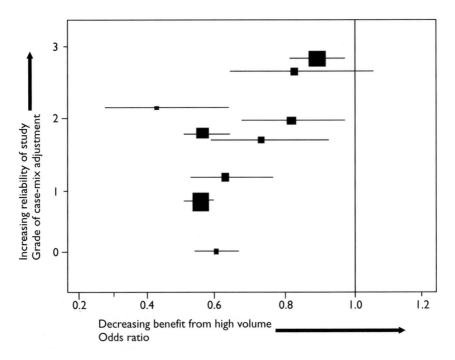

Figure 18.1 How estimates of the benefits of increased volume (> 200) of CABG vary by adequacy of adjustment of case mix.

significant volume effect (Ruby *et al.* 1996). Another recent study, while making some attempt at adjustment, failed to use well validated severity measures developed for use in studies of neonatal intensive care (Phibbs *et al.* 1996).

Less than a quarter of the analyses identified in our review took into account a significant number of the clinical factors that have been demonstrated to affect prognosis. Of these methodologically more reliable studies, nearly half found no statistically significant association between volume and measured outcome (NHS Centre for Reviews and Dissemination 1997). Adjustment based on data from clinical databases – which provide more detailed physiological and clinical information on which to base indicators of prognosis than administrative databases – are more likely to give unbiased results (Shroyer *et al.* 1996). However, even with clinical databases, all relevant prognostic factors may not be known, or captured accurately, or adjusted for properly, because the way in which they affect outcome may be unclear.

A further refinement would be to use clinical data from sites participating in a randomised trial of a procedure to see whether the effectiveness of the procedure varies by volume. While the analysis would still need to adjust for case-mix because the patients would not have been randomly assigned to low and high volume providers, it is likely that the entry criteria used in the trial would ensure that the patients are more homogeneous than is usually the case in clinical databases.

In estimating the strength of association between volume and outcome by employing a trial in which patients are randomly allocated, for example, to either high volume or low volume, clinicians would probably be less susceptible to bias. Only one such study was identified, in which patients were randomly allocated to an operator who had performed more than 500 interventional procedures or to an operator who had performed fewer than 50 procedures (Talley *et al.* 1995). Measures of clinical success after coronary angioplasty in this relatively small study did not differ significantly between the different operators. Clearly, concerns may arise about the ethics of allocating patients to low volume operators when there is a consensus that better quality is achieved by those with higher volumes. However, there may be sufficient naturally occurring variation in volumes to make this feasible and acceptable in certain areas,

Cause and effect

Even if a clear association is reliably demonstrated, the direction of causality may not be obvious. Two of the theories put forward to explain the reported relationship between volume and outcome are 'practice makes perfect' and 'selective referral'. These have very different implications for policy and the degree of concentration of services. If providers of care improve outcome by doing more, then in principle any hospital could improve its outcome by expanding its level of activity in a clinical area. On the other hand, if higher volume reflects preferential referral to providers with good results, then increasing the level of activity is less likely to improve quality in that unit. However, it is possible that the average quality at the level of the local health care system might increase if two further conditions hold: patients not already being treated by the best providers are diverted there from units with lower quality care, and the resulting increased workload experienced by the best providers does not lower the quality of care.

The majority of studies compare hospitals at only one point in time. These cross-sectional data are unable to provide the evidence needed to show whether quality would improve if smaller hospitals increased their volume over time. Only by using longitudinal study designs can the effects of changes in volume be studied, but few such studies have been carried out. The problem of inferring potential for improvement over time from cross-sectional data is illustrated by a study that examined hospital volume and in-hospital mortality for several procedures (including hip replacement and cholecystectomy) using both cross-sectional and longitudinal analyses (Boles 1994). Although several of the cross-sectional analyses found that mortality was lower in higher volume hospitals, the longitudinal analyses in the same hospitals found that the mortality rate did not fall as hospitals increased their volume of activity. Similarly, a study of patients undergoing hip fracture surgery in Canada found that fluctuations of within-hospital volume over time had no significant effect on mortality even though there was an association between outcome and volume between hospitals (Hamilton and Hamilton 1997). This finding is more consistent with the 'selective referral' hypothesis than the 'practice makes perfect' hypothesis.

Hospital or clinician?

Another problem with research in this area is the level of analysis. Most of the studies have only examined hospital volume data, when it may be at the level of the clinician that volume is important. Therefore, the hospital effect may be a poor substitute for an untested clinician effect.

In order to better understand the contribution that hospital volume, clinician volume and indeed other factors (such as quality of facility and supporting team) might have upon outcome, it is necessary to be able to consider each separately. Ideally, multi-level or hierarchical modelling techniques should be employed which allow patient, clinician and hospital level effects and possible interactions to be analysed appropriately (Rice and Leyland 1996).

Measuring and interpreting clinician volume is in itself problematic. For example, it may be unclear whether the clinician identified in a database actually undertook the procedure, supervised the operation or was simply the leading member of the clinical team. New members of staff will only have data for a relatively short period but their start date may not be recorded, while other staff may only be full-time for some of the year. This should be taken into account when calculating annual volume figures. In some clinical areas, volume may only be important in order to gain sufficient experience to become competent but have little effect thereafter.

Measures of outcome

Most of the research in this area uses the hospital mortality rate as the measure of patient outcome. For various reasons, this measure is unlikely to be a valid indicator of quality of care. First, hospital mortality is unlikely to be a good proxy for longer-term survival, and differences in short-term survival may simply reflect hospital discharge policies. Second, and more fundamental, morbidity and quality of life can be equally important outcomes, particularly in conditions with low mortality rates. Apparent improvements in quality due to modest increases in survival may mask unmeasured reductions in health status.

Conclusions

Previous surveys have acknowledged many of these problems such as inadequate case-mix (Black and Johnston 1990; Luft *et al.* 1990). However, this appears not to have significantly affected the interpretation of the evidence. It is our contention that most research in this area is insufficiently reliable to inform policy on the use of volume as an indicator of quality for credentialing purposes or as the basis for the reconfiguration of services (Crawford *et al.* 1996). However, studies investigating the volume–outcome relationship continue to be published, many of which display the same weaknesses identified in research published over the last 15 years.

Access to large datasets can encourage the suspension of disbelief in researchers, and the administrative databases, particularly in North America, that contain a huge amount of data for analysis have provided fertile ground for people seeking PhDs. However, perhaps the time has come for a moratorium on such potentially biased and uninformative analyses. Editors should now be less tolerant of these methodologically flawed and potentially misleading studies, which are being used by policy-makers as a justification for the re-configuration of some services and as a basis for some credentialing criteria. The trend towards more research-based health policy requires more methodologically rigorous studies as a basis for policy.

Attention should now be focused on developing more reliable approaches to exploring these types of questions. This could include the further testing of improved case-mix measures (Wray *et al.* 1997), exploration of innovative statistical techniques such as instrumental variables to deal with selection biases (McClellan *et al.* 1994), use of appropriate hierarchical modelling techniques to take into account factors operating at clinician and hospital levels with prospectively collected clinical data (Rice and Leyland 1996) and, where feasible, the use of experimental designs. This would go some way towards providing the evidence needed to assess the degree to which volume of activity can be used as a variable to improve the quality of health care.

References

American College of Surgeons (1984) 'Guidelines for minimal standards in cardiac surgery', *Bulletin of the American College of Surgeons*, January: 67–9.

Banta, D. and Bos, M. (1991) 'The relation between quantity and quality with coronary artery bypass graft (CABG) surgery', *Health Policy*, 18: 1–10.

Black, N. and Johnston, A. (1990) 'Volume and outcome in hospital care: evidence, explanations and implications', *Health Services Management Research*, 3: 108–14.

Boles, M.D. (1994) A causal model of hospital volume, structure and process indicators and surgical outcomes, PhD dissertation, Richmond, Virginia Commonwealth.

Crawford, F.A., Anderson, R.P., Clark, R.E., Grover, F.L., Kouchoukos, N.T., Wauldhausen, J.A. and Wilcox, B.R. (1996) 'Volume requirements for cardiac surgery credentialing: a critical examination', *Annals of Thoracic Surgery*, 61: 12–16.

Davenport, R.J., Dennis, M.S. and Warlow, C.P. (1996) 'Effect of correcting outcome data for case-mix: an example from stroke medicine', *British Medical Journal*, 312: 1503–5.

Ferguson, B., Sheldon, T. and Posnett, J. (1997) *Concentration and Choice in London*, London: Royal Society of Medicine Press.

Hamilton, B.H. and Hamilton, V.H. (1997) 'Estimating surgical volume-outcome relationships applying survival models: accounting for frailty and hospital fixed effects', *Health Economics*, 6: 383–95.

Jones, J. and Rowan, K. (1995) 'Is there a relationship between the volume of work carried out in intensive care and its outcome?', *International Journal of Technology Assessment in Health Care*, 11: 762–9.

Luft, H.S., Garnick, D.W., Mark, D.H. and McPhee, S.J. (1990) *Hospital Volume, Physician Volume and Patient Outcomes. Assessing the evidence*, Michigan: Health Administration Press.

McClellan, M., McNeil, B.J. and Newhouse, J.P. (1994) 'Does more intensive treatment of acute myocardial infarction in the elderly reduce mortality? Analysis using instrumental variables', *Journal of the American Medical Association*, 272: 859–66.

NHS Centre for Reviews and Dissemination (1997) *Concentration and Choice in the Provision of Hospital Services. The Relationship between Hospital Volume and Quality of Health Outcomes*, CRD Report 8 (part 1), York: University of York.

Phibbs, C.S., Bronstein, J.M., Buxton, E. and Phibbs, R.H. (1996) 'The effects of patient volume and level of care at the hospital of birth on neonatal mortality', *Journal of the American Medical Association*, 276: 1054–9.

Rice, N. and Leyland, A. (1996) 'Multilevel models: applications to health data', *Journal of Health Services Research and Policy*, 1: 154–64.

Ruby, S.T., Robinson, D., Lynch, J.T. and Mark, H. (1996) 'Outcome analysis of carotid endarterectomy in Connecticut: the impact of volume and speciality', *Annals of Vascular Surgery*, 10: 22–6.

Sagar, P.M., Hartley, M.N., MacFie, J., Taylor, B.A. and Copeland, G.P. (1996) 'Comparison of individual surgeon's performance', *Diseases of the Colon and Rectum*, 39: 654–8.

Shroyer, A.L.W., Marshall, G., Warner, B.A., Johnson, R.R., Guo, W., Grover, F.L. and Hammermeister, K.E. (1996) 'No continuous relationship between veterans affairs and hospital coronary artery bypass grafting surgical volume and operative mortality', *Annals of Thoracic Surgery*, 61: 17–20.

Sowden, A.J., Deeks, J.J. and Sheldon, T.A. (1995) 'Volume and outcome in coronary artery bypass graft surgery: true association or artefact?', *British Medical Journal*, 311: 151–5.

Talley, J.D., Mauldin, P.D., Leesar, M.A. and Becker, E.R. (1995) 'A prospective randomised trial of 0.010" versus 0.014" balloon PTCA systems and interventional fellow versus attending physician as primary operator in elective PTCA: economic, technical and clinical end points', *Journal of Interventional Cardiology*, 8: 623–32.

Wray, N.P., Hollingsworth, J.C., Peterson, N.J. and Ashton, C.M. (1997) 'Case-mix adjustment using administrative databases: a paradigm to guide future research', *Medical Care Research and Review*, 54: 326–56.

A complete, unedited version of this article can be found as Sowden, A.J. and Sheldon, T.A., 'Does volume really affect outcome? Lessons from the evidence' in the *Journal of Health Services Research and Policy* (1998) Volume 3, Number 3, pages 187–90.

Chapter 19

Consequences of discharges from intensive care at night

Caroline Goldfrad and Kathy Rowan

Abstract

Background: It is generally believed that pressure for beds on intensive care units (ICUs) has increased in the UK. This study used discharge at night as a proxy measure to investigate pressure.

Methods: Night was defined in two ways: 'out of office hours' from 22.00 to 06.59h and 'the early hours of the morning' from 00.00 to 04.59h. The rate of discharge at night was compared for 21,295 adult admissions to 62 ICUs covering the period 1995–98 with 10,806 admissions to 26 ICUs covering the period 1988–90. With data solely from 1995–98, the consequences of discharge at night and premature discharge were investigated.

Findings: Overall, 2269 (21.0%) admissions did not survive the ICU in 1988–90 compared with 4487 (21.1%) in 1995–98. Of ICU survivors, 2.7% were discharged at night (22.00–06.59h) in 1988–90 compared with 6.0% in 1995–98. In 1995–98, night discharges (22.00–06.59h) had a higher crude (odds ratio 1.46, 95% CI 1.18–1.80) and case-mix adjusted (1.33, 1.06–1.65) ultimate hospital mortality. Higher odds ratios were observed when the definition of night was 00.00–04.59h. Premature discharge was commoner at night, 42.6% vs 5.0% and its importance was apparent when incorporated into the logistic-regression model (premature discharge 1.35, 1.10–1.65; night discharge 1.17, 0.92–1.49).

Interpretation: Night discharges from ICU are increasing in the UK. This practice is of concern because patients discharged at night fare significantly worse than those discharged during the day. Night discharges are more likely to be 'premature' in the view of the clinicians involved. The implication of these results is that many hospitals have insufficient intensive-care beds. In deciding whether or not to invest more resources in intensive care we must, however, consider the cost-utility of this particular service compared with other ways that additional resources could be used.

Source: *The Lancet*, 355, 2000, 9210, 1138–42.

Introduction

It is generally believed that pressure for beds on intensive care units (ICUs) has increased. Although no rigorous research evidence exists, the increasing number of reports and correspondence related to this subject does suggest that the pressure on bed availability in ICUs may be greater now than before.

Increasing numbers of admissions with a concomitant decrease in length of stay in the ICU have been reported (Mitchell *et al.* 1995). Occupancy rates have been described as very high. The shortage of available ICU beds in London, UK, and elsewhere (Mitchell *et al.* 1995) has been detailed and a wide variation in provision of facilities has been recorded (Smith *et al.* 1995; Metcalfe *et al.* 1997). Cancelled operations due to the lack of available ICU beds (Smith *et al.* 1995) and high rates of refused admissions have been reported, both regionally (Working Party 1994) and nationally (Metcalfe *et al.* 1997). The transfer of patients over long distances in search of an ICU bed has also been reported (Bion 1995; Chadda 1995) and the potential dangers of transferring critically ill patients has been highlighted (Bion 1995). Premature discharge of patients has been described (Ryan *et al.* 1997; McQuillan *et al.* 1998).

A national bed register covering England was introduced in 1996 by the Department of Health to ease the problem of finding a suitable bed for a critically ill patient (Warden 1996). In addition, the Intensive Care Society, the professional organisation of intensive care doctors, has called for both an increase in ICU facilities in areas of low provision and a formal transport system (Wallace and Lawler 1997).

With the results of the Intensive Care Society's UK APACHE II study from July 1988 to September 1990, which indicated a high death rate on the ward after discharge from ICU (variation 6–16 per cent across ICUs) (Rowan *et al.* 1993), and the belief that discharging patients from ICUs at night does not constitute good quality care, our study used discharge at night as a proxy measure to investigate pressure on ICUs. The aim was to investigate the change, over time, in the rate of discharge at night from ICUs and to find whether there were any adverse consequences following discharge at night.

By the use of two high-quality clinical databases, the UK APACHE II study database (Rowan *et al.* 1993a, 1993b) and the Intensive Care National Audit and Research Centre's Case Mix Programme Database (CMPD) (Rowan 1996), the rate of discharge at night for 1988–1990 was compared with the rate for December 1995 to April 1998. We used data solely from the CMPD to compare the consequences of discharge at night with discharge during the day.

Methods

Database

Data were extracted for the 10,806 admissions to 26 ICUs in the UK APACHE II study database, covering 1988–1990, and for the 22,059 admissions to 62 ICUs in the CMPD, covering 1995–1998. All these data had been collected prospectively. Age exclusion criteria (age <16 years) used in the UK APACHE II study were applied to the CMPD, resulting in 21,295 adult admissions. Deaths in ICU were excluded from the analyses.

Data

We defined night firstly as 'out of office hours' (22.00–06.59 h) and secondly as 'the early hours of the morning' (00.00–04.59 h).

Solely by the use of the CMPD, the APACHE II probability of hospital death, defined as death before discharge from hospital after intensive care, was used to describe case-mix overall. Probabilities of hospital death were estimated by the UK APACHE II model (Rowan 1992).

Subsequent readmissions to ICU were identified. For discharges directly transferred to another ICU, in either the same or another hospital, survival data (alive/dead) at final discharge from ICU or hospital were extracted. For deaths at final discharge from hospital, the time to hospital death, in days, was calculated.

Data were also extracted for the variables 'reason for discharge from ICU' and 'destination following discharge from ICU'. The former was based on a clinician's subjective assessment of a patient's readiness for discharge in the light of the needs of other patients for the available ICU beds. No attempt was made to impose standard explicit criteria for this variable.

For all discharges, we used data for the variable 'date of ultimate discharge from hospital' to calculate the length of stay in hospital after discharge from the original ICU. In order to verify whether patients were being discharged at night due to pressure on ICU beds, the time, in hours, to the next admission (turnover time for the bed) was calculated.

Analyses

The overall proportion of discharges at night, and the proportion, by hour, were compared for the two periods for all ICUs and, additionally, for the ICUs common to both databases. For 1995–1998 solely (CMPD), discharges at night were compared with discharges during the day for case-mix, readmission rates and crude and case-mix adjusted, ultimate hospital mortality. Time to death, reason for discharge and time to next admission, destination after discharge, length of stay in the original ICU, in subsequent ICUs and in hospital were also compared.

Results

Trend in night discharges

There were 2269 (21.0 per cent) admissions who did not survive the ICU during 1988–1990 compared with 4487 (21.1 per cent) during 1995–1998. Overall, 2.7 per cent of discharges occurred at night in 1988–1990 compared with 6.0 per cent in 1995–1998 (Table 19.1), a 2.2-fold increase. The proportion of discharges at night varied 16-fold across ICUs in 1988–1990 compared with 25-fold in 1995–1998. Similar results were seen when the definition for discharge at night was restricted to discharge from ICU between 00.00h and 04.59h. When the ICUs common to both databases, denoted 'same ICUs', were compared ($n = 9$), similar results were seen. The proportion of discharges were consistently greater from 16.00h to 07.00h for 1995–1998 compared with 1988–1990 (Figure 19.1).

Table 19.1 Proportion of discharges at night from ICUs participating in UK APACHE II study compared with CMPD

	APACHE II		CMPD	
	All ICUs	Same ICUs	All ICUs	Same ICUs
ICUs	26	9	62	9
Adult (≥16 years) admissions	10,806	4131	21,295*	4064[†]
ICU survivors (% adult admissions)	8528 (78.9)	3219 (77.9)	16,789 (78.8)	3255 (80.1)
Discharges 22.00–06.59 h (% ICU survivors)	234 (2.7)	94 (2.9)	1009 (6.0)	182 (5.6)
Range of discharges at night across ICUs (%)	0.6–9.6	1.9–4.0	0.7–17.2	2.2–15.0
Discharges 00.00–04.59 h (% ICU survivors)	91 (1.1)	43 (1.3)	433 (2.6)	81 (2.5)
Range of discharges at night across ICUs (%)	0–4.0	0–2.3	0–9.4	1.1–7.0

Admissions before applying age exclusion criteria (admissions <16 years) used in APACHE II study = *22,059 and [†]4206.

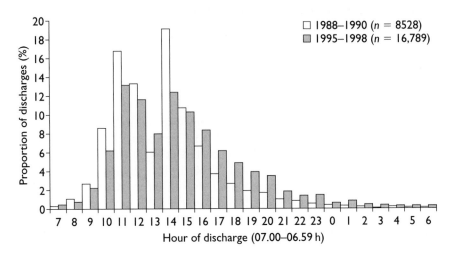

Figure 19.1 Proportion of discharges by hour for ICUs in UK APACHE II study compared with CMPD.

Case-mix for night versus day discharges

For 1995–1998, the case-mix of discharges at night compared with discharges during the day are presented in Table 19.2. Mean age was similar, the proportion with a severe past medical history was slightly lower for discharges at night and the acute severity of illness, measured by the mean APACHE II score, was higher, as was the median probability of hospital death.

Table 19.2 Case-mix for night (22.00–06.59 h) versus day discharges

	Night discharges (n = 1009)	Day discharges (n = 15,747)
Mean (95% CI) age (years)	57.5 (56.4–58.7)	58.2 (57.9–58.5)
Admissions (≥85 years) (%)	29 (2.9)	386 (2.5)
Admissions with medical history (%)	127 (12.6)	2259 (14.3)
Admissions eligible for calculation of APACHE II scores (% of total)	792 (78.5)	14,792 (93.9)
Mean (95% CI) APACHE II score	15·5 (15.1–16.0)	14.6 (14.5–14.7)
Admissions eligible for calculation of APACHE II probabilities (% of total)	706 (70.0)	13,293 (84.4)
Median (interquartile range) APACHE II probability (%) of hospital death	16.2 (7.6–32.1)	13.7 (6.7–26.7)

Outcome for night versus day discharges

The proportion of admissions discharged at night who were subsequently readmitted for intensive care was similar to the proportion discharged during the day (7.9 per cent vs 6.4 per cent, Pearson $\chi^2 = 3.65$, $P = 0.06$). Ultimate ICU mortality was 2.5-fold greater for night discharges ($\chi^2 = 21.96$, $P = 0.00$) and the ultimate hospital mortality was 1.4-fold greater ($\chi^2 = 23.05$, $P = 0.00$). The time to death in hospital after discharge from the ICU was similar for night and day discharges. The population eligible for case-mix adjustment using the APACHE II method was $n = 12,951$. The odds of hospital death for discharges at night compared with discharges during the day were significantly increased both for crude (odds ratio 1.46 [95% CI 1.18–1.80]) and for case-mix adjusted ultimate hospital mortality (1.33 [1.06–1.65]). When the definition of discharge at night was restricted to discharges between 00.00h and 04.59h, higher odds ratios were seen, 1.62 (1.19–2.21) and 1.53 (1.11–2.13), respectively.

The variation in the proportion of night discharges (0.7–17.2 per cent) and in ultimate hospital mortality (5.0–24.8 per cent), across the 62 ICUs, suggested heterogeneity. To address the hypothesis that high ICU night discharge was associated with high ICU ultimate hospital mortality, potential clustering was accounted for by robust estimates of variance (Huber 1967). After adjusting for a possible cluster effect of ICUs, night discharge remained significant ($P = 0.036$). Graphical representation of mortality ratios (observed hospital deaths divided by APACHE II expected hospital deaths) for each ICU ordered by proportion of night discharges showed no relation between excess case-mix-adjusted ultimate hospital mortality and increasing proportion of night discharges.

Reason for discharge

Only 44.1 per cent of discharges at night were judged by clinicians to be fully ready for discharge compared with 86.3 per cent of discharges during the day (Table 19.3). Premature discharge ('early discharge due to shortage of ICU beds') was judged to be much commoner at night (42.6 per cent) than during the day (5.0 per cent). In contrast, only a small proportion of discharges at night were judged to be 'delayed due to shortage of ward beds'. These clinical judgements were corroborated by the finding that the median time to the next admission at night was less than half that during the day (2.3h vs 5.5h) and was halved again for those for whom clinicians judged the discharge to be premature (1.2h).

Ultimate hospital mortality was greater for patients who were discharged prematurely (18.9 *vs* 13.3 per cent, $\chi^2 = 29.4$, $P < 0.01$). The difference remained significant after adjustment for case-mix (odds ratio 1.41

Table 19.3 Reason for discharge for night (22.00–06.59 h) versus day discharges

Reason for discharge	Night discharges (n = 1009)	Day discharges (n = 15,747)
Fully ready for discharge (%)	445 (44.1)	13,593 (86.3)
Early discharge due to shortage of ICU beds (%)	430 (42.6)	780 (5.0)
Current level of care continuing in another unit (%)	94 (9.3)	632 (4.0)
Delayed discharge due to shortage of ward beds (%)	18 (1.8)	387 (2.5)
Discharge for palliative care (%)	17 (1.7)	322 (2.0)
Self-discharge against medical advice (%)	5 (0·5)	31 (0.2)
Median (interquartile range) time to next admission (h)	2.3 (0.8–15.3)	5.5 (2.0–20.5)
Median (interquartile range) time to next admission for premature discharge (h)	1.2 (0.5–5.4)	2.3 (0.9–10.3)

[95% CI 1.17–1.71]). The importance of premature discharge was apparent when it was incorporated into the logistic regression model: premature discharge odds ratio 1.35 (1.10–1.65); night discharge odds ratio 1.17 (0.92–1.49; Table 19.4). Premature discharge and night discharge were correlated (Pearson correlation coefficient = 0.55, $P < 0.01$).

Discussion

Night discharges from ICU doubled in the UK over the past decade – a worrying trend because patients discharged at night fare significantly worse than those discharged during the day. Before considering possible explanations for these findings, it is important to recognise a potential methodological limitation – the adequacy of the UK APACHE II model for case-mix adjustment. While we can never be certain that all potential

Table 19.4 Outcome for night versus day discharges – impact of premature discharge

Definition of night	OR (95% CI)
22.00–06.59 h	
Crude*	1.46 (1.18–1.80)
Case-mix adjusted*	1.33 (1.06–1.65)
After adjustment for premature discharge	1.17 (0.92–1.49)
00.00–04.59 h	
Crude*	1.62 (1.19–2.21)
Case-mix adjusted*	1.53 (1.11–2.13)
After adjustment for premature discharge	1.33 (0.95–1.87)

*Ultimate hospital mortality for night versus day discharges.

risk factors have been taken into account, the model used was developed and extensively validated in the UK (Rowan *et al.* 1993b). There could be unknown confounders, such as will-to-live or genetic predisposition, and this uncertainty can only be resolved by a randomised trial. However, it is hard to imagine such a trial ever being done.

The rising proportion of night discharges reflects increasing demand on intensive care beds. Given that the level of need (as measured by the median probability of hospital mortality which was 19.6 per cent in 1988/90 vs 20.1 per cent in 1995/98) has not changed significantly, the increase in demand seems to have arisen from an increase in the incidence of severely ill patients identified by clinicians as suitable for intensive care. One contributor will be the rising rate of surgical procedures; for example, coronary artery bypass grafting rose by 10 per cent per year in the period in question (Black *et al.* 1996).

The main reason why night discharges do worse than day discharges is that they are more likely to be premature in the view of the clinicians involved. Their judgements were validated by the shorter bed turnover interval seen after discharge. Indeed, while night was still associated with an increased risk of subsequent death, the risk ceased to be significant with premature discharge in the model. Other factors that might account for a worse outcome for night discharges include poorer quantity and quality of care available at night both during transfer and at the destination. Transfers in the middle of the night may be traumatic both physically and psychologically for patients.

What are the implications of these findings? From the point of view of clinical audit, it may seem that the incidence of premature discharges (whether at night or during the day) would be a useful measure of unmet need. We would caution against the use of this, because it depends on clinical judgement and is, therefore, vulnerable to manipulation. Instead, given the correlation between the proportions of premature and of night discharges, we would recommend the latter be adopted as it is most unlikely to be manipulated by clinicians. It also has the practical advantages of being a process rather than an outcome measure.

The implications of our findings for the health system are that many hospitals do not have enough intensive care beds. In deciding whether or not to invest more resources in intensive care we must, however, consider the cost-utility of this particular service compared with other ways that additional resources could be used. Meanwhile, it is important that all ICUs ensure that they are making best use of their facilities.

References

Bion, J. (1995) 'Rationing intensive care: preventing critical illness is better, and cheaper, than cure', *British Medical Journal*, 310: 682–3.

Black, N.A., Langham, S., Coshall, C. and Parker, J. (1996) 'Impact of the 1991 NHS reforms on the availability and use of coronary revascularisation in the UK (1987–1995)', *Heart*, 1996; 76: 131.

Chadda, D. (1995) 'Intensive care units are overloaded, inquiry finds', *Health Services Journal*, July 20: 4.

Huber, P.J. (1967) *The behaviour of maximum likelihood estimates under non-standard conditions*, *Proceedings of the Fifth Berkeley Symposium on Mathematical Statistics and Probability*, Berkeley: University of California Press, 221–3.

McQuillan, P., Pilkington, S., Allan, A., Taylor, B., Short, A., Morgan, G., Nielsen, M., Barrett, D., Smith, G. and Collins, C.H. (1998) 'Confidential inquiry into quality of care before admission to intensive care', *British Medical Journal*, 316: 1853–8.

Metcalfe, M.A., Sloggett, A. and McPherson, K. (1997) 'Mortality among appropriately referred patients refused admission to intensive-care units', *Lancet*, 350: 711.

Mitchell, I., Grounds, M. and Bennett, D. (1995) 'Intensive care in the ailing UK health care system', *Lancet*, 345: 652.

Rowan, K.M. (1992) Outcome comparisons of intensive care units in Great Britain and Ireland using the APACHE II method, DPhil thesis, University of Oxford.

Rowan, K. (1996) 'Need for a national arthroplasty register. Intensive Care Society has set up a centre for national audit', *British Medical Journal*, 313: 1007–8.

Rowan, K.M., Kerr, J.H., Major, E., McPherson, K., Short, A. and Vessey, M.P. (1993a) 'Intensive Care Society's APACHE II study in Britain and Ireland – I: variations in case mix of adult admissions to general intensive care units and impact on outcome', *British Medical Journal*, 307: 972–7.

Rowan, K.M., Kerr, J.H., Major, E., McPherson, K., Short, A. and Vessey, M.P. (1993b) 'Intensive Care Society's APACHE II study in Britain and Ireland – II: outcome comparisons of intensive care units after adjustment for case mix by the American APACHE II method', *British Medical Journal*, 307: 977–81.

Ryan, D.W., Bayly, P.J.M., Weldon, O.G.W. and Jingree, M. (1997) 'A prospective two-month audit of the lack of a high-dependency unit and its impact on intensive care', *Anaethesia*, 52: 265–75.

Smith, G.B., Taylor, B.L., McQuillan, P.J. and Nials, E. (1995) 'Rationing intensive care – intensive care provision varies widely in Britain', *British Medical Journal*, 310: 1412–13.

Wallace, P.G.M. and Lawler, P.G. (1997) 'Bed shortages – regional intensive care unit transfer teams are needed', *British Medical Journal*, 314: 369.

Warden, J. (1996) 'Emergency bed register announced', *British Medical Journal*, 313: 575.

Working Party (1994) *Review of Intensive Care Services in the West Midlands*, Birmingham: NHS Executive West Midlands.

A complete, unedited version of this article can be found as Goldfrad, C. and Rowan, K., 'Consequences of discharges from intensive care at night' in *The Lancet* (2000) Volume 355, Number 9210, pages 1138–42.

Chapter 20

System-induced setbacks in stroke recovery

Elizabeth Hart

Abstract

This study reports research on the experiences of stroke survivors and their informal carers who are receiving stroke services in the community. Several survivors had suffered setbacks that were a direct consequence of their interactions with health and social care services and were system induced. This paper introduces and discusses the concept of the system-induced setback.

Introduction

In a review of the sociology of chronic illness, Bury called for a recognition not only of the problems people face but of the positive actions people take to 'mobilise resources and maximise favourable outcomes' (Bury 1991: 462). Bury argued that the way in which people respond to the disruptive effects of chronic illness involves a 'greater degree of consciousness and calculation in everyday life, whether at home or work, than is normally experienced': to define such actions as merely 'coping strategies' is to underestimate the extent to which people engage in the 'strategic management' of their illness (Bury 1991: 462).

Drawing on Bury's argument, and applying it to stroke, Pound *et al.* (1995, 1999) challenge the popular image of people as passive 'victims' of stroke, for whom the NHS and the state shoulders the financial 'burden of care', while individual families bear also the emotional, social and physical burdens. As such they are critical of the pervasive 'burden of care' paradigm, which they see as problematic in that it 'distracts attention away from the person with the stroke at the same time as casting her or him negatively as an encumbrance'. (Pound *et al.* 1999: 120). Instead of

Source: *Sociology of Health and Illness*, 23.1, 2001, 101–23.

focusing on the mental processes that people deploy to cope with their condition, this approach focuses on *what people do* in terms of the actions taken to maintain key relationships over time, set and achieve realistic goals, and maintain a sense of hope for the future.

The present paper draws on this earlier work, and in particular on Pound *et al.*'s research on stroke, a field in which, in contrast to other chronic conditions, 'there has been little interest in exploring the ways in which ... people actively respond to their condition ... ' (Pound *et al.* 1999: 121). This paper similarly recognises the need for a more positive focus on stroke survivors which takes account of the fact that, far from being passive victims, people take an active and creative role in managing their lives in the months following their stroke' (Pound *et al.* 1999: 126). However, the present paper argues that people's responses to living with a stroke involve far more than simply a response to their condition, however creative and active, but also involve a response to the way health and social care services are organised and delivered. The findings of the present study indicate that the misery that is a common and well-known characteristic of stroke cannot be explained solely in terms of the injury that the stroke has caused to the brain, nor in terms of a natural depressive reaction to the event. Instead, in a significant number of families, this misery is related to failures in the health and social care services that are put in place in the aftermath of stroke. More broadly, the paper is a contribution to discussions of the limitations of biomedicine in respect of understanding the impact of chronic illness and disability on people's lives in the longer term (Popay and Williams 1996): it shows that knowledge of the *causes* of disease can obstruct an understanding of the disease *process* because the medical model screens out social, professional and organisational factors. In turn the sociological focus on disability as a social process rather than a physical condition has tended to draw attention away from the fact that social processes can have physical consequences which further restrict what the body can do, irrespective of how society constructs disability.

The study

In the present study, 57 survivors had been interviewed. The in-depth, qualitative nature of the study meant that, in addition to ethical considerations, it was necessary to restrict the sample, since ultimately it would not be possible to interview in-depth more than about 60 stroke survivors.

Evaluating the Pilot Community Stroke Service: setbacks as an emerging theme

The main aim of the Pilot Community Stroke Service was to provide rehabilitation in people's homes and local communities, to improve co-ordination between existing services and to 'top up' others, thereby making better use of what was already available, as well as enabling survivors and professionals to access a range of other health and social care services.

The findings from the whole study showed that for many survivors and their families the pilot service was a 'lifeline', confirming both the need for, and the relevance of, a patient-focused and multi-disciplinary approach to stroke rehabilitation in the community. Nevertheless, the findings also show that setbacks occurred both before *and after* the advent of the Pilot Community Stroke Service, and that the new service could not prevent people from falling through the gaps between services, or through the gaps between practitioners within its own multi-disciplinary team. This was after all a pilot service, which by its very nature was attempting to pioneer a new way of working with people in their homes and local communities, and during the course of this evaluation the team was in the process of learning how to work together as well as how to work with other professionals in other agencies, across health and social care, hospital and community. As already noted it sought to enable survivors and informal carers, as well as professionals, to gain better access to what services were already available. However, this proved far from straightforward, and well over 18 months into the Pilot Community Service, the problems within social services about the respective roles of social care workers and occupational therapists in assessment of clients was impeding the service, as were some 'difficult' GPs (Peggs 1997). That people in this study who accessed the pilot service still experienced system-induced setbacks, despite the best efforts of the team, underlines the extent and complexity of the problems facing stroke services in the community, and the enduring impact of fragmentation and poor co-ordination on service provision (Wade *et al.* 1985; King's Fund 1988).

Categories of setback and stroke profiles

Of the 13 survivors in the study who experienced system-induced setbacks, four had suffered one stroke, and the other nine people had had two or more strokes. It was possible to group the 13 accounts of system-induced setbacks under five broad categories as follows:

1 Pre-stroke/nothing can be done.
2 Hospital stay acute phase/nothing can be done.
3 Discharge (including discharge from hospital, outpatients, and being referred on from one service or professional to another such as social services, housing and GP).
4 Fall.
5 Re-admission (to hospital or to a nursing home for respite care).

System-induced setbacks: a description

Mrs Morton had some warning of a stroke. Mrs Morton presented to her GP on two occasions: the first time her GP diagnosed a 'mild TIA', sent her home and told her to take an aspirin. The second time, some months later, she again presented to the same GP with weakness down one side, and as before was sent home and told to take an aspirin but this time when her blood pressure was 200/110. As on the first occasion, a few hours after seeing her GP, the family had to call an ambulance and she was admitted to hospital as an emergency.

Mrs Morton was frustrated by the system: she twice ended up in hospital as an emergency admission only a few hours after seeking help from her GP. She also encountered negative attitudes akin to those arising from the belief that 'nothing can be done' which Hoffman (1974)[1] found to be widespread among general hospital staff.

Hospital stay acute phase/nothing can be done

Of the 13 survivors who had system-induced setbacks, three people experienced these in the acute phase while in hospital.

After his second stroke, Mr Cornwell was also admitted to a general medical ward (formerly care of the elderly) at a local hospital. Far from feeling reassured that all that could be done was being done, this family came up against the belief that 'nothing could be done' (Hoffman 1974)[1], which was at odds with their own belief that Mr Cornwell was capable of much more than staff seemed to expect of him.

It emerged from the interviews that in the early days following the stroke the hospital experience reinforced their feelings of hopelessness and despair. Faced with a situation in which the hospital stay was making matters worse, the family of Mr Cornwell had to become 'management strategists' in the way that Bury (1991) suggests. They intervened in a downward spiral of events to try and protect the patient from the system. However, they were assisted by a health professional who knew the system and supported them in their efforts.

---

[1] In a study of nurses on a general medical ward caring for stroke patients, Hoffman (1974: 51) identified a widespread belief that 'nothing can be done' to help such patients, which was in contrast to the patients 'very hopeful prognosis'. Hoffman argued that nurses' negative beliefs arose in the context of the hospital's commitment to the 'classical medical goals of curing and healing'. In such a context the needs of stroke patients were perceived as inconsistent with what the institution regarded as 'doing something' (1974: 53): 'Thus we discover that "nothing can be done" is not so much dependent on the physiological condition of the patients, as it is upon the goals and orientations of the people who treat them' (1974: 53).

Discharge from hospital/referred on

This category is very broad because it encompasses setbacks of the kind to which survivors are particularly vulnerable when they are discharged or referred on from one service or one professional to another, whether this be from hospital to social services, from consultant to GP, or from physiotherapist to physiotherapist.

Of the 13 survivors, eight experienced setbacks in this category. Mr Denison (who, in addition to the stroke, suffered heart problems and had one leg amputated below the knee) spent over a thousand nights sleeping in a chair downstairs waiting for the housing department to convert his garage into a bedroom, and it was only when, after exhausting every other avenue, his daughter took direct action and threatened to go to the local newspapers with the story that anything was done. Mr and Mrs Denison had the support of the Pilot Community Stroke Service. The team member involved described her role as 'helping them [Mr and Mrs Denison] to keep their heads above water' because 'an awful lot of his reactive depression was about other services and not getting things done, and things weren't being done, so that was a difficult situation'.

The reactive depression experienced by Mr Denison was systemic in two senses: because it was avoidable had professionals behaved differently, and because it had a 'knock-on' effect on other professionals in other parts of the system, who expended time and effort in responding to problems created by colleagues elsewhere.

Falls

Of the 13 survivors, five had falls and, of these, three were living in nursing or residential homes at the time. Dealing first with the latter three people, all had had falls which resulted in system-induced setbacks. Mr Andrews was first interviewed in a residential home to which he had been discharged from hospital 'in a rush' and which he was desperate to leave. While there, he suffered a broken neck of his femur when he fell in his room. While in hospital for an operation to mend the fracture, he contracted a hospital-acquired infection, became very ill and had to have another operation to clean out the wound.

Because of his fall Mr Andrews was in hospital for over two months, during which time he became very ill, and lost much of the mobility which he had gained painstakingly over the previous months. However, his refusal to leave hospital to return to the residential home where he had fallen, and where he had been unhappy, meant that he was eventually found a place at a different one in which he felt more comfortable.

Re-admission to hospital/respite care

Under the 'readmission to hospital/respite care' category, five survivors experienced a system-induced setback. Mr Martin's setback provides an illustration of how an intervention, intended to support Mrs Martin as the full-time carer, made the situation worse for both of them.

The day before the researcher's visit Mr Martin had returned home from two weeks in a local nursing home for respite care, during which time, as his wife explained, he had been left in his wheelchair, and had not been helped to stand 'or anything'. At home, before he went in for respite care, 'he had been stood up three times a day at the bar or to get to the commode'. But since coming back from respite he had not been able to stand. Every time she had visited he had been 'wet through' [with urine] and left that way. While he was in respite care his spectacles had been broken, the foot plate on the wheelchair appeared to have been damaged (someone came to repair it while the researcher was there), and the special sheepskin cover on which Mr Martin sat to prevent pressure sores 'had not come back from respite – he's been without it for a week'. Mrs Martin had a list of other belongings which had not been returned.

Several stroke survivors and families in this study were treading a fine line between being able to manage and not being able to manage and, as both Kleinman (1988) and Charmaz (1991) have observed, this means that for people with chronic illness even very small changes can have far-reaching consequences. This was certainly true for Mr and Mrs Martin because if he could not even stand, then Mrs Martin could no longer care for him at home, and there would be no choice but for Mr Martin to live permanently in a nursing home.

Discussion

In organising the data into five broad categories of setback, and showing how setbacks were induced by the system, the aim has been to illuminate underlying patterns of experiences which appear, from the perspective of survivors and their families, to be specific to them. But when connected in this way, the data present us with a genuine paradox: the findings show that what stroke survivors and their families share is the uniqueness of their experience. Just as with other chronic illnesses (Charmaz 1991: 135), what happens in the aftermath of stroke appears to the survivor and his/her family to be individual to them, uncertain and idiosyncratic. Such feelings are reinforced by the structure of medical and social care, as survivors develop innovative ways of managing their lives, as they deal with the consequences of poor co-ordination and fragmentation of services (Charmaz 1991; Thorne 1993).

As already noted, because it renders visible underlying social and organisational processes in recovery which are normally obscured, the concept of system-induced setback can be used as an overall framework from which to extend the medical sociological literature on stroke. It is also useful as a way of reframing (Doolittle 1992) the way we think about the process of recovery and the consequences of stroke: it enables account to be taken of the impact on recovery from stroke of the way services are organised and delivered, while at the same time recognising the active role that survivors and families play in managing their lives. This enables a more appropriate allocation of responsibility for some of the misery associated with stroke, drawing attention to the way that failures in the system may be obscured, explained away and indeed accepted as inevitable, given stroke's poor prognosis.

References

Bury, M. (1991) 'The sociology of chronic illness: a review of research and prospects', *Sociology of Health and Illness*, 13: 451–68.

Charmaz, K. (1991) *Good Days, Bad Days: The Self in Chronic Illness and Time*, New Brunswick: Rutgers University Press.

Doolittle, N.D. (1992) 'The experience of recovery following lacunar stroke', *Rehabilitation Nursing*, 17: 122–5.

Hoffman, J.E. (1974) "'Nothing can be done': social dimensions of the treatment of stroke patients in a general hospital', *Urban Life and Culture*, 3: 50–70.

King's Fund (1988) 'Treatment of stroke', *British Medical Journal*, 297: 126–8.

Kleinman, A. (1988) *The Illness Narratives: Suffering, Healing and the Human Condition*, New York: Basic Books.

Peggs, S. (1997) *Final Evaluation of the Nottingham Pilot Community Stroke Service*, [unpublished report] Nottingham: Nottingham Community Health NHS Trust.

Popay, J. and Williams, G. (1996) 'Public health research and lay knowledge', *Social Science and Medicine*, 42: 759–68.

Pound, P., Bury, M., Gompertz, P. and Ebrahim, S. (1995) 'Stroke patients' views on their admission to hospital', *British Medical Journal*, 311: 18–22.

Pound, P., Gompertz, P. and Ebrahim, S. (1999) 'Social and practical strategies described by people living at home with stroke', *Health and Social Care in the Community*, 7: 120–8.

Thorne, S.E. (1993) *Negotiating Health Care: the Social Context of Chronic Illness*, London: Sage.

Wade, D.T., Hewer, R.L., Skilbeck, C.E. and David, R.M. (1985) *Stroke: A Critical Approach to Diagnosis, Treatment and Management*, London: Chapman & Hall.

A complete, unedited version of this article can be found as Hart, E., 'System induced setbacks in stroke recovery' in *Sociology of Health and Illness* (2001) Volume 23, Number 1, pages 101–23.

Part 5

Change management

Introduction

The focus on improving the quality and performance of health services through a range of different mechanisms and the challenge of managing the associated change is a common theme throughout health care systems.

Numerous change strategies are being used in health systems at a range of levels to improve performance. These include incentives at the individual level such as performance-related pay, or organisational performance assessments; organisational restructuring, such as mergers: attempts to change organisational culture, for example, using total quality management: or attempts at radical organisational transformation, such as business process re-engineering.

In this section we have selected five articles that study different strategies to improve performance and quality – some more narrowly defined than others – drawing on a range of disciplines and approaches, and using a range of research methods. The articles also illustrate the contrasting ways in which different disciplines and approaches consider change management issues.

The first article by Goddard *et al.* uses economic theory, in particular principal/agency theory, as the basis for a qualitative study, to analyse potential unintended consequences of using information to control health systems. Their focus is the NHS performance assessment framework and its attempt, as the authors see it, to redress the information imbalance. Using principal/agent theory they predict a number of problems that may arise from using information to control health systems. These include: measurement issues (indicators may be incomplete measures of outcomes leading to focus on short-term rather than long-term issues); attribution issues (indicators used are result of joint efforts of a number of agencies and/or agent can manipulate reports of indicators to misrepresent actual performance); and reward issues (potential for 'gaming' on the part of the agent to obtain advantage). These issues were tested by the authors in eight case study hospitals. They found evidence for each of the potential problems they had predicted and conclude that 'the unintended consequences of some measures may actually encourage agents to behave in ways which are directly contradictory to what was expected'.

The second article, by Shortell and colleagues, analyses the impact of a method that has been used to attempt to improve the quality and out-comes of patient care, total quality management (TQM). Taking an epi-demiological approach, the authors assess the impact of TQM and organisational culture on a number of process and outcome measures for patients following coronary artery bypass graft surgery (CABG). The study is based on a prospective cohort of 3045 CABG patients from 16 hospitals using risk-adjusted clinical outcomes, functional health status, patient satisfaction and costs. TQM and organisational culture were meas-ured using a two-part questionnaire administered to health care profes-sionals and managers involved in the care of CABG patients. While the authors found two- to four-fold differences in many of the quality and outcome indicators among the study hospitals, consistent among other studies, they found that TQM implementation and a supportive organisa-tional culture contributed little to this variation. The authors argue that their study underlines that 'medical care is a complex, highly interdepen-dent process influenced by multiple variables', as TQM implementation and a supportive organisational culture were not enough on their own to affect patient care.

The next two articles, by Pettigrew *et al.* and Harrison *et al.*, take a very different approach to Shortell and colleagues, and focus on different aspects of a particular change which was introduced in the NHS in the 1980s, the introduction of general management, in very different ways. Pettigrew *et al.* analyse eight case studies of strategic service change in 'high change' districts ('those processing high change agendas' such as reconfiguration of acute services or closure of Victorian asylums) in order to draw out 'receptive and non-receptive contexts for change', while Harrison *et al.* analyse the impact of general management more directly. Pettigrew *et al.*, using the method of 'longitudinal and processual compara-tive case study', identify eight factors derived inductively from their case studies which represent 'a pattern of association rather than a simple line of causation'. These factors include interlocking issues such as key people leading change, environmental pressure, and quality and coherence of policy. Harrison *et al.*, drawing on institutional theory, analyse the impact of the introduction of general management in 11 health authorities. Based on interviews, observations, analysis of documents and performance indi-cators, the authors suggest that although the Griffiths reforms had an impact particularly on managers and nurses, it fell short of facilitating 'a major cultural shift'. They explain this in a number of ways including the failure of the Griffiths model to take into account the political con-text within which the NHS is situated and its failure to address medical autonomy.

Our final article looks at possible challenges to the role of research evidence as a change strategy in health care. Rosen, using three case studies of the introduction of new medical technologies, analyses the different way in which doctors and managers conceptualise 'effectiveness' and therefore use different types of evidence. Based on 51 interviews in nine hospitals and health authorities and documentary analysis in four of these, Rosen shows how decision-makers from different professional backgrounds place different priority on clinical, financial, organisational and personal objectives in their use of 'evidence'. This has important implications for initiatives, such as clinical governance in the NHS, which encourage the use of effectiveness research in practice and policy but which fail to recognise the complexity of objectives held by decision-makers and therefore overestimate what such initiatives can achieve.

Chapter 21

Enhancing performance in health care: a theoretical perspective on agency and the role of information

Maria Goddard, Russell Mannion and Peter Smith

Abstract

This paper examines the role of information in securing control of health care systems. The paper shows the importance of serious dysfunctional consequences arising from the use of information as a means of control.

Introduction

In the 1997 White Paper, *The New NHS: Modern, Dependable* (Department of Health 1997) (and its Scottish and Welsh equivalents) the UK government set out a new framework for managing and assessing the performance of the National Health Service. The Performance Framework (NHS Executive 1998) will focus on six key areas of activity and outcome: health improvement, fair access, effectiveness, efficiency, patient/carer experience, and the health outcomes of NHS care.

The discipline of economics played a key role in inspiring and informing the nature of the internal market reforms of 1991 (Culyer *et al.* 1990). In particular, the 'quasi-market' in health care was intended to mimic the function of markets in more conventional commodities, and deliver the professed concomitant benefits of increased competition, improved efficiency and extension of consumer choice.

The principle underlying the 'New NHS' reforms is that 'what counts is what works'. That is, elements of the existing system that were perceived to be working are to be retained, while those that have failed will be discarded. In particular, the distinction between provider and purchaser of health care is retained, keeping in place much of the structure of the internal market, albeit with an increased emphasis on long-term agreements (rather than short-term contracts) and on trust and co-operation

Source: *Health Economics*, 9, 2000, 95–107.

(rather than competition) (Goddard and Mannion 1998). In this light, the key role afforded the Performance Framework can be viewed as an attempt to redress the lack of attention given to informational issues in the 1991 reforms, and to seek to make good the poor informational base on which the internal market has hitherto been expected to function.

In examining the expected impact of the Performance Framework, it is essential to have a proper understanding of the strengths and limitations intrinsic to the use of information in a quasi-market.

We take it as given that – from a neoclassical perspective – the improved information base afforded by the Performance Framework will lead to substantial direct benefits. Among other benefits, it will enable purchasers to formulate more complete agreements with providers and therefore to secure performance more in line with national and local objectives. However, notwithstanding the improvement on previous arrangements, the new information base will remain severely limited in its scope and usefulness. Many information asymmetries between purchasers and providers will be perpetuated, yet the increased emphasis on using this imperfect database may lead to serious unintended and dysfunctional consequences.

The purpose of this paper is to examine the potential for such unintended consequences implicit in the new arrangements.

The role of information in the NHS

Following the internal market reforms the emphasis shifted to the collection of comparative information on which purchasers of health care could base their purchasing decisions and to waiting times information on which citizens could assess the performance of local health services.

In England, performance information such as the Patient's Charter indicators and Health Service Indicators have focused almost entirely on processes rather than outcomes.

An adequate information base is fundamental to the efficient functioning of an economic system, and the NHS is no different in this respect. Table 21.1 sets out the information bases for three contrasting modes of

Table 21.1 Modes of governance and information

Mode of governance	Information requirements	Use of information
Clan	Traditions	Peer review
Market choices	Prices	Purchaser/user
Hierarchy	Rules	Bureaucratic

Adapted from Ouchi (1979).

governance, based on the typology developed by Ouchi (1979), which is in turn an extension of the transactions costs framework developed by Williamson (1975). Ouchi puts forward three modes of governance: clan control, market control and hierarchical control, each with its own information requirements and modes of using information.

Ouchi posits that the choice over the most efficient governance structure for a given transaction is linked to the ease by which outputs can be measured and the degree of clarity of understanding of the transformation process by which inputs are transformed into outputs (Table 21.2). Where outputs are easily measurable, but knowledge of the transformation process is imperfect, it is deemed efficient to use an information system that is concerned with output measurement and Ouchi views this as most economically dealt with by the market where all relevant information including performance is captured by the clearing price. Where outputs are not easily measured but the transformation process is well understood, knowledge of the behaviour of those involved in the transformation process is the key informational requirement. In this case the most efficient mode of control is the hierarchy. A hierarchical mode of control relies on a set of rules or targets which are enforced by a system of hierarchical surveillance where each superior sets standards to which output of subordinates is compared. Performance is assessed in terms of rule compliance and the meeting of specified targets.

In the case where it is possible to measure outputs easily and where the transformation process is well understood, Ouchi states that either markets or hierarchies are suitable modes of governance. Where the opposite scenario exists and it is not easy to measure outputs and the transformation process is not well understood he identifies the usefulness of self or social and cultural controls, and the associated clan governance.

In the ideal type system of clan control, members share a common (professional) culture. Individuals are socialised into particular traditions regarding appropriate behaviour and a high commitment to a code of conduct. Rewards are attached to displaying the correct attitudes and values and these may take the form of some ritual or ceremony that serves to reinforce these same attitudes and values. Control is achieved through

Table 21.2 Most efficient governance and antecedent conditions

		Knowledge of transformation process	
		Perfect	Imperfect
Ability to measure outputs	High	Markets/hierarchies	Markets
Clan hierarchies	Low	Hierarchies	Clan

Adapted from Ouchi (1979).

the alignment of the objectives of principal and agent rather than through legal or bureaucratic sanctions. Performance information is transmitted via soft and informal channels and is closely associated with the standards and norms of professional behaviour.

It is conventional to argue that, before the 1991 reforms, control in the NHS was dominated by the medical profession or clan (Bourn and Ezzamel 1986). Clinicians, through their professional training and specialised knowledge, were best placed to understand the transformation process. It has also been widely perceived that the NHS has a predominantly hierarchical mode of governance. The organisational form of the NHS, and many of the management structures put in place, such as general management and performance review, reflected the sorts of practices traditional to a hierarchy, so that it might be more correct to characterise the 'old' NHS as a mixture of clan and hierarchy.

One reading of the 1991 market reforms is that they signalled a belief that advances in information transmission had rendered obsolete such modes of control, with their manifold inefficiencies. According to this line of thought, it could be argued that, now that there was a better understanding of the clinical transformation process and – more importantly – improved measurement of outcomes, a system of market control had become the most effective form of governance. In the event, such hopes have proved excessively optimistic. Although the market reforms remain impervious to definitive evaluation, it is difficult to argue that they have led to unambiguous improvements in performance.

Thus, the new policy for the NHS can be viewed as an attempt to find a governance structure that strikes the right balance between the various forms of control posited by Ouchi. With its emphasis on trust and co-operation it signals a move back towards a modified form of clan control and a retreat from the pseudo-market model. At the same time, the emphasis on the Performance Framework signals a determination to improve the information base in order to avoid the worst consequences of a reliance on clan control, and a move back towards hierarchical control. In the context of Table 21.2, it perhaps signals an attempt to position the NHS somewhere towards the centre of the table.

Theoretical context

There are three fundamental potential weaknesses of the principal/agent model of control. First, the *measurement* of desired outcome may be poor or incomplete. Second, knowledge of the relationship between the agent's effort and outcome may be incomplete, which we term the problem of *attribution*. And third, the chosen *reward* schedule may imply unintended incentives.

Measurement issues

The chosen outcome measure may be only a partial measure of outcome, and important aspects of desired outcome may not be captured. This may lead to *tunnel vision* – concentration on areas that are included in the performance indicator scheme, to the exclusion of other important areas.

A particularly important incompleteness associated with many performance measurement schemes is the absence of consideration of long-term outcomes. This can lead to *myopia* on the part of the agent: concentration on short-term issues to the exclusion of long-term outcomes.

Attribution issues

It may be the case that some of the outcomes are actually the results of the joint efforts of a number of agencies. Where the variance of unattributed outcome is large it becomes very difficult to design incentive schemes that encourage co-operation and progress towards improvement in joint outputs. This can lead to a form of *sub-optimisation*: the pursuit by agents of narrow local objectives, at the expense of the objectives of the organisation as a whole.

An important attribution issue arises if it is in the power of the agent to manipulate the reported performance measure in a way that improves reported behaviour without any concomitant improvement in actual behaviour, giving rise to *misrepresentation* of reported performance.

Reward issues

The setting of the reward schedule (either implicit or explicit) is crucial to the development of principal/agent relationships. In practice, rewards are often set on the basis of the agent reaching some target, the basis for such targets frequently being some improvement on past performance. This gives rise to the potential for *gaming* on the part of the agent, in which behaviour is altered so as to obtain strategic advantage.

This system gives rise to a phenomenon known as the ratchet effect, which may arise whenever multi-period systems of targets and rewards are put in place. The essence of the ratchet effect is that, although the agent may be rewarded for achieving or exceeding current targets, the penalty for securing good performance in any one year is that a high feasible level of performance has been revealed to the principal. The principal's expectations may therefore have been permanently raised, and the agent can expect to be 'rewarded' with tougher performance targets in the future. Its targets have been irreversibly 'ratcheted' up. Under these circumstances, given that performance levels are positively related to the agent's effort, the agent has a strong incentive to report persistently low levels of performance. This may result in low productivity bonuses in the current year. The reward to the agent, however, will be modest performance targets in future years, with the concomitant reduced effort requirement and increased bonuses.

Qualitative evidence from the NHS

The overall aim of our study was to investigate the types of information used to assess the performance of NHS hospital trusts (providers). An important objective was to identify any unintended and dysfunctional behavioural consequences of the range of performance measures used in the NHS in force at the time of the new proposals, in the context of the theoretical framework set out above.

The research was based on case studies of eight hospital trusts. We limited the choice to non-teaching District General Hospitals in order to make our sample as homogeneous as possible.

The empirical component of the study involved an analysis of published and confidential statistics relating to the performance of each trust. In addition, qualitative methods were used to explore – for a range of stakeholders – the nature of their objective functions, and the perceived incentives, benefits and drawbacks intrinsic to current systems. Within each trust semi-structured interviews were undertaken with the Chief Executive, the Medical Director, a nurse manager and a junior doctor. We interviewed the Finance Director of the local health authority for each trust (the trust's main purchaser). At the regional offices, we interviewed staff responsible for provider finance and performance. The study is based on the results from 41 interviews.

We now consider the behavioural consequences predicted by the principal/agent models set out in the previous section.

Tunnel vision

We found clear recognition by all staff that the current indicators did not give a 'rounded' view of the performance of a trust and that the specific focus of indicators often diverted attention from equally legitimate (but unmeasured) aspects of trust performance.

The current priority given to waiting times targets was frequently cited as diverting attention and resources away from other important spheres of trust performance. In particular, the lack of measures relating to clinical outcomes was mentioned frequently in our study.

Sub-optimisation

We found that although each trust had corporate objectives, these object-ives were not always aligned with the specific incentive structures for dif-ferent staff within the organisation. In particular, it was clear that it was often difficult to align the trust financial objectives with specific clinical priorities.

Strategies for dealing with sub-optimisation were discerned. We found that setting devolved budgets and formal appraisal schemes were the two main mechanisms for transmitting trust-level objectives down to staff at various levels within the organisational hierarchy.

Myopia

There was a general feeling among respondents that many of the current performance indicators are short-term in nature and actions taken now may not show up in indicators for several years. The perspective of those people responsible for taking actions which influence long-term outcomes will be influenced by the likelihood that they will still be in post when the outcomes are revealed.

Misrepresentation

The scope for misrepresentation of data within a trust environment is particularly broad because many of the data used to measure performance and hold staff to account are under the direct control of those staff. A mixed picture emerged in our study, with some people citing specific instances of misrepresentation, while others said they were aware of the potential for such practices but were confident that they did not happen within their organisation.

Gaming

The most frequently cited example of gaming in our study concerned the efficiency index. This gives a target for the year-on-year improvement in costs to be achieved by a trust. Many respondents indicated they would be reluctant to achieve high gains one year for fear that they would be expected to deliver the same or higher gains in the future.

The financial regime in which trusts operate was also felt to encourage some gaming. It was noted that trusts which fail to meet their financial duties will often get 'bailed out' by the region and thus there may be an incentive to fail to meet these targets.

Discussion

In this paper we have considered the role of information in securing control of health care systems. We have shown that a principal/agent framework can provide rich insights into predicting potential economic consequences of current government policy. The theoretical predictions generated by this literature are supported by the findings of our empirical study into the behavioural outcomes of the current system of performance indicators.

It is clear from our theoretical and empirical work that the publication of performance measures does not always secure the desired changes in behaviour. The unintended consequences of some measures may actually encourage agents to behave in ways which are directly contradictory to what was expected. This was true of both clinicians and managers in our study.

Smith (1995) sets out a number of possible approaches to mitigating the sorts of dysfunctional consequences arising from the agency problem in health care. These include:

- involving staff at all levels in the development and implementation of performance measurement schemes;
- retaining flexibility in the use of performance indicators, and not relying on them exclusively for control purposes;
- seeking to quantify every objective, however elusive;
- keeping the performance measurement system under constant review;
- measuring client satisfaction;
- seeking expert interpretation of the performance indicator scheme;
- maintaining careful audit of the data;
- nurturing long-term career perspectives among staff;
- keeping the number of indicators small;
- developing performance benchmarks which are independent of past activity.

Clearly, the specific policy solutions adopted to overcome the problems identified will need to be carefully planned, as some of the measures potentially conflict with each other. The key will be to identify those problems most likely to jeopardise the success of the initiative and to focus on the appropriate measures to overcome them.

Within Ouchi's framework, the discussion above emphasises the potentially dysfunctional consequences of excessive reliance on a hierarchical form of governance such as the NHS Performance Framework. The importance of our findings suggests that emphasis on this single mode of governance in health care is unlikely to be optimal, and that the additional controls contributed by markets and clans will offer some useful counterbalances to the hierarchy.

References

Bourn, M. and Ezzamel, M. (1986) 'Organisation culture in the National Health Service', *Financial Accountability and Management*, 2: 203–23.

Culyer, A., Maynard, A. and Posnett, J. (1990) *Competition in health care: Reforming the NHS*, Houndmills: Macmillan.

Department of Health (1997) *The New NHS: Modern, Dependable*, London: HMSO.

Goddard, M. and Mannion, R. (1998) 'From competition to co-operation: new economic relationships in the NHS', *Health Economics*, 7: 105–19.

NHS Executive (1998) *A National Framework for Assessing Performance. Consultation document*, Leeds: NHS Executive.

Ouchi, W.G. (1979) 'A conceptual framework for the design of organizational control mechanisms', *Management Science*, 25: 833–49.

Smith, P. (1995) 'On the unintended consequences of publishing performance data in the public sector', *International Journal of Public Administration*, 18: 277–310.

Williamson, O.E. (1975) *Markets and Hierarchies: Analysis and Antitrust Implications*, New York: Free Press.

A complete, unedited version of this article (containing the economic models underlying the theoretical predictions) can be found as Goddard, M., Mannion, R. and Smith, P., 'Enhancing performance in health care: a theoretical perspective on agency and the role of information' in *Health Economics* (2000) Volume 9, pages 95–107.

Chapter 22

Assessing the impact of total quality management and organisational culture on multiple outcomes of care for coronary artery bypass graft surgery patients

Stephen Shortell, Robert Jones, Alfred Rademaker, Robin Gillies, David Dranove, Edward Hughes, Peter Budetti, Katherine Reynolds and Cheng-Fang Huang

Abstract

This study assessed the impact of total quality management (TQM) and organisational culture on a set of endpoints of care for coronary artery bypass graft surgery (CABG) patients, including risk-adjusted adverse outcomes, clinical efficiency, patient satisfaction, functional health status, and cost of care. It used a prospective cohort study of 3045 CABG patients from 16 hospitals using risk-adjusted clinical outcomes, functional health status, patient satisfaction and cost measures. Implementation of TQM and organisational culture were measured using validated instruments. It found little effect of either TQM or culture on the endpoints of care for CABG patients.

Introduction

Total quality management (TQM) is a process increasingly used by hospitals to improve the quality and outcomes of care. It is defined as the systematic involvement of health care teams in identifying the underlying causes of unnecessary variation in processes and outcomes of care, and taking corrective and preventive action with the goal of continuous quality improvement in patient care delivery (Deming 1986; Juran 1990). While specific TQM interventions to improve quality and outcomes of care have met with some success, most of them have been limited to a single site and a narrow set of outcome indicators (Shortell *et al.* 1998).

Source: *Medical Care*, 38.2, 2000, 207–17.

The purpose of this investigation was to examine the mortality, other adverse clinical outcomes, clinical efficiency, patient functional health status, patient satisfaction and costs of care of coronary artery bypass graft (CABG) surgery performed in hospitals, using TQM as a strategy to improve quality and outcomes of care. CABG was selected because it is a high-cost, high-volume procedure with known cause-and-effect relationships. In addition, the culture of each hospital was assessed to document the degree to which providers delivering care believed they were involved in decision-making processes, and were supported to make the changes necessary for improvement. We hypothesised that patients would experience more positive clinical outcomes, greater clinical efficiency, higher functional health status, higher patient satisfaction and lower costs the greater the extent to which the hospitals providing their care have implemented TQM and have a supportive organisational culture.

Methods

Overview of research design

A prospective cohort study of 3045 patients receiving CABG at 16 selected hospitals was undertaken. Hospitals were selected to ensure variability in baseline TQM implementation, CABG-specific patient risk adjusters were used to control for differences in severity, and generalised estimating equations were used to take into account the correlated patient observations within hospitals.

Hospital selection

A screener questionnaire was sent to 760 hospitals to determine their volume of annual discharges and approach to quality improvement. The 245 (32 per cent) hospitals that responded were significantly larger, more urban, more likely to be teaching hospitals and more likely to be members of a system than the 515 non-responders. Responding hospitals that reported an annual CABG volume of at least 200 procedures ($n = 76$) were invited to participate in this study, because better outcomes are known to be associated with this criterion (Grumbach et al. 1995).

Ensuring baseline variability in TQM

Data from the screener questionnaire and from the 1993 National Survey of Hospital Quality Improvement Efforts (Barsness et al. 1993) were used to categorise the 76 eligible hospitals that were also willing to participate in the study as high (41 hospitals) or low (35 hospitals) in regard to TQM experience and maturity. This was based on two scales involving (1) the clinical application of TQM such as the extent of quality improvement deployment, including the use of data to improve quality; and (2) training and participation, including the percentage of physicians and others working on quality improvement teams. Sixteen hospitals were randomly selected. Over the five years 1989–1994 before the study, risk-adjusted CABG mortality averaged 4.28 per cent for the high-TQM and 4.16 per cent for the low-TQM hospital groups ($P = $ NS).

Evidence that initial variance existed between the high- and low-TQM groups was indicated by data on the two TQM scales. These scales provided meaningful distinction between the high- and low-TQM groups of hospitals with respective scores of 1.19 versus 0.38 ($t = 2.95$; $P \le 0.01$) for the clinical application scale and 0.51 versus −0.40 ($t = -3.72$; $P \le 0.006$) for the training and participation scale. Despite these initial differences in TQM experience and maturity, all study hospitals engaged in specific targeted interventions to improve the quality and outcomes of care for CABG patients during the study period.

Patient eligibility and recruitment

The protocol defined all patients undergoing CABG during the study interval to be eligible for inclusion except those with (1) preoperative length of stay >3 days, (2) dialysis-dependent renal failure, (3) need for concomitant valve replacement, or (4) haemodynamic decompensation at catheterisation or percutaneous transluminal coronary angioplasty. Study protocol also required completion of a baseline functional health status questionnaire before or soon after the operation.

Measures of patient outcomes and costs

Baseline clinical, cardiac catheterisation, surgical and clinical outcome data were entered during 1995 and 1996 by data co-ordinators at each site into standardised collection forms. *CABG mortality* was defined as death in hospital or within 30 days of discharge. A variable termed *any adverse outcome* was also defined to include any occurrence of (1) death, (2) return to operating room, (3) postoperative stroke, (4) mediastinitis or (5) postoperative atrial fibrillation. Measures of *clinical efficiency* included length of stay >10 days, operating room time and postoperative intubation time.

The RAND Short Form 36 (SF36) (Ware 1988) was obtained at baseline to measure *functional health status* in all patients. The study protocol called for repeating this measure six months after discharge, and this was accomplished in 79 per cent of surviving patients. *Patient satisfaction* questionnaires were completed at four weeks or less after discharge by 81 per cent of patients. Detailed data on all *costs* associated with inpatient hospitalisations were collected for 97.4 per cent of patients.

Measures of TQM and organisational culture

At each of the 16 hospitals, an average of 54 clinicians (surgeons, anaesthesiologists, nurses, technicians) and administrative support staff directly involved in the care of CABG patients completed a two-part questionnaire to assess the hospital's TQM implementation and culture. Response rates were 78 per cent for management support personnel, 58 per cent for other health professionals, 55 per cent for nurses, 43 per cent for surgeons and anaesthesiologists, and 55 per cent overall.

The quality management section of the questionnaire involved a 58-item instrument based on the National Malcolm Baldridge Quality Award criteria (GAO 1991). This instrument assessed seven major areas of quality management work: (1) *leadership*, the extent to which senior executives and physician leaders were personally involved and committed to quality improvement efforts (Weiner *et al.* 1997); (2) *information and analysis*, the extent to which accurate, reliable and timely data were used to improve the quality of care and services provided; (3) *strategic quality planning*, the strength of efforts to involve all relevant staff in developing and implementing plans to improve quality; (4) *human resource utilisation*, the level of staff education and training to improve quality; (5) *quality results*, assessment of the effectiveness of hospital efforts to improve quality; (6) *quality management*, the extent to which all work units contribute to overall quality and operational performance requirements; and (7) *customer satisfaction*, the hospital's ability to determine and satisfy patient and provider needs.

The *organisational culture* section of the questionnaire used a 20-item instrument previously applied in other studies of both health care and non-health care organisations to define the beliefs, norms, values and behaviours of organisation members relative to the characteristic way in which work is approached and conducted (Dennison 1990; Zamutto and Krakower 1991). The results of this instrument are based on an assignment of 100 total points by each respondent to four culture dimensions: (1) *group culture*, emphasising affiliation, teamwork, co-ordination and participation; (2) *developmental culture*, emphasising risk-taking, innovation and change; (3) *rational culture*, emphasising efficiency and achievement; and (4) *hierarchical culture*, emphasising rules, regulations and reporting relationships.

Statistical analysis

Unit of analysis/enrolment issues

Given that variation in enrolment rates could have introduced selection bias, individual patient data were used as the primary unit of analysis. This approach permitted the baseline clinical characteristics of each patient to be used to adjust all observed outcomes using statistical models developed for each endpoint. Adjusted individual patient data were also aggregated by each individual hospital to provide performance results on each end-point that was used to compare hospitals with each other and as groups. Selection bias was also assessed in several additional ways.

Risk adjustors

Risk adjustments were made by using population-averaged generalised estimating equations (Liang and Zeger 1986) on all clinical endpoints, with adjustment for baseline differences on patient age, gender, previous cardiac bypass operation, acuteness of clinical presentation (elective, or urgent/ongoing ischaemia or haemodynamic instability), ejection fraction (capped at 60) and a co-morbidity index pre-modelled for each dependent variable.

Generalised estimating equations

The identity link (comparable to multiple linear regression analysis) was used to analyse the continuous variables of functional health status, patient satisfaction and cost. The logit link (comparable to multiple logistic regression analysis) was used to analyse all the other dependent variables, which were dichotomous. Independent variables (TQM, Baldridge scale and group culture) and all risk-adjusting variables were in the model for each dependent variable. Hospital-specific averages were used for the Baldridge and group culture scales. For six-month func-tional health status, baseline functional health status was included in the model. Compound symmetry within hospital and independence between hospitals was assumed for the covariance structure to address issues of repeated measures and intra-class correlation. By selection of different link functions, all outcome measures could be analysed with the same method.

The ratio of the model parameter estimate to its standard error is the standard normal variate (z statistic) used for hypothesis testing. Between-group comparisons of 1437 persons in eight TQM hospitals versus 1608 persons in eight non-TQM hospitals were done by testing the z statistic for the TQM variable in the model. All analyses used the person as the unit of analysis and were two-tailed. For variables that were hospital-specific, all persons at the same hospital had the same value.

The coefficients in the model may be interpreted as follows. For adverse clinical outcomes and length of stay >10 days, the exponentiated TQM coefficient is the odds ratio of these outcomes for the TQM group relative to the non-TQM group. The exponentiated Baldridge and group coefficients are the odds of these outcomes for a given value of the independent variable relative to the odds for a value 1 unit less. For the other outcomes, the TQM coefficient is the mean difference in outcome between the TQM and non-TQM groups. The Baldridge and group coefficients are the mean difference in outcome for a 1-unit difference in the independent variable.

Taking into account the within-hospital correlation of outcomes, the sample size had 80 per cent power to detect an effect size (mean difference between TQM and non-TQM hospitals/standard deviation) of ≤ 0.30 for each continuous outcome except operating room time (effect size $= 0.91$) and cost (effect size $= 0.47$). There was 80 per cent power to detect an odds ratio of 2.0 for outcomes between TQM and non-TQM hospitals. Two-tailed tests at the 0.05 level were done.

Results

Overall, 41 per cent of all eligible patients undergoing CABG at the 16 study hospitals were enrolled into the study. Enrolment ranged from 29 to 78 per cent. Compared with these 3045 patients, patients undergoing CABG at study sites but not enrolled in the study tended to be sicker and were more likely to have undergone surgery on an emergency basis, were urgent transfers from other institutions, or were weekend admissions. The in-hospital mortality rate for CABG at all 16 hospitals was 4.21 per cent for patients not enrolled (range 0–11.5 per cent) and 1.55 per cent for patients enrolled (range 0–4.60 per cent).

Table 22.1 summarises the baseline clinical characteristics of the 3045 study patients used to develop a model to risk-adjust observed study endpoints. The coefficients indicate the relative importance of each variable (based on z statistics) in the risk-adjustment model for the endpoint of adverse clinical outcome. The wide range among the 16 hospitals in mean values for patient data grouped by site emphasises the importance of risk adjustment on an individual patient basis.

Table 22.2 presents the descriptive statistics of the endpoints and the TQM variables. As observed with the baseline clinical characteristics, many of the endpoints (especially unadjusted) demonstrate wide variation. Two- to four-fold differences are observed for adverse clinical outcomes, length of stay >10 days, operating room time, postoperative intubation time and cost.

Multivariate models based on the generalised estimating equations that included the initial TQM categorisation, the Baldridge score or the group culture score, along with all risk adjusters, were performed to assess the relationship between these three separate indexes of hospital quality efforts and the various endpoint measures described previously (Table 22.3). The hospital categorisation as a high- or low-TQM site on study

Table 22.1 Baseline clinical characteristics of 3045 patients

Baseline clinical characteristics	Mean (SD)	No. (%)	Individual range	Hospital range	Z coefficient
Age (years)	64.3 (10.4)		24–90	62.4–67.5	12.9
Ejection fraction (%)	50.0 (10.5)		10–60	40.8–54.7	–4.1
Priority (% emergent, urgent, ischaemia, haemodynamic instability)		1081 (35.5)		9.0–75.9	0.3
Previous bypass (%)		115 (3.8)		0.6–11.6	1.5
Sex (% male)		2338 (76.8)		68.8–83.1	2.1
Co-morbidity variables (%)					3.8
Creatine ≥2		56 (1.8)		0.6–8.3	4.5*
Diabetes		711 (23.3)		17.4–30.4	0.05*
Severe COPD		324 (10.6)		1.4–42.9	3.9*
Carotid artery disease		249 (8.2)		2.3–18.5	11.1*
Peripheral vascular disease		329 (10.8)		4.2–22.1	4.1*
Other severe co-morbid disease		2323 (76.3)		35.8–95.0	0.6*

COPD, chronic obstructive pulmonary disease.
*Coefficients for the co-morbidity variables are based on a separate premodelling analysis and are independent of the other risk-adjusting variables.

Table 22.2 Outcome endpoints and total quality management variables

Outcome endpoints	n	*No. (%)*		*Hospital range*	
				Unadjusted	*Adjusted*
Death in hospital or within 30 days of discharge	3045	45 (1.5)		0.4–4.6	1.5–2.0
Any adverse clinical outcomes* (%)	3045	681 (22.4)		10.1–36.1	20.2–25.8
Length of stay >10 days (%)	3044	295 (9.7)		3.3–14.9	8.0–13.0
		Mean (SD)	*Individual range*		
Operating room time (hours)	3026	4.69 (1.33)	0.7–11.5	3.2–6.0	4.6–4.9
Postoperative intubation time (hours)	2819	13.8 (20.0)	0.1–610.9	8.2–18.9	12.7–17.8
Overall patient satisfaction	2297	1.85 (0.62)	1–4.8	1.7–2.0	1.8–1.9
Patient satisfaction with doctors	2295	1.65 (0.72)	1–5	1.4–1.9	1.6–1.7
Patient satisfaction with nurses	2296	1.74 (0.76)	1–5	1.5–2.1	1.7–1.8
Needs of heart patients	2241	2.36 (0.74)	1–4	2.2–2.6	2.3–2.4
Six-month functional health (physical)	2308	46.4 (10.6)	13.8–69.2	43.3–49.3	44.7–47.1
Six-month functional health (mental)	2308	48.3 (8.9)	12.0–67.7	45.6–50.4	46.4–49.1
Cost (dollars, adjusted by market wages)	2539	18,166 (8664)	252–142,083	12,014–26,065	17,661–19,374
TQM variables	n	*No. (%)*	*Individual range*	*Range*	
Baseline TQM	3045	1437 (47.2)	0 or 1	0 or 1	
		Mean (SD)			
Baldridge scale	3045	3.26 (0.22)		2.72–3.65	
Group culture score	3045	21.0 (6.1)		11.3–31.6	

*Includes death in hospital or within 30 days of discharge, return to operating room, postoperative stroke, mediastinitis and postoperative atrial fibrillation.

Table 22.3 Risk-adjusted* generalised estimation equation analysis of patient outcomes

	n	TQM	Baldridge	Group
Any adverse clinical outcomes	3045	−0.12 (0.27) (−0.65–0.41) $P = 0.66$	−0.16 (0.48) (−1.10–0.78) $P = 0.74$	−0.02 (0.02) (−0.06–0.03) $P = 0.52$
Clinical efficiency				
Length of stay > 10 days	3044	−0.30 (0.17) (−0.63–0.02) $P = 0.07$	1.77 (0.49)[‡] (0.81–2.72) $P = 0.0003$	−0.02 (0.01) (−0.05–0.005) $P = 0.11$
Operating-room time	3026	−0.60 (0.37) (−1.33–0.13) $P = 0.11$	−1.04 (0.60) (−2.21–0.13) $P = 0.08$	0.06 (0.02)[‡] (0.02–0.10) $P = 0.004$
Postoperative intubation time	2819	−0.23 (1.32) (−2.82–2.36) $P = 0.86$	−1.87 (2.17) (−6.13–2.39) $P = 0.39$	−0.24 (0.10)[‡] (−0.43 to −0.05) $P = 0.01$
Patient satisfaction				
Overall	2297	0.05 (0.06) (−0.07–0.18) $P = 0.40$	−0.14 (0.11) (−0.35–0.07) $P = 0.18$	−0.003 (0.003) (−0.09–0.04) $P = 0.46$
With doctors	2295	0.001 (0.07) (−0.14–0.14) $P = 0.99$	−0.02 (0.13) (−0.29–0.24) $P = 0.85$	−0.002 (0.005) (−0.01–0.01) $P = 0.69$
With nurses	2296	0.17 (0.09) (−0.01–0.34) $P = 0.07$	−0.44 (0.16)[‡] (−0.76 to −0.13) $P = 0.005$	0.002 (0.005) (−0.01–0.01) $P = 0.75$
Needs of heart patients	2241	−0.007 (0.06) (−0.12–0.11) $P = 0.90$	−0.10 (0.12) (−0.34–0.14) $P = 0.42$	−0.002 (0.005) (−0.01–0.01) $P = 0.63$
Functional health status				
Six-month functional health (physical)[†]	2284	−0.05 (0.99) (−1.99–1.89) $P = 0.96$	−0.68 (2.07) (−4.74–3.38) $P = 0.74$	0.19 (0.07)[‡] (0.06–0.33) $P = 0.005$
Six-month functional health (mental)[†]	2284	0.34 (0.66) (−0.96–1.64) $P = 0.61$	−2.41 (1.31) (−4.99–0.16) $P = 0.07)$	0.12 (0.04)[‡] (0.03−0.20) $P = 0.01$
Cost (market wage index adjusted)	2539 2539	156 (2006) 156 (2006) (−3775–4089) $P = 0.94$	−2930 (4061) −2930 (4061) (−10,890–5030) $P = 0.47$	13 (165) 14 (165) (−309–336) $P = 0.94$

Values shown are coefficient (standard error), (95% confidence interval) and P value.
*Adjusted for age, gender, previous bypass, priority of operation, ejection fraction and a co-morbidity index premodelled for each dependent variable.
[†]Also adjusted for baseline physical or mental functional health scores.
[‡]$P < 0.05$.

entry had no measurable impact on any study endpoint. A higher Baldridge scale was associated with higher patient satisfaction with nursing care ($P = 0.005$), with a coefficient of -0.44. This means that if the scale increased by 0.93 units (the hospital mean range for the scale) the patient satisfaction scores decreased (improved) by 0.41 units (0.44×0.93) on the 1–5 patient satisfaction scale. But the scale was also associated with a greater percentage of patients with a length of stay >10 days ($P = 0.0003$), with a coefficient of 1.77. This means that if the scale increased by 0.93 units, the odds of there being a length of stay >10 days increased by exp (1.77×0.93), or 5.2-fold.

A higher group culture score was associated with shorter postoperative intubation times ($P = 0.01$), with a coefficient of -0.24, resulting in a postoperative intubation time decrease of (0.24×60) = 14 minutes for every 1-unit change in the group culture scores. But group culture was also associated with longer operating-room times ($P = 0.004$), with a coefficient of 0.06 resulting in an operating-room time increase of (0.06×60) = 3.6 minutes for a 1-unit change in the culture score. A higher group culture was also associated with higher six-month physical function (coefficient = 0.19; $P = 0.005$) and mental function (coefficient = 0.12; $P = 0.01$) health status scores.

The range for the physical function scale was 43.3–49.6, or 6 points, and that for the group culture scale across hospitals was 11.3–31.6, or 20.3 points. Thus, if the hospital group culture mean moved from the lowest to the highest hospital, a distance of 20.3 points, then the expected change in the *physical health* scale would be 0.19 (the coefficient in Table 22.3) $\times$ 20.3 = 3.9 points, which represents 65 per cent of the 6-point hospital range for physical health. Similarly, in regard to *mental health* functioning, the range was 45.6–50.4, or 4.8 points, with the group culture range of 20.3 points. Thus, if the hospital group culture mean moved from the lowest to the highest hospital, a distance of 20.3 points, then the expected change in the mental health functional scale would be 0.12 (the coefficient in Table 22.3) $\times$ 20.3 = 2.4 points, representing 50 per cent of the 4.8 hospital range for mental health.

Selection bias analysis

The enrolment of eligible patients varied from 29 to 78 per cent. Several analyses were conducted to assess the potential bias of differential enrolment. Each outcome endpoint was adjusted on individual patient data using a comprehensive set of baseline characteristics known to indicate disease severity and to influence observed outcomes. This approach tends to reduce variation observed among institutions by eliminating that caused by differences in disease severity among patients entered into the study at each institution. To evaluate the influence of this method on study results, all analyses were also done without risk adjustment, and the conclusions were unchanged.

We also conducted the analyses eliminating the three hospitals with the most erratic enrolment. The findings remained the same except that group culture was significantly associated with fewer adverse clinical outcomes ($P = 0.001$) and a lower percentage of patients with length of stay >10 days ($P = 0.03$). Also, the Baldridge TQM scale was significantly associated with greater overall patient satisfaction ($P = 0.049$) but a lower six-month mental health functional health status score ($P = 0.006$). Adjusting directly for different enrolment rates at each hospital did not substantively change the results shown in Table 22.3.

The above analyses support the internal validity of the study findings. However, the sickest CABG patients were not able to be included in this study, and this compromised the external validity or generalisability of the findings to other CABG patient populations. One could argue that the sickest patients have the most to gain from efforts to improve the quality and outcomes of care; TQM efforts to improve quality for these patients may have a larger effect than we found with the composition of patients enrolled in this study.

Discussion

The present findings showing a two- to four-fold difference in many quality and outcome variables among the study hospitals are consistent with recent reviews and assessments. However, TQM implementation and a supportive organisation culture, for the most part, are not associated with these differences. It is important to remember that the provision of medical care is a complex, highly interdependent process influenced by multiple variables. Blumenthal and Epstein (1996) note that methods are now available for 'changing the processes of care to achieve better outcomes'.

These results suggest the complexity and challenge involved. A positive organisational culture and perceived progress in implementing TQM practices appear to have little influence by themselves. There is a need to further examine the relationships between individual professional skill and motivation, group-level micro-system team processes, and specifically tailored interventions, along with larger organisation-wide issues involving culture, leadership, decision support systems and incentives (Weiner *et al.* 1997). This will require simultaneous multi-level interventions (individual, group and organisation) that address significant opportunities to reduce variation and improve quality and outcomes.

References

Barsness, Z.I., Shortell, S.M., Gillies, R.R., Hughes, E.F.X., O'Brien, J.L., Bohr, D., Izui, C. and Kralovec, P. (1993) 'National survey of hospital quality improvement activities', *Hospital Health Networks*, December 5: 52–5.

Blumenthal, D. and Epstein, A.M. (1996) 'Quality of health care, part 6: the role of physician in the future of quality management', *New England Journal of Medicine*, 335: 1328–31.

Deming, W.E. (1986) *Out of the Crisis*, Cambridge: Massachusetts Institute of Technology Center for Advance Engineering Study.

Dennison, D.R. (1990) *Corporate Culture and Organizational Effectiveness*, New York: John Wiley & Sons.

GAO (General Accounting Office) (1991) *Management Practices: US companies Improve Performance through Quality Efforts*, GO/NSIAD-91–190, Washington, DC: US Government Printing Office.

Grumbach, K., Anderson, G., Luft, H.S., Roos, L.L. and Brook, R. (1995) 'Regionalization of cardiac surgery in the United States and Canada: geographic access, choice, and outcomes', *Journal of the American Medical Association*, 274: 1282–8.

Juran, J.M. (1990) *The Juran Road Map to Total Quality*, Wilton, CT: The Juran Institute.

Liang, K.L. and Zeger, S.L. (1986) 'Longitudinal data analysis using generalized linear models', *Biometrika* 73: 13–22.

Shortell, S.M., Bennett, C.L. and Byck, G.R. (1998) 'Accelerating the impact of continuous quality improvement on clinical practice: assessing the evidence and recommendations for 'improvement'', *Milbank Quarterly* 76: 593–624.

Ware, J.E. (1988) *How to Score the Revised MOS Short-form Health Scales*, Boston: Institute for the Improvement of Medical Care and Health, New England Medical Center.

Weiner, B.J., Shortell, S.M. and Alexander, J.A. (1997) 'Promoting clinical involvement in hospital quality improvement efforts: the effects of top management, board, and physician leadership', *Health Services Research*, 32: 491–510.

Zamutto, R.F. and Krakower, J.Y. (1991) 'Quantitative and qualitative studies of organizational culture', *Researching Organizational Change and Development*, 5: 83–114.

A complete, unedited version of this article can be found as 'Assessing the impact of Total Quality Management and organizational culture on multiple outcomes of care for coronary artery bypass graft surgery patients' in the *Medical Care*, Volume 38, Number 2, pages 207–17. The authors are Shortell, S., Jones, R., Rademaker, A., Gillies, R., Dranove, D., Hughes, E., Budetti, P., Reynolds, K. and Huang, C.

Chapter 23

Receptive and non-receptive contexts for change

A. Pettigrew, E. Ferlie and L. McKee

Abstract

This report focuses on progress in implementing service changes at District Health Authority level in the UK. The key questions guiding the study include, did the top-down changes of the 1980s secure change at local levels, and if so, why and how? Was there evidence of variability in the rate and pace of change in districts facing broadly similar change objectives? What features of the outer and inner context of each district caused change to occur, and how did those features of context interweave with the change strategies used in the different localities? What mixture of top-down and bottom-up pressure provided momentum and energy for change, and how was early progress maintained, increased or lost?

Introduction

The questions raised about why, how and when change occurs are of universal significance at all levels in both the private and public sectors.

Comparative case study analyses have demonstrated that districts addressing the same strategic change problem display both differences and similarities in their experience of the strategic change process. Therefore we need to confront the key generic question: why is it that the rate and pace of strategic change differs across districts? (See Appendix for research aims and methodology.)

The starting point was that the rate and pace of change could be explained by a subtle interplay between the content, context and the process of change. Context may therefore be a critical shaper of process (Pettigrew 1985). We conclude that the management of change is likely to be contextually very sensitive; that there is no one way of effecting change in such a pluralist organisation as the NHS, where the introduction of

Source: *Shaping Strategic Change*, London, Sage, 1992.

general management has not been at all general, and there seemed almost as many general managements as general managers.

Is it possible to begin to see any patterns in the way that strategic service change occurs? A good focus for this analysis is the distinction between receptive and non-receptive contexts for change where by the term 'receptive context' we mean that there are features of context (and also management action) that seem to be favourably associated with forward movement. On the other hand, in non-receptive contexts there is a configuration of features associated with blocks on change.

Receptivity and change in the NHS: the eight
factors (Figure 23.1)

There are some intellectual caveats to be made about the structure of our argument.

First, the eight factors outlined in Figure 23.1 should be seen as providing a linked set of conditions which provide high energy around change. The factors represent a pattern of association rather than a simple line of causation (Pettigrew 1990).

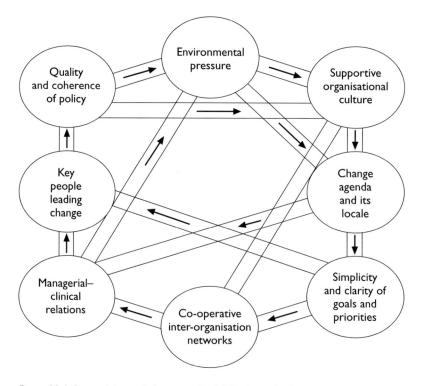

Figure 23.1 Receptivity and change in the NHS: the eight factors.

Secondly, notions of receptivity and non-receptivity are dynamic not static concepts. Receptive contexts for change can be constructed through processes of cumulative development but such processes are reversible, either by the removal of key individuals or ill-considered action.

Thirdly, in the way that continued processes are reversible so they are also indeterminate in their outcomes and implications. We are presenting a view of change processes which recognises emergence and iteration.

Factor 1: the quality and coherence of 'policy' – analytical and process components

In our study the quality of 'policy' generated at local level was found to be important, both from an analytic and a process perspective. Analytically, data played a major role in substantiating a solid case, and we would not generally support the argument of 'paralysis by analysis' (Peters and Waterman 1982).

Perhaps analytical considerations represent necessary conditions, while sufficient conditions relate to attention to processes of negotiation and change. A broad vision seemed more likely to generate movement than a blueprint, allowing interest groups to buy into the change process, and top-down pressure to be married with bottom-up concern.

The role of broad, imprecise visions in stimulating change processes has also been reported. Baier *et al.* (1986) note that policy support may increase with the ambiguity of proposed policies, but at the cost of administrative complications.

Finally, long-term issues (such as psychiatry) needed to be kept on change agendas, which could be difficult in the NHS where there is a tendency for every issue to be famous for 15 minutes.

Factor 2: availability of key people leading change

An important factor which makes change highly contextually sensitive is the availability of key people in critical posts leading change. We do not here refer to heroic and individualistic 'macho managers', but rather leadership exercised in a much more subtle and pluralist fashion. There was a critical role for continuity: paradoxically there is a requirement for a substantial degree of stability in the effective management of strategic change.

The link between the unplanned movement of key personnel and the draining of energy, purpose, commitment and action from major change processes has now been established from a whole series of research studies (Kanter 1985; Pettigrew 1985). What is rarely mentioned as a corollary of the problem is that the change process or programme then goes into a period of regression, leaving the newcomer manager to start again but now possibly in a soured and non-receptive context for change.

The diversity of leadership was also apparent both in terms of its occupational base (clinicians as well as managers) and hierarchical level. Often it was personalities not posts that were important: personal skills were more important in managing change than formal status or rank within the organisation. Research (Pettigrew and Whipp 1991) in private sector strategic change processes also points to the need to broaden and deepen the leadership cadre if long-term results are to be achieved in change processes.

Pettigrew and Whipp (1991) specifically use the term 'leading change' rather than 'leadership' to denote the collective, complementary and multi-faceted aspect of leading change. Leadership, they suggest, has too many connotations of individualism and one-dimensional heroism. The need appears to be for a combination of planning, opportunism and the adroit timing of interventions

Factor 3: long-term environmental pressure – intensity and scale

Studies of strategic change outside the NHS (Pettigrew 1985) have highlighted the significant role of intense and large-scale environmental pressure in triggering periods of radical change. The picture in the NHS is more complex, as in some instances excessive pressure can drain energy out of the system. In some of our districts, financial crises produced a wide range of pathological organisational reactions such as delay and denial, collapse of morale and energy and the scapegoating and defeat of managers. Financial crisis was here seen as a threat to the organisation, rather than as an opportunity for radical reconfiguration. In others, financial crisis was even played up and skilfully orchestrated by management in order to accelerate the process of rationalisation.

Factor 4: a supportive organisational culture

'Culture' refers to deep-seated assumptions and values far below surface manifestations, officially espoused ideologies, or even patterns of behaviour. The past weighs a heavy hand in shaping these values, setting expectations about what is and what is not possible. This may be a strength or a weakness, as difficult experiences in the past are projected forward.

Broadly our studies in both the public and the private sector conclude that tremendous energy is required to effect cultural change. One avenue is through the use of leaders as role models for a wider diffusion process. Another feature is the attempt to create a general managerial cadre as opposed to a small number of general managers. We know that rewards may be important, and that there is an important role for human resource management policies and practices.

If we concentrate on the managerial subculture, we can select out some features of a district culture associated with a high rate of change:

- Flexible working across boundaries with purpose-designed structures rather than formal hierarchies.
- Open, risk-taking approach.
- Openness to research and evaluation.
- Strong value base which helps give focus to what otherwise might be a loose network.
- Strong positive self-image and sense of achievement.

Such features of local culture develop characteristically from the values and change experiences of key leaders, interlinked with environmental pressure and effective managerial–clinician relations.

Factor 5: effective managerial–clinical relations

The managerial–clinical interface was obviously critical. The pattern found was one of wide variation in the quality of such relations, and when clinicians had gone into opposition, they could exert a powerful block on change. Perhaps more surprisingly managers varied in the extent to which they saw relationship-building and trading with clinicians as a core part of their brief.

Manager–clinician relations were easier where negative stereotypes had broken down, perhaps as a result of the emergence of mixed roles or perspectives. For managers, it was important to understand what clinicians valued and hence what they had to do to engage in effective trading relations.

From a clinical perspective, there is an important group of clinicians who think managerially and strategically. Clinical directors are clinicians who think across the patch, and may even be able to speak for the medical community as a whole. Considerable managerial acumen was needed to foster positive alliances and managers sometimes had to enter into deals, offering incentives while holding on to the core objective, and enforcing penalties where this was seen as politically possible.

Factor 6: co-operative inter-organisational networks

Many changes in the priority group sector in particular were underscored by the development and management of inter-organisational networks with such agencies as Social Services Departments and voluntary organisations. Districts had little power in such settings, but rather had to win influence. A number of features could enrich these networks, such as the existence of boundary-spanners who crossed agency divides, and clear referral and communications points.

The most effective networks were both informal and purposeful, but also fragile and vulnerable to turnover. But at their best such networks provided opportunities for trading and education, for commitment and for marrying top-down and bottom-up concerns. The significance of purposeful networks and their role as arenas for trust building and deal making is a key part of Kanter's (1985) perspective and data on how substantial change occurs.

Factor 7: simplicity and clarity of goals and priorities

Managers varied greatly in their ability to narrow the change agenda down into a set of key priorities, and to insulate this from the short-term pressures apparent in the NHS. So managers may be wise to ignore or minimise some of the ever-changing sources of pressure, while using others to amplify their pre-existing change objectives.

The question of simplicity and clarity of goals and priorities is one aspect of a much more general analytical and practical problem of how the nature of the context of change influences the rate and pace of change. Van Meter and Van Horn (1976) argue that the implementation process is likely to be influenced by the amount of change involved and the extent of goal consensus among the participants.

Factor 8: the fit between the district's change agenda and its locale

Private sector research on, for example, human resource change, has indicated that various features of the locale where change is to occur may inhibit or accelerate change. Thus Hardy's studies (1985) of organisational closures demonstrate how and why climate building for such changes is linkable to high levels of unemployment and consequential changes in the power balance between managers and trade unionists.

In the NHS the nature of the locale also had an impact on how easy it was to achieve change:

- The degree of co-terminosity with Social Services Departments (SSDs).
- Whether there is one large centre of population or two or more major towns.
- Whether there is a teaching hospital presence.
- The strength and nature of the local political culture.
- The nature of the local NHS workforce.

While many of these factors may appear beyond management control, awareness of their influence could nevertheless be important in anticipation of potential obstacles to change. Some of them may also be reshaped in the long term by higher tiers or locally through human resource management activities.

Some implications of the findings

Turning problems and panics into sustainable action

In the NHS 'panics' and 'crises' are legion. There is a developing tradition in the social sciences (e.g. Barrett and Hill 1984) which explains the culture of panics as symbolic decision making. Crisis-as-opportunity (Starbuck *et al.* 1978) as distinct from the consequences of crisis-as-threat (Jick and Murray 1982) is a crucial mechanism for turning problems into live issues.

Looking across our cases a range of factors helped with energy mobilisation. These include: mobilisation of crisis, articulation of broad visions, role of leadership in challenging old behaviours, encouragement of deviants and of early action to signal new changes of direction, building of complementary teams and networks of leaders; and positive reinforcement of early successes in the change process. However, in the way that the NHS finds it difficult to disentangle panics and problems from issues, and to turn the former into the latter, there is the additional difficulty that issues themselves may have an attention cycle (Hogwood 1987). Public, media and organisational attention may shift to newer issues, and old ones may fade even if unresolved.

Managing incoherence

The NHS is an extremely large and complex organisation. Managing incoherence remains the most wide-ranging challenge in producing change in the NHS, as indeed it was in our high performing private sector organisations (Pettigrew and Whipp 1991). We can signal some of the inputs and dynamics of producing that coherence by focusing on the role of incentives and of combining top-down pressures and bottom-up concerns in change processes.

Incentives and the politics of exchange

It has long been recognised that incentives and rewards of various kinds have a role in reinforcing and sustaining change processes (Kanter 1985). More recent research (Pettigrew *et al.* 1990) has also established that the selective use of a variety of human resource factors, such as performance review criteria and systems, career development pathways, and reward and recognition systems, can help to reinforce early behavioural change in cultural change processes.

However, this research on service change demonstrates the critical role of incentives and the politics of exchange in both the mobilisation and sustaining aspects of change processes.

Combining top-down pressure and bottom-up concerns

It is apparent that top-down pressures have not produced similar shifts in this balance of power, across all localities and change processes. Top-down pressure has been evident in our districts, and most fundamentally where that pressure has been selectively and astutely orchestrated at local level and linked in a coherent fashion to bottom-up concerns. However, all this requires considerable managerial skill.

Conclusions

The results of this research on managing service change also point to critical organisational and managerial skills. Our findings signal the importance of analytical and conceptual skills in policy analysis, political and negotiating skills, and skills of networking and managing across inter-organisational boundaries.

Leading change calls for the resolution of not so much great single issues but rather a pattern of interwoven problems (Whipp and Pettigrew 1990). The skill in leading change therefore centres on managing a series of dualities and dilemmas. The broadest, of course, relates to the need to handle what Berman (1978) calls the macro and micro aspects of implementation.

For central government, policy has to influence local delivery organisations to behave in desired ways and in response to central actions; the local organisations have to devise and carry out their own internal policies (Berman 1978). The dual task is to build a climate of leading change while at the same time raising energy and tension levels and setting out new directions *before* precise action is taken.

There is also the duality of simultaneously managing continuity and change. The development of a receptive context for change has to share its influence with needs for continuity.

Finally, there is the requirement to build commitment, energy and action from hierarchies and networks. Contrary to a current management fad (e.g. Kanter 1989), large bureaucratic organisations will not be able to switch from hierarchies to networks, rather they will have to build and use both. Our case studies have demonstrated that in a pluralistic and multi-level system like the NHS, change can arise from the generalised pressure of hierarchies linking up to the customised needs and solutions coming out of local networks. But there is no respite from the ever-present duality of holding together an organisation while simultaneously re-shaping it.

Appendix: Research aims and methodology

Research aims

The project aims were formally described as follows:

- *To study strategic service change in the NHS.* The approach adopted was to track the influence of general management on strategic service change processes.
- *To focus on 'high change' districts.* A second decision was to select districts tackling many of the major strategic issues. Our sample therefore may not reflect the 'average' district but rather those processing high change agendas, and therefore one should be cautious in extrapolating from the sample to the whole population. The decision to select 'high change' districts was made for two reasons. First, questions of managerial capacity to handle change would stand out in much sharper relief in these districts where changes of major substantive importance were proceeding. Secondly, the closure of Victorian asylums and the construction of new District General Hospitals are societal processes of great importance where general management faces a visible test.
- *To identify motors of, and barriers to, change.* Case studies of strategic service change in these 'high change' districts should not only be descriptive. This is not only a question of assessing the impact of general management, which may represent only one source of change, or may play no role in the case at all, or indeed have a negative role.

Case study methodology – comparative, longitudinal and processual

The basic methodology used has been that of longitudinal and processual comparative case study.

The methodological approach adopted here has allowed for the analysis of retrospective change, real-time analysis and prospective or anticipated change. Historical antecedents and the chronology of change are considered vital. The design choice in this study has been to conduct intensive analyses of relatively few cases, rather than a more superficial analysis of a larger number.

A variety of data sources has been used in these case studies. Archival material was often used most in the early stages, supplying a chronology of change. Routinely available statistics were also used. Meetings were attended (between five and ten per district) in order to observe group dynamics. Semi-structured interviews were undertaken with about 50 respondents per district (400 altogether), with respondents selected either because of their lead position in the organisation or because they were involved directly in the change process. Finally, there was informal observation while the researcher was in the district.

Sample selection

Acute sector and priority group changes were chosen as the substantive basis of the research after a comprehensive literature review, discussion with key academics and regional personnel, and a survey of the 1984–1985 Regional Strategic Plans. We selected two change issues in each district as a minimal means of forcing the question of the competing pressures on the managerial agenda (see Table 23.1).

The second task was to select the districts. Regions were asked

Table 23.1 District–issue matrix

District Health Authority	Acute sector		Priority groups	
	Development	Rationalisation	Development	Rationalisation
St Helens and Knowsley		Across two-sited DGH		Mental illness closure by 1992
Paddington and North Kensington	AIDS*	Closure, achieved 1986		
Preston	DGH – 5 years on: overspend			Mental illness reduction
Bloomsbury	AIDS*	General strategy Also Accident and Emergency closure		
Bromsgrove and Redditch	New DGH New DGH		Mental handicap community provision	
Milton Keynes			Mental illness community provision	
Mid Downs			Mental handicap community provision	Mental handicap closure by 1990
Huddersfield			Mental handicap community provision	Mental handicap reduction/ closure

DGH, District General Hospital.
*This issue subsequently acquired a community- as well as a hospital-based focus.

to provide some documentation on a shortlist of three, after which the final decision would be made in order to avoid too heavy a regional steer. Additionally we tried to 'pair' districts at least to some extent to facilitate comparison.

References

Baier, U.E., March, J.G. and Saetren, H. (1986) 'Implementation and ambiguity', *Scandinavian Journal of Management Studies*, 2: 197–212.

Barrett, S. and Hill, M. (1984) 'Policy, bargaining and structure in implementation', *Policy and Politics*, 12: 218–39.

Berman, P. (1978) 'The study of macro and micro implementation', *Public Policy*, 26: 157–85.

Hardy, C. (1985) *The Management of Organizational Closure*, Aldershot: Gower.

Hogwood, B. (1987) *From Crisis to Complacency*, Oxford: Oxford University Press.

Jick, T.D. and Murray, V.V. (1982) 'The management of hard times: budget cutbacks in public sector organizations', *Organisation Studies*, 3: 141–69.

Kanter, R.M. (1985) *The Change Masters: Corporate Entrepreneurs at Work*, London: Allen and Unwin.

Kanter, R.M. (1989) *When Giants Learn to Dance*, New York: Simon and Schuster.

Lorsch, J. (1986) 'Managing culture: the invisible banner to strategic change', *California Management Review*, 28: 95–109.

Peters, T.J. and Waterman, R. (1982) *In Search of Excellence: Lessons from America's Best Run Companies*, New York: Harper and Row.

Pettigrew, A.M. (1985) *The Awakening Giant: Continuity and Change in ICI*, Oxford: Basil Blakewell.

Pettigrew, A.M. (1990) 'Is corporate culture manageable?', in D. Wilson and R. Rosenfield (eds) *Managing Organizations: Text, Readings and Cases*, London: McGraw Hill.

Pettigrew, A.M. and Whipp, R. (1991) *Managing Change for Competitive Success*, Oxford: Basil Blackwell.

Pettigrew, A.M., Hendry, C. and Sparrow, P.R. (1990) *Corporate Strategy Change and Human Resource Management*, Research and Development Paper no. 63, Sheffield: Department of Employment.

Starbuck, W.H., Greve, A. and Hedberg, B.L.T. (1978) 'Responding to crisis', *Journal of Business Administration*, 9: 111–37.

Van Meter, D.S. and Van Horn, C.E. (1976) 'The policy implementation process: a conceptual framework', *Administration and Society*, 6: 445–88.

Whipp, R. and Pettigrew, A.M. (1990) 'Leading change and the management of competition'. Paper presented to Strategic Management Society Workshop on Leadership and the Management of Strategic Change, Robinson College, Cambridge University, December.

A complete, unedited version of this article can be found as Chapter nine (Receptive and non-receptive contexts for change) and Appendix (Research aims and methodology) in Pettigrew, A., Ferlie, E. and McKee, L. (1992) *Shaping Strategic Change*, London: Sage.

Chapter 24

General management in the NHS: assessing the impact

S. Harrison, D.J. Hunter, G. Marnoch and C. Pollitt

Abstract

In this chapter we describe, and present the results of, a major study into post-Griffiths management which we conducted between 1987 and 1989.

Introduction

Aims and design of the research

In undertaking the research our principal aims were to:

- describe the work that general managers were doing, as research into their behaviour was surprisingly limited (Hunter 1985);
- map the perceptions of senior NHS managers (and other senior staff) concerning the impact, or impacts, of general management;
- ascertain whether there were systematic differences in the impact of general management between one health authority and another, and to explain such differences;
- review and develop theories of organisation within the NHS.

We adopted a research design that was primarily ethnographic. Our ability to conduct a 'before-and-after' study was limited by the variety of reliable descriptions of what had happened 'before'. An experimental approach was ruled out by our inability to control the relevant variables, and by the absence of any control group. Finally, the objectives of the reform had in any case only been specified in a loose, qualitative manner.

The research was conducted in 11 health authorities. We decided to pitch most of our investigations at district level (serving a total population of approximately 300,000) and at unit (service-provider) levels, but also to

Source: *General Management in the NHS*, Chapter 3, London, Macmillan, 1992.

strengthen our contextual understanding by conducting selected interviews at regional levels and with senior officials and ministers in central government.

We selected the districts in which the interviews were to take place according to a variety of criteria. We chose a mixture of large and small, urban and rural, northern and southern and, perhaps most importantly, 'well-resourced' and 'under-funded'.

Methods

In each of the eight districts and two boards we carried out an average of 37 long, loosely structured interviews, averaging more than one hour in duration. We supplemented the interviews with observation of a number of meetings, and with extensive study of documents, both published plans and internal memoranda. We also compared the format and content of the minutes of key management committees before and after the arrival of general management. Finally, we collected performance indicator data for each English district for 1984–1985, 1985–1986 and 1986–1987.

Implementing Griffiths: what worked and what didn't

The first step was to record the views of NHS staff on the degrees to which certain features of (Griffiths-type)general management appeared to them to be working in the ways that the 'official line' had suggested they should (Department of Health 1983). The particular features on which we concentrated our questioning, observations and documentary analysis were:

- the setting up of new management structures within districts;
- speed of decision making and implementation;
- the clearer allocation of responsibilities to individual managers;
- the usefulness of the individual performance review (IPR) system for managers;
- the development of greater responsiveness to the preferences of consumers of NHS services;
- the use of management budgets and resource management as a key management tool;
- increased use of performance indicator data and other types of formal, comparative data.

One of the most striking features to emerge from our data is the way in which views on several of these issues show acute variation between different groups and levels of staff. For example, most of the nurses we spoke to thought that decisions were now taken more quickly (and generally approved of that), while most of the consultants thought the opposite. This suggests that the 'improvements' generated by general management are very unevenly distributed.

In all the authorities studied there had been changes in formal organisational structures attendant upon the introduction of general management, and in most of them these changes had been substantial. Appropriate formal structures do not, by themselves, produce good decisions, but they can contribute to reducing overlap and delay, and to the grouping together of highly interdependent functions. They can also carry a symbolic significance, for example, when clear organisational equality is granted to a community function relative to an acute function. We encountered a great variety of local structures, but only isolated protest or criticism.

Senior managers were equally divided on the question of the speed of decision making and implementation. Unit general managers (UGMs) emerged as a group particularly likely to think that acceleration had occurred, while district-based planners and administrators tended to be more sceptical. Consultants were the most pessimistic category – very few of them could see any speeding up, while the great majority of nurses believed that decisions were being arrived at more quickly, giving as their main reason the elimination of one or more tiers of nursing hierarchy.

Most of our respondents thought that the introduction of general management had resulted in more precise allocations of personal responsibility. However, many of them also believed that this greater clarity did not yet extend very far down this hierarchy. Again, consultants were the most pessimistic group, a majority claiming that they could not see that the allocation of responsibilities between managers was any clearer at all.

IPR plans are one important way in which an individual's responsibilities can be clarified. In general we found that the IPR system was well received. Senior nurses and managers who were ex-nurses appeared the most enthusiastic. About half the UGMs, however, were critical. These managers experienced IPR as a rather top-down, time-consuming bureaucratic 'game'.

The development of greater consumer responsiveness is not an issue that emerged well from our research. A heavy majority of both the nurses and (particularly) the consultants thought that little or nothing of real significance was yet going on. There was widespread cynicism concerning what were seen as rhetorical or superficial gestures by management towards 'consumerism', while there remained glaring inadequacies in basic service provision.

Our findings concerning the use of management budgeting (MB) and resource management (RM) are reported in greater detail elsewhere (Pollitt *et al.* 1988). Briefly, we found a few enthusiastic managers, but many cautious ones, and a handful of enthusiastic consultants but a large majority of determined sceptics. The sceptics included quite a number of consultants with extensive experience of MB – few of these had found the information they received to be particularly interesting or useful.

Finally, we enquired into the use of comparative performance data. Use of these indicators is now quite widespread. However, use of performance indicators (PIs) at a district level by district general managers (DGMs) and planning and finance staff appears to be far more frequent than use by medical or nursing staff. In so far as they are aware of them medical staff tend to question their accuracy and/or claim that they are not sufficiently detailed or sensitive to case-mix to be of much use. 'We don't particularly trust them', as one consultant told us.

Clinical quality was still regarded as professional territory – or as one (rather pro-Griffiths) consultant put it, 'management stops at the consulting room door'. On the whole post-Griffiths managers continued to accept this demarcation, although there were naturally occasional exceptions where the local cocktail of personalities was such that a respected manager was allowed at least to raise questions with the medical staff.

The content of general management agendas

One of Griffiths' criticisms of the consensus management team concept was that decision making was insufficiently proactive. For Griffiths, general management implied a more strategic orientation and devolved responsibility for action. How far did general managers' agendas in our selected health authorities comply with this view?

Management agendas comprised a number of inputs of varying significance. Local priorities jostled with national priorities for attention and looming over them all was the centralty of finance. At one level, the management agenda was long and complex. At another it was deceptively simple – keeping within budget. With 47 national priorities awaiting attention, the agenda was unmanageable for general managers. As one health authority chair remarked, 'in business if I had more than 10 priorities my business was going down the drain'.

Without exception, general managers believed that agendas were dominated by financial considerations. At best, general managers were obliged to balance a 'here and now' issue, that is not over-spending, with the achievement of the long-term strategy, for example, dispersing patients from long-stay hospitals into the community.

Clinicians were the most outspoken group in terms of criticising what appeared to them to be the dominant concern of general managers.

A key aspect of the Griffiths changes was that general managers had been singularly unsuccessful in confronting clinicians. As one senior official put it, general managers 'are playing around the periphery'. Changes were taking place but mainly through attention to support services. Little attention was being given to clinical developments. Many general managers believed that Griffiths had grossly underestimated the power of consultants.

Given the shape of the managerial agendas, the extent to which the general managers were seen, or saw themselves, as handmaidens of the government was often a matter of some concern. There was a fear that involvement in a controversial issue like competitive tendering could damage a good manager's credibility with certain staff groups and make it more difficult to secure progress in other areas.

Coupled with IPRs and short-term contracts, general managers faced overwhelming pressures to conform to and accept a narrow, finance-driven agenda. For many managers, their immediate objective was to secure their future and have their contracts renewed. These pressures seemed at odds with the Griffiths prescription for managers who would think and act proactively.

The impact of hierarchy

Griffiths urged the creation of a strong central management body committed to pushing responsibility down the line. Managers were also expected to exercise a new authority. In spite of this commitment to delegation, other pressures (e.g. the desire for financial control at the centre) were making for a highly centralised system of management.

Our research in the regions uncovered a consistent view to the effect that the Management Board (subsequently renamed the NHS Executive) did not provide a strong central management influence on the organisation.

In six out of nine English districts there was a consistent view among district officers and clinicians that regions adopted an overbearing posture with too much detailed interference. Region was therefore both a 'paternalistic and distant body'.

A strong feeling prevailed that regions undermined authority in the districts. Several managers questioned the region's capacity effectively to intervene in detail: 'region tries to meddle in affairs of detail which are beyond its capacity for understanding'.

We now move on to *district–unit* relations. On the whole UGMs said that they enjoyed a greater authority and autonomy of decision making. Yet the evidence also suggests that the basis of these claims is questionable. UGMs in certain districts under financial strain complained about the contributions which were demanded of them by the district to help meet the overspend problem.

In general, workable relations had been established between authorities and their units over respective responsibilities. However, the research did reveal a well-founded dilemma over 'contesting loyalties'. UGMs are clearly not wholly sure as to where their primary loyalty should lie – with the unit or the district/board.

Changes in the post-Griffiths manager's status had not in general resulted in a restructuring of the relationships between managers and doctors. As one unit officer put it when asked how doctors had reacted to Griffiths, 'consultants are all right as long as it doesn't bother them'. At unit level where the relationship between managers and clinicians is perhaps the most crucial, there was a widely held view among the consultants and nurses that UGMs had not found any substantial new authority.

Differences between authorities

Our prediction of finding substantial differences between authorities was fulfilled, but our expectation that this would be related to measurable differences in the tightness of resource constraints was not.

In so far as we could find a general explanation of the differences between districts under general management, it seemed that many of these had evidently existed before general management. They had merely continued, or been amplified, under the new regime.

One tentative observation was that management/doctor relations had perhaps undergone the most marked changes in the two districts where the DGM had come from outside the NHS. The staff in these districts tended to explain this in terms of the new DGM feeling less bound by cultural assumptions specific to the NHS. For a honeymoon period, at least, they were able to innovate more freely. Furthermore, their previous careers outside the NHS may have afforded them some initial status in the eyes of the consultants, status which the doctors would not necessarily accord to 'just another administrator'. It should be emphasised, however, that this breathing space could be misused. While the two examples in our study had used their 'innocence' creatively, there were contemporary cases elsewhere which resulted in 'outsider' general managers leaving the service very quickly after colliding with local doctors or politicians.

A changing culture?

The concept of an organisational 'culture' is a subtle one. There has been a recent tendency to regard 'culture' as something that top management can mould and remould at will. This assumption has been fashionable in business circles and has frequently influenced the language of those advocating general management in the NHS (see, for an example, Barbour 1989). Others, however, have argued that this approach is both conceptually and empirically over-ambitious (e.g. Meek 1988; Politt *et al.* 1990).

Our fieldwork yielded little suggestion that general managers were indulging in 'cultural management' as a conscious process. No new sets of 'key values' were in evidence – rather there was plenty of evidence of the old NHS 'tribalism', with each professional group displaying its own particular attitudes and priorities. Doctors still held to a predominantly 'diplomatic' view of the role of management – that it was the principal duty of managers to oil the wheels and seek out compromises between the various groups and interests comprising the service (Harrison 1988). The model of a proactive management, setting goals, implementing plans for

with a sense of professional accomplishment. NHS managers work in an arena where a profuse and unstable range of values and priorities must be taken into account. The Griffiths model seems to view the manager as a technician whose practice consists in applying the principles derived from management science to the problems of his/her organisation. In its adherence to a different theory of management, the Griffiths report was flawed.

There are consequences of such failure of analysis. Without clear objectives, *effectiveness* cannot be measured and therefore cannot function as one of the main criteria for organisational performance. Thus the kind of performance assessment envisaged within managerialism begins to slide towards a lop-sided emphasis on narrower notions of *efficiency* and *economy*.

Without objectives it is also very hard to discuss the kind of programme (as opposed to structural) reforms which might ease some of the pressures on the NHS. Business managers may ask 'what business should we be in?', but without guiding objectives it is hard for health authorities and NHS managers to do the same. The aims and purposes of the NHS remain grand, but vague.

Finally, our research has pointed towards the pervasive importance of two structural features of the NHS. The first of these is medical autonomy. The power of the medical profession has formed a central theme in the massive literature on health services organisation. Even among professions, doctors are unusual in the scope of their autonomy. In the NHS hospital consultants can, broadly speaking, admit whichever patients they choose, treat them in whatever way they wish, discharge them when they see fit, and leave it to others to sort out the resource and staffing consequences of these 'clinical' decisions. They cannot be instructed to alter any of these decisions by a manager, and the Griffiths reforms did nothing to alter this.

Many consultants thus continue to maintain a semi-detached relationship with NHS management. In his studies of the implementation process Sabatier (1986) has demonstrated the importance of basing reforms on sound casual assumptions. In particular he has emphasised the jurisdiction component within such assumptions – to what extent are implementing agencies given jurisdiction over the organisational linkages vital for the achievement of the proposed reforms? In these terms the Griffiths model again appears deficient. General managers were not given sufficient fresh authority to do more than make very cautious, incremental progress towards harnessing consultants to management objectives.

The second structural feature which has limited the implementation of Griffiths is the fiscal situation of the NHS. The marginally constrained ability of doctors to commit resources becomes even more problematic in a situation where central government is determined to restrain overall expenditure, yet both the demand for and the supply of health care are increasing.

Our final conclusion is, therefore, that implementation of the Griffiths model has been handicapped by tensions and limitations which were inherent in the original report, by flawed understanding of the management problem in the NHS and by wider developments (the failure of government to set clear priorities plus the deteriorating financial situation), which were beyond its remit. Despite this, its impact has been considerable, especially among managers and administrators themselves, and also with nurses. We would hesitate, however, to describe this as a major cultural shift: the diversity of NHS subcultures ('tribalism') remains, and the Griffiths model has not yet become dominant. In the words of a unit general manager: 'It has been a partially funded palace revolution, not a thorough-going, fully-funded management revolution'.

References

Alvessson, M. (1987) *Organization Theory and Technocratic Consciousness: Rationality, Ideology and Quality of Work*, Berlin: de Gruyter.

Barbour, J. (1989) 'Notions of "success" in general management', *Health Services Management Research*, 2: 53–7.

Department of Health. (1988) *NHS Management Inquiry (The Griffiths Report)*, London: Department of Health.

Habermas, J. (1971) *Towards a Rational Society*, London, Heinemann.

Harrison, S. (1982) 'Consensus decision-making in the National Health Service: a review', *Journal of Management Studies*, 19: 377–94.

Harrison, S. (1988) *Managing the National Health Service: Shifting the Frontier?*, London: Chapman & Hall.

Hunter, D.J. (1984) 'NHS management: is Griffiths the last quick fix?', *Public Administration*, 62: 91–4.

Meek, V.L. (1988) 'Organisational culture: origins and weaknesses', *Organization Studies*, 9: 453–73.

Pollitt, C.J., Harrison, S., Hunter, D. and Marnoch, G. (1988) 'The reluctant managers: clinicians and budgets in the NHS', *Financial Accountability and Management*, 4: 213–34.

Pollitt, C.J., Harrison, S., Hunter, D. and Marnoch, G. (1990) 'No hiding place: on the discomforts of researching the contemporary policy process', *Journal of Social Policy*, 19: 169–90.

Sabatier, P.A. (1986) 'What can we learn from implementation research?', in F.-X. Kaufman, G. Majone and V. Ostrom (eds) *Guidance, Control and Evaluation in the Public Sector*, Berlin: de Gruyter, 313–25.

Siedentopf, H. (1982) 'Introduction: government performance and administrative reform', in G.E. Caiden and H. Siedentopf (eds) *Strategies for Administrative Reform*, Lexington, MA: Lexington Books.

A complete, unedited version of this article can be found as Harrison, S., Hunter, D.J., Marnoch, G. and Pollitt, C., 'General management in the NHS: assessing the impact' (Chapter 3) in *Just Managing: Power and Culture in the NHS* (1992) London: Macmillan.

Chapter 25

Applying research to health care policy and practice: medical and managerial views on effectiveness and the role of research

Rebecca Rosen

Abstract

Objectives: This study explores the way in which doctors and managers think about the effectiveness of health care interventions and how this shapes the evidence they use to support decision making.

Methods: Case studies of the introduction of three new medical technologies in nine National Health Service (NHS) hospitals and health authorities.

Results: Effectiveness research provides essential evidence on clinical and cost-effectiveness and is used primarily by clinicians and public health doctors for this purpose. However, research fails to provide the 'evidence' required by managerial decision makers, who are interested as much in the effect of a technology on organisational performance as on patient health and well-being. The evidence used to inform technology adoption decisions reflects the professional role and objectives of different decision makers.

Conclusions: The assumed relationship between 'research' and 'evidence' for the purpose of promoting effective health care does not take account of the wide range of objectives pursued by different health care decision makers and the varied sources of 'evidence' they use to support their decisions.

Introduction

This paper describes a study to explore the application of research to decisions about the introduction of three contrasting new medical technologies. Despite mechanisms to control their early use, new technologies often diffuse widely before well designed effectiveness research is

Source: *Journal of Health Services Research and Policy*, 5.2, 1990, 103–8.

available. As a result, case studies of technology adoption offer a useful vehicle to study how medical and managerial decision makers use research to inform practice and policy, to question assumptions about the link between research and 'evidence-based' health care and to consider the implications of these observations for implementing the concept of 'clinical governance' in the National Health Service (NHS).

The term 'effectiveness research' is used here to describe studies to evaluate the clinical effectiveness and cost-effectiveness of specific health care interventions. In their discussion of 'clinical governance', Scally and Donaldson (1998) emphasise that the application of such research is central to the concept of 'clinical governance', be it in relation to individual treatment decisions (evidence-based medicine) or to health policy decisions (evidence-based policy). Furthermore, Gray has argued the case for 'evidence-based' health care organisations which should be obsessed with 'finding, appraising and using research-based knowledge in decision-making' (Gray 1997).

There are important assumptions underlying these approaches to health care practice and policy. First, that effectiveness research *is* the fundamental element of evidence-based decisions and that initiatives to apply research are the key to improving effectiveness. Second, that research can be applied equally to all forms of health care decision, despite differences between the individual patient focus of evidence-based medicine, the population perspective taken by most health planners and the organisational viewpoint of most hospital managers. Such differences raise questions about the appropriate influence of research in different health care contexts. Third, advocates of evidence-based policy and organisations expect that managers will become involved in the application of effectiveness research in health care decisions.

Greer's study of decisions on technology adoption in American hospitals illustrates the varied objectives pursued by health professionals in different settings (Greer 1998). She identified three different systems operating in a cluster of mid-Western community hospitals. The 'medical individualistic' system was seen within the clinical consultation and the primary objectives were the promotion of patient welfare and reduction of risk. The 'fiscal–managerial' decision system was seen at departmental level and focused on the impact of a technology on the efficient running of the hospital. In the hospital-wide 'strategic-institutional' system, the primary objective pursued by decision makers was to maintain a hospital's status and competitiveness.

The implications of the varied aims of decision makers for the development of evidence-based practice and policy have been little explored. The following case studies allow consideration of the extent to which research is used as evidence for decision making and the ways in which different health professionals conceptualise 'effectiveness' and the 'evidence' they use to support their decisions.

Methods

The case study method was used to study the adoption of three contrasting new medical technologies by NHS acute hospitals. The technologies were selected to include both new equipment and new 'practice' technologies (medical practices such as blood tests or surgical techniques which are not 'embodied' in equipment are called practice technologies) and to maximise contrast in terms of cost and complexity. This reflects the observation that the processes for, and people involved in, decision making on technology adoption vary with different sorts of technology (Battista and Hodge 1995; Greer 1998). Each technology was studied in three different hospital/health authority sites, with data collection taking place during 1995–1996.

The technologies studied were:

- Vascular stenting, which can be provided to patients by a single clinician without immediate need for complex clinical support systems (stents are small metal tubes that can be used to support arteries after angioplasty).
- The triple test, which is a three-factor blood test to assess the risk that a foetus is affected by Down's syndrome. The triple test is a low-cost, simple technology for individual patients, but high-cost and complex to organise when applied to whole populations.
- The excimer laser, which is used for the treatment of short-sightedness and some corneal disorders and is a high-cost embodied technology.

Semi-structured interviews were conducted with individuals who had been involved in the introduction of case study technologies. Initial interviews were conducted with the clinical director of the relevant hospital department and a public health consultant in the related purchasing authority. (Within the UK NHS, public health doctors advise purchasers of health care on the impact of their purchasing on population health and may thus be involved in policy-making on new technologies.) A mixture of purposive and snowball sampling was used to identify further interviewees. Purposive sampling aimed specifically to include departmental business managers, more senior general managers and doctors within hospitals. Within purchasers, public health doctors and contract managers were included. Snowball sampling involved conducting further interviews with individuals described by earlier interviewees as being involved in decision making on the case study technologies. Interviewees granted access to documentary records (archive material, business cases, letters and memos) in four of the nine study sites and these were examined for consistency with verbal reports. A fieldwork diary was also kept to record the researcher's impressions about the interviews.

Interviews were taped and transcribed, and confidentiality was assured. They were guided by an aide mémoire of subjects, aiming primarily to explore how effectiveness research was used for decision making, while allowing flexibility to 'talk around' the subject.

Analysis of case study data

Analysis was based on the methods of constant comparison and analytical induction (Glaser and Strauss 1967). Interview text was coded and categorised, and data in each category were examined to develop hypotheses about the link between available research and technology adoption and use. The analysis was iterative, and as new data became available from each case study the whole dataset was re-analysed both to generate new hypotheses and to ensure that previous hypotheses were sustained by new data. Documents were assessed through content analysis based on the categories and hypotheses developed from interview data, and the consistency of verbal accounts with documentary records was examined.

Results

The study was conducted in a total of nine NHS hospitals and their associated purchasers. The study sites included four teaching hospitals, four district general hospitals and an eye infirmary. Fifty-one interviews were conducted with doctors and managers from both sides of the purchaser–provider split, and lasted an average of 70 minutes.

Data are presented below to support the hypothesis that decision makers from different professional backgrounds – specifically, clinicians and managers – conceptualise effectiveness in different ways and, therefore, obtain evidence to support their decisions in different ways and from different sources.

The many meanings of effectiveness

Understanding how interviewees conceptualised the idea of 'evidence' requires prior consideration of the meanings they attributed to the idea of 'effectiveness'. The comments suggest that clinicians, general managers, clinical managers and public health doctors attribute different meanings to the term 'effectiveness', reflecting the range of objectives associated with their professional role. Comments addressed clinical and economic effects as well as the impact of the technology on the hospital as an organisation. These have been clustered together to illustrate the various meanings of effectiveness held by different interviewees.

Clinical effectiveness and cost-effectiveness

The conventionally accepted meanings of clinical effectiveness and cost-effectiveness were evident in comments from clinicians, public health doctors and managers. Medically trained interviewees described assessing the mortality and morbidity associated with stents and lasers or the sensitivity and specificity of the triple test. Clinicians also shared a more general meaning of effectiveness – about ensuring that patients feel better and recover quickly – with hospital managers arguing that use of stenting and the excimer laser were 'in the best interests of patients' or involved 'doing the best for patients' as they were minimally invasive. A hospital manager interviewed for the triple test study argued that she would support the introduction of a new technology which was 'in the best interest of patients, which would let them go home quicker or be treated in a nicer environment'. They also emphasised 'obvious' aspects of clinical effectiveness, with another hospital manager explaining that 'any fool could see that it is obviously better to treat a blocked artery with a balloon and a stent than to open them up'. Purchaser managers tended to depend on their public health colleagues for advice about the clinical effectiveness of new interventions, focusing their own attention more on costs.

The way in which interviewees judged the 'cost-effectiveness' of the technologies illustrated a varied understanding of the term, ranging from the cost reduction associated with a technology through to cost-benefit assessments. Both consultants and hospital managers argued that stenting was cheaper than open surgery without referring to any comparison of effects and the costs associated with re-occlusion and re-treatment, and one consultant commented that the triple test was provided 'cost-effectively' because no extra medical staff were required for the service.

'Administrative' 'accountancy' and 'strategic' effectiveness

Alongside the clinical and economic meanings of effectiveness associated with evidence-based medicine, comments from hospital general managers in particular, and to a lesser degree from clinical directors, demonstrated a range of additional reasons for deciding that a new technology was worth using. For these interviewees, the 'effectiveness' of a technology was judged partly by its potential contribution to the smooth running of the hospital.

The idea of 'administrative effectiveness' relates to the contribution of a technology to the fulfilment of contracts between health care purchasers (i.e. health authorities) and providers. It is illustrated by a comment from a manager interviewed for the triple test study who explained a new system for early pregnancy assessment: '... the service is really popular and it means women get treated much quicker. We're seeing some switching of care now. GPs at X who used to refer to [Hospital A] are switching to us and it's meant a rise of 400 referrals'.

The desirability of technologies that generate income or reduce the cost of care reimbursed through the block contract – as seen in some of the stenting and excimer study sites – illustrates the idea of 'accountancy effectiveness'. This is seen in a comment from a general manager from the stenting study: 'If the clinicians want to use a technique that is proven, then that's a clinical decision. I have to make sure we can pay for it and it is still cheaper to do a [stent] on a patient than keep them in for 10 days after an operation'. The money they were paid for each patient was fixed, so a cheaper procedure generated income for the department.

'Strategic effectiveness' encompasses the idea of keeping hospital services at the cutting edge of medicine and able to attract high-quality staff – an idea evident in the words of a teaching hospital manager from the triple test study: 'There is no point in [the obstetricians] doing amniocentesis here if every district general hospital in the country can do the same thing'.

Sources of 'evidence of effectiveness'

Given the range of meanings of effectiveness described above, the sources of 'evidence' used by decision makers were necessarily more varied than the effectiveness research that is commonly associated with evidence-based practice and policy. Clinicians described using published research, although the way in which they did so varied considerably, from 'pulling out a couple of papers' to '[writing] a two side summary of all the studies which had been published at that time'. They also described using other sources of evidence relating to outcomes that are not typically reported in published research. All the other hospital and purchaser general managers relied on clinicians or public health doctors to obtain and review research on the clinical effects of the technologies. They drew their 'evidence' from general reports about the potential role of new technologies, hospital activity data, local analysis of general practitioner (GP) referral rates and management accountancy information.

A senior teaching hospital manager explained that, 'We're not usually looking for piles of research paper to ... you know ... to support the case. We're more interested in evidence that this is the direction in which the speciality is moving'. Comments from clinical managers tended to combine reference to discussion with doctors about effectiveness research on the case study technologies with comments about their organisational impact.

Discussion

The case studies presented here used decisions about technology adoption as a vehicle to examine the way health professionals from different professional backgrounds understand the concept of effectiveness and use research evidence in their decisions. They were conducted during the period of the NHS 'internal market', when the use of contracts between health authorities and health care providers (hospital and community trusts) was intended to create incentives for efficiency in health care provision (Robinson and Le Grand 1993). The case studies nevertheless provide insights into approaches taken by different health professionals to clinical effectiveness and evidence-based practice.

Responsibility for clinical governance has been placed on the shoulders of senior managers, and a key part of this responsibility lies in ensuring the provision of effective services. There is a general expectation that improving clinical effectiveness will involve identifying and applying available research evidence, but the case studies suggest that this view is not shared by all relevant decision makers. Interviewees from all professional groups stated their commitment to improving the health of patients. However, medical interviewees focused primarily on assessing clinical impact through research use and, for practising clinicians, through personal experience and collegial opinion. Managers reported developing their views on clinical effectiveness on the basis of discussions with clinicians, focusing their own attention on assessing the effects of the technologies on their organisation on the basis of non-research evidence.

These observations highlight the different combinations of clinical, financial, personal and organisational objectives pursued by different decision makers which may affect how different players become involved in implementing clinical governance. The use of research evidence, by clinicians is focused primarily on maximising health improvement in individual patients – typifying the practice of evidence-based medicine. However, the case studies suggest that managers in an 'evidence-based organisation' would be likely to pursue a combination of health improvement in patients and hospital performance improvement, informed mainly by clinicians' opinions of clinical effectiveness and local studies of administrative data. This is not to say that they do not or will not participate in work to enhance clinical effectiveness, but that such work is unlikely to be their main priority.

The observation that different decision makers pursue different but overlapping objectives has been reported in other studies. Greer's conclusions about the different decision systems operating within hospitals were noted earlier (Greer 1998), and similar observations have been made in studies by Weingart (1993) and Luce and Brown (1995) on the introduction of new technologies in America.

What might be the implications of these findings for involving managers in those aspects of clinical governance which relate to promoting clinical effectiveness? Despite recent efforts to encourage evidence-based management and the participation of managers in promoting clinical effectiveness, important differences remain between the involvement of doctors and general managers in this area of work. This is perhaps unsurprising given the repeated exclusion of general managers from issues of clinical decision making. Harrison (1988) argued that prior to the 1983 NHS Management Inquiry (the Griffiths Report) managers were cast in the role of 'diplomats' who were never intended to have any influence over clinical matters (Department of Health 1983), and Strong and Robinson (1990) described their role as predominantly administrative. The subsequent 1991 NHS reforms further developed the role of hospital managers, involving them in areas of work that had previously been medically dominated, such as consultant appointments, and enabling them to reform some services by using the threat of the effects of competition to achieve change. Crucially, however, control of clinical audit was left in the hands of doctors. General managers were largely excluded from an area of work that would have given them direct input into improving effectiveness and clinical quality. So, with responsibility for the development of clinical governance systems now placed on chief executive officers, what is the prospect for managerial involvement in the promotion of clinical effectiveness?

Packwood (1997) proposes that the role of NHS managers has changed in that they now exert tighter control over activities performed at the lower levels of the NHS, but Harrison et al. (1992) argue that they are still preoccupied with the consequences of the financial constraints under which the NHS operates and that they have little time left for the strategic development of services. Papers by Long and Harrison (1996) and Murphy and Dunning (1997) illustrate that general managers can become involved in needs assessment, guideline development and the use of evidence-based practice. However, the current case studies suggest that interest in such matters is far from universal and that the application of research to health care practice and policy is largely seen as the role of clinicians and public health doctors. Clinical managers, however, described a more balanced assessment of both the clinical and organisational impact of the case study technologies. They described judging clinical and administrative effectiveness and potential financial impact, combining the use of clinical and administrative 'evidence' to inform their decisions.

The relevance of research to the information needs of policy-makers has been questioned in both non-medical and medical contexts (Higgins 1980; Coyle 1993). Williamson (1992) notes that clinical effectiveness research addresses very precise questions and often fails to provide the broader answers needed by decision makers. The case studies highlight the fact that effectiveness research rarely addresses the organisational effects of new technologies against which hospital performance is measured. Other forms of information are therefore required which can be used by decision makers in conjunction with research.

A central theme of clinical governance is to improve effectiveness, and it is assumed that this will involve applying effectiveness research to practice and policy. This view fails to recognise the complex mixture of personal and professional objectives held by decision makers and leads to unrealistic expectations of what can be achieved. This is not to say that there is no scope to enhance the impact of research in clinical and policy decisions and to encourage greater participation by managers. However, recognition of the need to meet a range of objectives other than improving clinical outcome will promote more realistic expectations of the potential of clinical governance work to enhance clinical effectiveness.

Acknowledgement

Thanks are offered to Nick Black for his advice and many useful comments during the conduct of the research.

References

Battista, R. and Hodge, J. (1995) 'The development of health care technology assessment', *International Journal of Technology Assessment in Health Care*, 11: 287–300.

Coyle, D. (1993) *Increasing the Impact of Economic Evaluations on Health Care Decision Making*, Discussion paper 108. York: Centre for Health Economics, University of York.

Department of Health (1983) *NHS Management Inquiry (The Griffiths Report)*, London: Department of Health.

Glaser, B. and Strauss, A. (1967) *The Discovery of Grounded Theory*, Chicago: Aldine.

Gray, M.J. (1997) *Evidence Based Health Care*, London: Churchill Livingstone.

Greer, A. (1998) 'The hospital's three decision making systems', *International Journal of Technology Assessment in Health Care*, 1: 669–80.

Harrison, S. (1988) *Managing the NHS: Shifting the Frontier?*, London: Chapman & Hall.

Harrison, S., Hunter, D., Marrocer, G. and Pollitt, C. (1992) *Just Managing: Power and Culture in the NHS*, London: Macmillan.

Higgins, J. (1980) 'The unfulfilled promise of policy research', *Social Policy and Administration*, 14: 195–208.

Long, A. and Harrison, S. (1996) 'Evidence-based decision making', *Health Service Journal*, 106 (Suppl 6).

Luce, B. and Brown, R. (1995) 'The use of technology assessment by hospitals, health maintenance organisations and third-party payers in the United States', *International Journal of Technology Assessment in Health Care*, 11: 79–92.

Murphy, M. and Dunning, M. (1997) 'Implementing clinical effectiveness: time for a change of gear', *British Journal of Health Care Management*, 3: 23–6.

Packwood, T. (1997) 'Analysing changes in the nature of health services management in England', *Health Policy*, 40: 91–102.

Robinson, R. and Le Grand, J. (1993) *Evaluating the NHS Reforms*, London: King's Fund Institute.

Scally, G. and Donaldson, L.J. (1998) 'Clinical governance and the drive for quality improvement in the new NHS in England', *British Medical Journal*, 317: 61–5.

Strong, P. and Robinson, J. (1990) *The NHS Under New Management*, Milton Keynes: Open University Press.

Weingart, S. (1993) 'Acquiring advanced technology decision-making strategies at twelve medical centres', *International Journal of Technology Assessment in Health Care*, 9: 530–8.

Williamson, P. (1992) 'From dissemination to use: management and organisational barriers to the application of health services research findings', *Health Bulletin* 50: 78–87.

A complete, unedited version of this article can be found as Rosen, R., 'Applying research to health care policy and practice: medical and managerial views on effectiveness and the role of research' in the *Journal of Health Services Research and Policy* (1990) Volume 5, Number 2, pages 103–8.

Part 6

Studying health care organisations

Introduction

The study of the way that health care organisations function and their relationships with other organisations is central to the study of the organisation and delivery of health services. This section contains a series of studies illustrating the broad range of issues which this topic can encompass, as well as the broad range of disciplines and research methods which can be applied to studying those issues.

The first paper (The reforms: success or failure or neither?) is an extract by Le Grand *et al.* taken from the conclusions drawn from a survey the authors undertook of the empirical evidence concerning the internal market introduced into the English National Health Service (NHS) in the 1990s. It uses policy analysis and economics to discuss whether the evidence indicates if the NHS internal market was a success or a failure. On the whole, it concludes that the internal market had little effect due to the weakness of the incentives and the strength of the constraints operating on both organisations and individuals. It then considers the lessons that can be learnt from the experiment. A key lesson is that it is unlikely that competition can be used as a major force for change inside the NHS. Finally it discusses if the lessons are apparent in the proposals for the internal market's successor, as laid out in the Labour Government's 1997 White Paper, *The New NHS: Modern and Dependable*.

The second paper (Some interim results from a controlled trial of cost sharing in health insurance) by Newhouse *et al.* reports on some of the interim results from the RAND health insurance experiment in the United States. They use economic theory and quantitative econometric methods to examine the effect on use of health care of varying the cost to the patient. As predicted, they find that people consume less outpatient care if it costs them more. However, the amount of care given once a person is hospitalised does not seem to be affected by varying the type of insurance plan.

In the third paper (Strong theory, flexible methods: evaluating complex community-based initiatives), Judge and Bauld look at approaches to evaluating English Health Action Zones (which were designed to reduce health inequalities) to demonstrate the use of theory-based evaluation for complex health-related initiatives involving several organisations. The theory-based evaluation they carry out is based on the theory of change approach. This involves a systematic and cumulative study of the links between activities, outcomes and contexts of the initiative. The theory of change approach can help solve one of the perennial problems encountered when evaluating complex activities involving several organisations in the social realm: namely the attribution of causality between activities undertaken and the desired outcomes.

In the fourth paper (Working together: lessons for collaboration between health and social services), Higgins *et al.* write about partnerships between caring organisations. They first look at the literature concerning inter-agency collaboration between health and social care, showing a history in England of policy encouraging such collaboration dating back at least to the 1970s; and finding evidence about factors that facilitate collaboration. Then they provide an analysis of a local experiment in joint service delivery in northern England which, in addition to demonstrating some benefits of joint working, also illustrates many of the factors impeding collaboration. These factors are a mix of cultural, professional and organisational differences between the agencies involved. The paper concludes by setting out the lessons for effective joint working that can be learnt from the analysis. The methods used in the analysis of the local experiment are not included in this extract. The whole version of the paper gives a full description of various qualitative techniques, such as interviews and documentary analysis.

In the fifth paper (Size, composition and function of hospital boards of directors: a study of organisation environment linkage), Pfeffer looks at the relationship between aspects of boards of hospital directors in a Midwestern state of the USA and their organisational context. This is a classic study from the 1970s in the field of organisational studies, using quantitative methods. The paper sees boards of directors as linkages between the organisation and its environment. It explores the different functions that boards of hospital directors perform in the American context, and the different forms of linkage with the hospital's environment. They find that the function of the board (here being defined as fund-raising or internal administration of the hospital) is partly explained by issues such as the ownership of the hospital and its source of funds. If a hospital is heavily dependent on private donations from the local community it is more likely to need a board which has a fund-raising function. Conversely, hospitals with religious affiliations and hospitals that receive larger proportions of their resources from federal government tend to place less importance on the fund-raising function of the board, and more on its administrative expertise. Moreover, they found that having influence in the local community is a more important criterion for selecting board members where the hospital relies on that community for a substantial proportion of its funds, than for a hospital which has substantial funding from government.

Chapter 26

The reforms: success or failure or neither?

Julian Le Grand, Nicholas Mays and Jennifer Dixon

Abstract (Editors' note)

This paper discusses the evidence as to whether the English National Health Service internal market can be considered a success or a failure. It then considers the lessons that can be learnt from the experiment. Finally it discusses if the lessons are apparent in the proposals for the internal market's successor, as laid out in the Labour Government's White Paper, *The New NHS* (Secretary of State for Health 1997).

Success or failure

We begin by examining the record of whether the internal market was a success or a failure with respect to the criteria of *efficiency, equity, choice and responsiveness* and *accountability*.

Efficiency

With respect to overall efficiency, over the period since the reforms were introduced there was an increase in activity, as measured by the Cost-Weighted Activity Index (CWAI), that was greater than the increase in resources over that period. The cost per unit of activity went down and, hence, if the CWAI is accepted as a reasonable measure of NHS output efficiency increased.

This apparent improvement in efficiency in a crude sense happened despite well publicised increases in transactions costs and specifically in management costs. These increases certainly occurred, although their origins and magnitude are open to question.

Source: *Learning from the NHS Internal Market: A Review of the Evidence*, London, King's Fund, 1998.

There is some evidence concerning the relative efficiency of different kinds of purchasers derived from comparisons of general practices served by the two approaches. For example, there was an initial difference in the rate of growth of prescribing costs between fundholders and non-fund-holders, and the difference in levels persisted, although the differentials stopped growing. Fundholders also generated more 'savings' or surpluses than Health Authorities (HAs). On the other hand, of all the purchasing models surveyed, fundholding appeared to have the highest transaction costs.

Equity

The principal equity issue that worried many analysts at the start of the internal market was the danger of cream-skimming – the deliberate selection of patients by both hospitals and fundholding practices who were easier or less costly to treat in order to protect budgets (Scheffler 1989; Le Grand and Bartlett 1993). However, there is no evidence that this has been a problem.

Instead, the chief equity concern that exercised press, public and politicians was the so-called 'two-tier' issue, whereby the patients of GP fundholders apparently received preferential treatment over patients being paid for by HAs. That this did indeed occur is borne out by most studies of the question. The only area where there remains significant disagreement concerns the extent to which this arose because fundholders were better purchasers or because they were better resourced.

Quality

Our review of the evidence with respect to the principal providers of secondary care, hospital trusts, found no evidence of improved quality that could be attributed to trust status. However, the reviews of the evidence with respect to purchasing did find some improvements, mostly attributable to fundholding.

An indicator of quality is waiting lists. These were subject to a series of initiatives both before and after the adoption of an internal market. Waiting lists have continued to grow in the 1990s as they did in the 1980s. However, although waiting lists have been growing in length, mean waiting times have been falling. The Conservative Government was successful in eliminating the small group of people waiting for very long periods of time for treatment. And people waiting for NHS treatment have, on average, been waiting for shorter periods of time.

Choice and responsiveness

The evidence suggests that choice for patients has not increased. With respect to HAs and responsiveness, there is anecdotal evidence of user consultations, but no systematic information on the consequences of such activities for patients. Incentives for HAs to respond to individual patient preferences seemed to be weak. No 'exit' was possible by dissatisfied users, and methods of expressing patient 'voice' (e.g. through Community Health Councils, or HA non-executive directors) were limited and little altered, if at all, by the reforms.

Fundholders appeared more successful than other forms of purchaser in obtaining responsiveness from providers. However, there was little evidence of increased choice for their patients.

There is no evidence that trusts have increased patient choice.

Accountability

There is a general view that 'upward' accountability of HAs to the centre is high, and that for GP fundholders relatively low. Although trusts were clearly accountable to purchasers, there is no evidence that trusts have become more accountable to their local populations and there is some suggestion that trust boards were chosen in part for their political allegiances. There is no sense in which the decision making of either HAs or trusts has become more transparent to the public.

Overall: little change?

Perhaps the most striking conclusion to arise from this survey of the evidence is how little overall measurable change there seems to have been related to the core structures and mechanisms of the internal market.

This apparent absence of obvious change attributable to the internal market may be because there was indeed little change. Or it may be because there *was* change, but the studies concerned either focused on the wrong indicators or focused on the right indicators, but their deficiencies of technique were such that they could not pick up the relevant changes in those indicators.

It is clear that in some, possibly unmeasurable ways, the NHS *has* changed fundamentally since the 1991 internal market reforms. Purchasing has involved significant organisational change. The criteria we have used to evaluate the evidence have not related directly to measuring this type of cultural and managerial shift. Our sense is that there has been a considerable degree of cultural change involving HAs, fundholding and non-fundholding practices. This is especially in terms of the extra attention being paid to the concerns of GPs of all types and an alteration in GPs' standing within the system, if not always in their coercive power. Also, there seems to have been a considerable increase in cost-consciousness throughout the service. Finally, there appears to be a wide, but not total, agreement that the device of separately identifying the purchaser role from that of the provider has proved broadly successful and should remain in some form.

But why did these organisational and cultural changes not result in more demonstrable impacts in the areas that we have investigated? The explanation must, therefore, lie with the way in which the internal market was implemented. And here there is a ready economic answer: *the incentives were too weak and the constraints were too strong.* For markets of any kind to work, all the relevant agents must be motivated by the relevant market signals; and they must have freedom of action to respond to those motivations (Le Grand and Bartlett 1993). Yet most of the key actors in the NHS internal market had, for a variety of reasons, little direct incentive to move in the direction indicated by market developments, and both the actors and the market signals themselves were heavily constrained by central government intervention. So, HAs could not keep or invest any surplus they generated, leaving them with the sole incentive to come in exactly on budget. The investment and, even more significantly, the pricing policies of trusts were strictly controlled; as a consequence, the opportunities for competition between them were highly restricted. HAs could not switch providers easily without destabilising them; also they were instructed to bail out trusts in financial difficulties, with the consequence that for many trusts budget constraints became viewed as 'soft', rather than 'hard'. Again, this had implications for competition. Trusts not only had limited opportunities to compete with one another; they had little incentive to do so, knowing that they could not keep any surpluses if they succeeded and that they would be bailed out if they failed. More generally, both HAs and trusts were not really treated as independent agents, but viewed more as partially decentralised instruments of central government policy.

All this is reinforced by the evidence concerning the relative performance of HAs and the one agent not mentioned above: GP fundholders. Fundholders could retain their surpluses and use them to improve their facilities. But fundholders also had strong non-pecuniary incentives – arising both from their professional ethos and from direct patient pressure – to see that their patients were promptly and effectively treated. Equally significantly, they were less constrained than HAs; they were subject to a weak accountability regime and, being relatively small, could switch their purchasing without massively destabilising providers. Instead, they represented an attractive source of marginal income to trusts. It is no coincidence that the area where it has been easiest to detect some significant changes is where the incentives were strongest and the constraints the weakest.

Another way of characterising the limitations of the reforms from a market point of view is to point to the inherent contradictions in the notion of a 'managed market' in which policy-makers and managers have sought to reconcile the objectives of competitive efficiency with other NHS strategic goals such as equity of access (Flynn and Williams 1997; Spurgeon *et al.* 1997). Long before the change of government in May 1997, we find the Department of Health encouraging the service to find the appropriate balance between competition and 'constructive co-operation' while also acknowledging the pragmatic advantages of *contestability* – the *possibility* that alternative providers might displace the existing ones in the absence of current competition (Department of Health 1994).

Finally, a yet more fundamental explanation for the failure of the internal market to have the impact its proponents hoped may lie in the motivations of the actors concerned. For markets to work effectively, individuals need to be motivated by the furtherance of their own interests. However, those working in the service often continued to see themselves as engaged in the provision of public services based on relations of mutual trust (Flynn *et al.* 1996; Broadbent and Laughlin 1997). In part, contracting had less impact than was expected because of the difficulty of specifying the content of services with sufficient clarity for contracting without threatening the relations of trust, professional discretion and long-term co-operation on which the effective production of many services largely depended (Flynn et *al.* 1996). Checkland (1997) showed that the form of the contracts was not an important element in the way in which the contracting process was translated into the production of services. Relationships between purchasers and providers continued to develop alongside the formal contracting process as much as through it, according to Spurgeon *et al.* (1997). All in all, both purchasers and providers were not perhaps as single-minded in the pursuit of a narrowly defined self-interest as the internal market required; in the terminology of one of the authors, they continued to operate more like 'knights' than like 'knaves' (Le Grand 1997).

The lessons to be learned

Even though much of the evidence is inconclusive, there are some lessons to be learned from the British internal market experience. First, although we do not have direct evidence, because assessing the overall effect of the internal market in a definitive way is almost certainly impractical, most analysts of the internal market would agree on the following. The split between purchaser and provider, together with the development of contracts or service agreements between purchasers and providers that the market necessitated, were desirable innovations which should be retained in any future development of the system – despite the fact that, for some commentators, the extent of regulation excessively weakened the incentives inherent in the system. However, there would be less agreement on the desirability of the other key aspect of the internal market – the introduction of competition – and this is discussed below.

On the purchasing side, if the policy aims are to promote *quality, choice* and *responsiveness*, then it seems to be important to have devolved purchasing with some degree of GP (or other local) involvement in, or even leadership of, the purchasing or commissioning process. Further, the evidence seems to suggest that the best way to sustain productive GP involvement is for the agency to have a measure of budgetary control.

The conclusions with respect to *equity* and *efficiency* are not so clear-cut. Devolution of power to smaller purchasing and commissioning units inevitably means that some will do different things from others. This in turn, is likely to mean that the more effective purchasers may provide a better service overall and certainly better aspects of part of their service than others.

There are other efficiency problems that appear to arise with devolved purchasing. Smaller units may have problems of managerial capacity and support, and their risk pool may be too small to carry out effective purchasing. Also, smaller purchasing units can create problems for provider planning and stability; the provision and maintenance of expensive facilities may require guarantees of future income streams that are difficult to obtain from a host of small purchasers.

On the provider side, the principal lesson concerns the question of competition. For the reasons already outlined, the competitive element within the internal market was not actually as great as its proponents had hoped, although still apparent in some areas and for some services (Propper and Bartlett 1997). This may have been a major reason why the internal market did not have the dramatic consequences predicted.

The Labour White Paper: *The New NHS*

In December 1997, the Labour Government published a White Paper in England (Secretary for State for Health 1997) proposing a further re-organisation of the NHS. Do the new proposals suggest that the lessons of the internal market experience have been learned? Do they constitute, as the Government has claimed, a 'third way'?

The most relevant of the new proposals for this discussion are summarised below.

- The purchaser/provider split is to remain, but the emphasis is to be on co-operative relationships, not competitive or adversarial ones. As a last resort, purchasers can switch their purchasing away from their current providers.

- Purchasers are to become primary care groups (PCGs), led by GPs and community nurses. PCGs will include up to 50 GPs and cover around 100,000 population. PCGs will hold budgets; they will be able to retain surpluses, which can be spent on services or facilities of benefit to patients. All GPs will be required to join PCGs. The current trusts will remain and will also be able to retain surpluses.
- Fundholders will be absorbed into PCGs. HAs will lose their purchasing role, except for certain highly specialised services, but will become the lead for Health Improvement Programmes and instrument for PCG accountability.
- Annual contracts will be replaced by three-year service agreements.
- A new performance 'framework', with new performance indicators emphasising effectiveness and outcomes, will be put in place.
- There will be two new national bodies: one to set standards – the National Institute for Clinical Excellence (NICE); the other to enforce them – the Commission for Health Improvement (CHIMP).

The first striking point about these proposals is that, despite some rhetoric to the contrary, key elements of the internal market are to be retained. The purchaser/provider split remains. The negotiated arrangements between purchasers and providers are unlikely to differ significantly from current contracts, except perhaps in being rather more long-term. The new GP-led commissioning organisations will hold budgets. Trusts and PCGs are both to be allowed to retain their surpluses. And purchasers will be able to switch to other providers if they are dissatisfied with their existing ones: so competition, or at least contestability (the potential in *extremis* for competition), will remain.

All this seems consistent with the lessons to be learned from the internal market experience which were laid out above. As noted, the purchaser/provider split was generally thought to be one of the more successful elements of the internal market. The evidence on the experience of different purchasing models showed that GPs with budgets tended to be the most effective purchasers. We noted the importance of retention of surpluses for purchasers and trusts. And it would be impossible to retain the purchaser/provider split without some possibility of competition. If purchasers did not hold the ultimate sanction of being able to take their business elsewhere, they would have no lever over providers. However, we also noted that contestability was likely to be limited, in practice, in most settings and that the nature of health care meant that longer-term collaborative relations between purchasers and providers were frequently as, or more, important for service development – thereby supporting the proposals to move to longer-term service level agreements rather than annual contracts.

There are areas where problems might arise. For instance, is 100,000 the 'right' size for the PCGs? What incentives are there for GPs to take part and what sanctions will PCG leaders have over 'free-riding' colleagues?

Another potential problem with PCGs relates to the cost of managing the 500 devolved purchasing organisations in England which will result from the setting up of PCGs, given the fact that the vast majority of the purchasing responsibility is currently exercised by around 90 HAs.

There may also be problems concerning the 'replacement' of competition by co-operation. For co-operation to work, particularly between purchasers and providers, there have to be either no conflicts of interest (unlikely) or else mechanisms for resolving any conflicts which arise. It is possible that keeping the possibility of competition as a last resort is just such a mechanism; and, again, given the difficulties of ensuring a properly competitive environment, it may be that this is an appropriate compromise. However, the precise effects of the new shift of emphasis will depend on the detailed, day-to-day interpretation of the future guidance and regulations by managers throughout the NHS.

Perhaps the area of greatest worry concerns the role of the centre. The performance management framework in the Labour White Paper is quite centralist in tone with a large number of performance indicators (37 are currently proposed) and with the introduction of institutions (NICE and CHIMP) designed to monitor performance and, if necessary, to intervene. There will also be a series of nationally determined service frameworks which will govern the limits of the discretion permitted to the PCGs as commissioners of services. Care will have to be taken that the government does not make the mistakes of its predecessor in paying lip service to the ideal of decentralisation while at the same time trying to retain a strong grip from the centre.

Overall, the White Paper's proposals deserve a guarded welcome, not least because they have preserved some of the features of the internal market that, as best as can be determined, have been demonstrated to work, while dispensing with some of its less successful aspects.

References

Broadbent, J. and Laughlin, R. (1997) 'Contractual changes in schools and general practices: professional resistance and the role of absorption and absorbing groups', in R. Flynn and G. Williams (eds) *Contracting for Health: Quasi-markets and the National Health Service*, Oxford: Oxford University Press, 30–46.

Checkland, P. (1997) 'Rhetoric and reality in contracting: research in and on the National Health Service', in R. Flynn and G. Williams (eds) *Contracting for Health: Quasi-markets and the National Health Service*, Oxford: Oxford University Press, 115–34.

Department of Health (1994) *A Guide to the Operation of the NHS Internal Market: Local Freedoms, National Responsibilities*, Leeds: NHS Executive.

Flynn, R. and Williams, G. (1997) 'Contracting for health', in R. Flynn and G.

Williams (eds) *Contracting for Health: Quasi-markets and the National Health Service*, Oxford: Oxford University Press, 1–13.

Flynn, R., Williams, G. and Pickard, S. (1996) *Markets and Networks: Contracting in Community Health Services*, Buckingham: Open University Press.

Le Grand, J. (1997) 'Knights, knaves or pawns? Human behaviour and social policy', *Journal of Social Policy*, 26: 149–69.

Le Grand, J. and Bartlett, W. (1993) *Quasi-markets and Social Policy*, London: Macmillan.

Propper, C, and Bartlett, W. (1997) 'The impact of competition on the behaviour of National Health Service Trusts', in R. Flynn and G. Williams (eds) *Contracting for Health: Quasi-markets and the National Health Service*, Oxford: Oxford University Press, 115–34.

Scheffler, R. (1989) 'Adverse selection: the Achilles heel of the NHS reforms', *The Lancet*, 1: 950–2.

Secretary of State for Health (1997) *The New NHS – Modern Dependable*, CM 3807, London: HMSO.

Spurgeon, P., Smith, P., Straker, M., Deakin, N., Thomas, N. and Walsh, K. (1997) 'The experience of contracting in health care', in R. Flynn and G. Williams (eds) *Contracting for Health: Quasi-markets and the National Health Service*, Oxford: Oxford University Press, 135–52.

A complete, unedited version of this article can be found as Le Grand, J., Mays, N. and Mulligan, J., (eds) part of the concluding chapter of *Learning from the NHS Internal Market: A Review of the Evidence* (1998) King's Fund: London.

Chapter 27

Some interim results from a controlled trial of cost sharing in health insurance

Joseph P. Newhouse, Willard G. Manning, Carl N. Morris, Larry L. Orr, Naihua Duan, Emmett B. Keeler, Arleen Leibowitz, Kent H. Marquis, M. Susan Marquis, Charles E. Phelps and Robert H. Brook

Abstract

A total of 7706 persons are participating in a controlled trial of alternative health insurance policies. Interim results indicate that persons fully covered for medical services spend about 50 per cent more than do similar persons with income-related catastrophe insurance. Full coverage leads to more people using services and to more services per user. Both ambulatory services and hospital admissions increase. Once patients are admitted to the hospital, however, expenditures per admission do not differ significantly among the experimental insurance plans. In addition, hospital admissions for children do not vary by plan.

The income-related cost sharing in the experimental plans affects expenditure by different income groups similarly, but adults' total expenditure varies more than children's. Sufficient data are not available on whether higher use by persons with free care reflects overuse, or whether lower use by those with income-related catastrophe coverage reflects underuse. Both may well be true.

Introduction

Controversy over the desirability of cost sharing in health insurance policies has simmered for decades and has occasionally boiled over, in part because of the meagre quantitative evidence about the effects of cost sharing on the demand for services and on patients' health status. The limited information available prompted the federal government to sponsor a controlled trial, which will end in early 1982. Results concerning the

Source: *New England Journal of Medicine*, 305.25, 1981, 1501–7.

effects on health are not yet available; only interim results about the use of services are available.

On the basis of economic theory and prior empirical work, we expected use to increase as cost sharing diminished (Scitovsky and Snyder 1972; Newhouse et al. 1974; Scitovsky and McCall 1977; Newhouse 1978). However, the magnitude of this effect was uncertain, as was its possible variation among different types of people (e.g. poor and non-poor) (Phelps and Newhouse 1972; Enterline et al. 1973; Rosett and Huang 1973; Beck 1974; Newhouse and Phelps 1976; Feldstein 1977). A dispute has also lingered about whether reductions in cost sharing for ambulatory services would increase or decrease the demand for hospital services (Hill and Veney 1970; Lewis and Keairnes 1970; Roemer et al. 1975). Those who argue that free ambulatory care decreases hospitalisation characterise cost sharing for ambulatory services as penny-wise and pound-foolish (Roemer et al. 1975).

Methods

Selection of families and sites

A total of 2756 families consisting of 7706 persons have been enrolled in one of several different health insurance plans: 70 per cent of them for three years, and the rest for five years. The families come from six areas of the country.

The six sites were selected to represent all four census regions, in order to account for regional variation; to obtain a spectrum of city sizes, because the complexity of the medical care delivery system could vary with city size; to achieve variation in the degree of pressure on the ambulatory care delivery system (e.g. in waiting times for an appointment and in the proportion of primary care physicians accepting new patients), because the response to the type of plan could vary according to the pressure already on the system; to include both northern and southern rural areas, because these areas tend to differ in economic and racial characteristics; and to ensure that one site had a well established prepaid group practice.

Description of insurance plans

The insurance plans offered to the families varied along two dimensions; the co-insurance rate (the fraction of the bill paid by the family) and the maximum dollar expenditure (an upper limit on the family's annual out-of-pocket expenditure). The four co-insurance rates were 0 (free care) and 25, 50 and 95 per cent. The maximum dollar expenditure varied as a fraction of the family's income, either 5, 10 or 15 per cent, to a maximum of

$1000. The 95 per cent co-insurance plan, together with the limit on the family's expenditure, approximates an income-related catastrophe plan.

Most enrolled families were permitted to seek care from any provider. All insurance plans covered a wide variety of services, including hospital, physician, dental, mental health, visual and auditory services, prescription drugs and supplies.

With two exceptions, each policy covered all services at a single co-insurance rate. First of all, three plans required 50 per cent co-insurance for dental services and outpatient mental health services, but only 25 per cent for all other services. These plans are grouped with the 25 per cent co-insurance plans in our analysis. Secondly, the individual deductible plan applied cost sharing solely to outpatient services; inpatient services were free to the family. The individual deductible plan thus approximated the situation of many families who have complete or nearly complete insurance for inpatient services but poorer insurance for outpatient services. It was designed to test the hypothesis that failure to provide full coverage for outpatient services inflates total medical expenditures by inducing additional hospitalisation (Roemer *et al.* 1975).

Method of analysis

Because plan assignment in the study was designed to be unrelated to any known covariates, differences in mean values by plan will yield unbiased estimates of differences in expenditure among plans. For ambulatory expenditure per person by plan, such a procedure gives satisfactory precision. The standard errors associated with total expenditure per person by plan, however, are unacceptably large. The imprecision results from rare, very large claims that make the sample mean a relatively unreliable estimate of the population mean. For this reason we augmented our analysis with more sophisticated methods. These methods are described at greater length elsewhere (Duan *et al.* 1981).

Results

Total expenditure per capita (inpatient plus ambulatory, excluding dental services and outpatient mental health services) rises steadily as co-insurance falls (Table 27.1). Expenditure per person with full coverage is approximately 60 per cent greater than that under the 95 per cent co-insurance plan. Expenditure in the other plans falls between these two extremes. The effects of varying the maximum dollar expenditure were small, and thus for clarity all plans with the same co-insurance rate have been combined.

The estimated effect of the 'hold-harmless' payment is negligible. That its effect should be negligible is plausible: it is as if an employer increased

Table 27.1 Actual annual total and ambulatory expenditure per person by plan in nine site-years*

Plan	Total expenditure ($)	Ambulatory expenditure ($)	No. of person-years for total expenditure	No. of person years for ambulatory expenditure[†]
Free care	401 ± 52	186 ± 9	2825	2834
25% co-insurance	346 ± 58	149 ± 10	1787	1792
50% co-insurance	328 ± 149	120 ± 12	766	766
95% co-insurance	254 ± 37	114 ± 10	1763	1764
Individual deductible				
95% co-insurance[‡]	333 ± 74	140 ± 11	1605	1609

*95 per cent confidence intervals are presented with expenditure data. Amounts are in current dollars, beginning in late 1974 and extending through late 1978. The figures are uncorrected for price-level differences by site or for small differences in allocation to plan by site. Confidence intervals are corrected for inter-temporal and intra-family correlations; such a correction cannot be made without imposing strong assumptions about the nature of the correlation. Ignoring inter-temporal and intra-family correlation, the F value to test the null hypothesis of no differences among the plans in total expenditure with 4,8741 degrees of freedom is 3.14 ($P < 0.05$). The F value to test the null hypothesis of no differences among the plans in ambulatory expenditure is 33.4 ($P < 0.01$)
[†]The sample for ambulatory expenditure includes 19 persons with a known hospital admission for whom the amount of inpatient expenditure is unknown.
[‡]Co-insurance in this plan applies to outpatient care only; inpatient care is free.

the cost sharing in the health insurance plan, passed the savings in premiums to employees, and added a general wage increase of about 10 per cent. It does not seem likely that the use of medical services would be much affected by the wage increase.

Differences in use among plans

Expressing differences among plans in dollars is a natural method of aggregating various services, but it does not indicate whether observed differences in expenditure reflect differences in the actual quantity of services consumed or in the price per unit of service. Which of these two factors predominates clearly affects one's interpretation of differences in expenditure.

In fact, variation in quantities of services consumed appears to account for most of the differences among plans. With plan means from the four site-years for which data on both expenditures and visits are available (year 2 in each site), the coefficient of correlation between visits per person and ambulatory expenditure per person is 0.94.

The likelihood of a visit to a physician or a hospital admission during a year also differs markedly across plans, further demonstrating that differences in expenditure result from variation in actual quantities consumed. By contrast with likelihood of admission, annual expenditure per hospitalised patient shows no consistent or significant relation to the type of plan.

Use by subgroup

An important objective of the experiment is to judge the effect of cost sharing on various subgroups of the population. Of special interest is whether cost sharing differentially affects adults and children, poor and non-poor, and blacks and whites. Expenditure by adults shows greater responsiveness to variation in cost sharing than does expenditure by children, largely because the likelihood of admission to a hospital among children shows no significant response to plan, whereas that among adults is significantly higher in the free care plan.

Different income groups have relatively similar responses. In Dayton, families in the lowest third of the income distribution have somewhat more responsiveness to the type of plan (expressed as a percentage) than do those in the highest third, but in the other three sites the two groups respond almost identically. Moreover, in Dayton the absolute decline (expressed in dollars) as co-insurance rises is very similar between these two income tertiles.

Blacks in Dayton spend about 20 per cent less than whites do (with a variety of characteristics, including plan, self-assessed health status before enrolment and income, held constant), and the difference is significant ($P < 0.01$). Why blacks in Dayton spend less is not clear.

Discussion

The policy debate over cost sharing

One alleged shortcoming of cost sharing in health insurance is that cost sharing, especially for ambulatory services, raises overall costs by inducing persons to delay seeking care and encouraging physicians to hospitalise patients who could be treated on an outpatient basis (Roemer *et al.* 1975). The results involving the individual deductible plan tend to refute this argument. Under that plan, the incentives for inappropriate use of the hospital are stronger than in other plans, because inpatient services are free. Physicians thus have a greater incentive to perform procedures in the hospital, although they could have been performed in the office. However, the probability of hospitalisation is lower in the individual deductible plan than in the free care plan, and significantly so for adults. Evidently, given the reduced use of outpatient services under the individual deductible plan, physicians less frequently see illness that leads to hospitalisation.

The medical consequences of the decreased hospital use in the individual deductible plan are not clear.

Any adverse effect of cost sharing on total expenditure from delay in seeking care is more than outweighed by other forces. The 95 per cent co-insurance plan and the free care plan probably differ most in the incentive to delay, yet total expenditure in the free care plan is well above that in the 95 per cent co-insurance plan, and the difference is significant ($P < 0.01$) in each site and year studied.

Another negative argument about cost sharing is its alleged promotion of an inequitable distribution of services. This argument is difficult to address, because no consensus on an operational measure of equity exists. If, in fact, the poor responded more to cost sharing than did middle-income groups, some might argue that the proportion of services going to the poor when care is free is the equitable amount – and that the proportion going to the poor when services are not free, by implication, is too low.

Our interim results indicate that the poor are not more responsive to cost sharing if the cost sharing is less for low-income families, as in the experiment. However, our results do suggest that cost sharing unrelated to income would differentially affect lower-income families.

Another definition of equity requires minimal variation of use with income (Andersen 1975). In three of the four sites for which we have results, the estimated relation between expenditure and income is small and not significant. In the fourth site (Dayton), a 1 per cent increase in income (with other factors equal) elicits approximately a 0.2 per cent increase in expenditure in each of the three years, and the relation is significant ($P < 0.01$). However, we cannot detect any difference among the plans in this relation; thus, making care free does not appear to eliminate the variation income with Dayton.

Perhaps the most frequently made argument for eliminating cost sharing is that medical services are a right for all and should not be rationed by price. Although this argument is philosophical, it may be based on the premise that full coverage improves health, or that cost sharing induces persons to forego necessary services. By contrast, perhaps the most common argument in favour of retaining cost sharing is that its elimination will induce persons to consume unnecessary services or to seek care for trivial problems. Our data are not sufficiently complete for us to determine whether the additional services consumed by persons facing lower co-insurance rates affect health.

Cost sharing and hospital costs per patient

Whatever merits or demerits cost sharing may have as an abstract principle, the plans that we studied did not greatly affect patients once they were hospitalised. An effect on cost per hospitalised patient could have been absent because any additional hospital services that a physician ordered were usually not subject to cost sharing; 70 per cent of the hospitalised patients exceeded the maximum dollar expenditure.

Because the cost per hospitalised patient is the most rapidly rising component of hospital expenditure (American Hospital Association 1979), it has been a focus for efforts towards policy reform. Within the range of cost sharing encompassed by the experimental plans (up to $1000 in any one year), manipulating cost sharing had neither a systematic nor a statistically significant effect on the cost per hospitalised patient. Expanding the range of expenditure to which cost sharing applies might affect the cost per hospitalised patient, but it is an unattractive option, because persons would then probably face more financial exposure than they would wish.

Can the results be generalised?

This experiment has measured how the demands of a small number of consumers increased as cost sharing fell – that is, how many more services the participants sought, and their physicians delivered, as co-insurance decreased. Will the experimental results be generalised to a widespread health insurance plan of a similar nature? The consistency of the results with national averages suggests that they will, but certain circumstances could cause behaviour to differ.

First of all, if insurance for ambulatory services was suddenly expanded, the resulting increase in the entire population's demand could exceed the short-run capacity of the medical care delivery system. If so, the additional demand could be rationed in several possible ways (Newhouse *et al.* 1974). It is most likely that longer waits for an appointment would occur, as happened in Montreal when cost sharing was eliminated (Enterline *et al.* 1973). We do not yet have a good understanding of which services would not be delivered if appointment times lengthened.

Secondly, the delivery system might not be allowed to expand to meet any new demand; for example, it could be constrained by budget limits or rate and fee controls, so that only a certain proportion of the demand would be met. The experimental plan, in general, covered billed fees or charges, but regulations or fee schedules might not permit such a procedure. We cannot predict from experimental data who might receive what services if budgets were constrained sufficiently so that not all the demand would be met.

Thirdly, if present cost sharing levels increased so that demand fell, some argue that physicians would create additional demand to offset the decline (Barer *et al.* 1979). The evidence supporting this argument, however, has been sharply questioned (Sloan and Feldman 1978; Bureau of Health Manpower 1980). Moreover, recent evidence on physicians' location behaviour suggests that they cannot fully offset a decline in demand per physician (Schwartz *et al.* 1980).

In summary, unless budget limits or other regulations constrain the response, a reduction in cost sharing will expand the total volume of resources in medical care, and conversely. Would such expansion be worth the foregone opportunities for other desired goods and services? One may wish to reserve judgement on that issue until more is known about how the additional medical services affect health and well-being.

References

American Hospital Association (1979) *Guide to the Health Care Field*, Chicago: American Hospital Association (Table 1).

Andersen, R. (1975) 'Health service distribution and equity', in R. Andersen, J. Kravits and O.W. Anderson (eds) *Equity in Health Services: Empirical Analyses in Social Policy*, Cambridge, MA: Baffinger, 9–32.

Barer, M.L., Evens, R.G. and Stoddart, G. (1979) *Controlling Health Costs by Charges to Patients: Snare or Delusion?*, Toronto: Ontario Economic Council.

Beck, R.G. (1974) 'The effects of co-payment on the poor', *Journal of Human Resources*, 9: 129–42.

Bureau of Health Manpower (1980) *The Target Income Hypothesis and Related Issues in Health Manpower Policy*, Washington, DC: Government Printing Office, DHEW publication no. (HRA)80-27.

Duan, N., Manning, W.G., Morris, C.N. and Newhouse, J.P. (1981) *A Comparison of Alternative Models of the Demand for Medical Care*, Santa Monica, CA: Rand Corporation.

Enterline, P.E., Saltor, V., McDonald, A.D. and McDonald, J.C. (1973) 'The distribution of medical services before and after "free" medical care – the Quebec experience', *New England Journal of Medicine*, 289: 1174–8.

Feldstein, M.S. (1977) 'Quality change and the demand for hospital care', *Econometrica*, 45: 1681–702.

Hill, D.B. and Veney, J.E. (1970) 'Kansas Blue Cross/Blue Shield outpatient benefits experiment', *Medical Care*, 8: 143–58.

Lewis, C.E. and Keairnes, H. (1970) 'Controlling costs of medical care by expanding insurance coverage: study of a paradox', *New England Journal of Medicine*, 282: 1405–12.

Newhouse, J.P. (1978) 'Insurance benefits, out-of-pocket payments, and the demand for medical care: a review of the literature', *Health and Medical Care Services Review*, 1: 1, 3–15.

Newhouse, J.P. and Phelps, C.E. (1976) 'New estimates of price and income elasticities of medical care services', in R.N. Rosett (ed.) *The Role of Health Insurance in the Health Services Sector*, New York: National Bureau of Economic Research, 261–313.

Newhouse, J.P., Phelps, C.E. and Schwartz, W.B. (1974) 'Policy options and the impact of national health insurance', *New England Journal of Medicine*, 290: 1345–59.

Phelps, C.E. and Newhouse, J.P. (1972) 'Effects of coinsurance: a multivariate analysis', *Social Security Bulletin*, 35: 20–9.

Roemer M.I., Hopkins C.E., Carr, L. and Gartside, F. (1975) 'Copayments for ambulatory care: penny-wise and pound foolish', *Medical Care*, 13: 457–66.

Rosett, R.N. and Huang, L.F. (1973) 'The effect of health insurance on the demand for medical care', *Journal of Political Economy*, 81: 281–305.

Schwartz, W.B., Newhouse, J.P., Bennett, B.W. and Willams, A.P. (1980) 'The changing geographic distribution of board-certified physicians', *New England Journal of Medicine*, 303: 1032–8.

Scitovsky, A.A. and McCall, N. (1977) 'Coinsurance and the demand for physician services: four years later', *Social Security Bulletin*, 40: 19–27.

Scitovsky, A.A. and Snyder, N.M. (1972) 'Effect of coinsurance on use of physician services', *Social Security Bulletin,* 35: 3–19.

Sloan, F.A. and Feldman, R. (1978) 'Competition among physicians', in W. Greenberg (ed.) *Competition in the Health Care Sector: Past, Present, and Future,* Germantown, MD: Aspen Systems Corporation.

A complete, unedited version of this article can be found as Newhouse, J., Manning, W., Morris, C., Orr, L., Duan, N., Keeler, E., Liebowitz, A., Marquis, K., Marquis, S., Phelps, C. and Brook, R., 'Some interim results from a controlled trial of cost sharing in health insurance', in the *New England Journal of Medicine* (1981) Volume 305, Issue 25, pages 1501–7.

Chapter 28

Strong theory, flexible methods: evaluating complex community-based initiatives

Ken Judge and Linda Bauld

Abstract

Many countries are moving from acknowledging the existence of health inequalities to developing policies to reduce them. Many such policies consist of complex interventions operating at a number of levels. Evaluating the efficacy of such initiatives poses particular challenges. This paper argues that there is real potential in applying a theory-based approach to the evaluation of complex community-based initiatives. Using examples from the evaluation of Health Action Zones in England, the paper outlines the key components of the approach. It argues that theory-based evaluation can strengthen programme design and implementation, and promote policy and practice learning about the most effective interventions for health improvement.

Introduction

There is a growing recognition that health policies, practices and processes require clear evidence about effectiveness. When resources are scarce, claims on them are numerous, and the potential exists for interventions to do harm as well as good; there is a strong ethical case for requiring that new policies should be evidence-based. But in areas such as health promotion there are real questions to be asked about what constitutes an appropriate evidence base. In England, for example, the Health Development Agency has explicitly recognised the nature of the challenge posed by a determined attempt to make use of evidence to promote population health and to tackle health inequalities.

Gillies (1999) argues that the challenge is 'to proffer a "modern" view of evidence which crosses methodological and disciplinary boundaries, and

Source: *Critical Public Health*, 11, 2001, 19–38.

which is grounded in theory whilst cognisant of political practicalities. This view requires a new consensus on a wider range of credible study methods and indicators for measuring the success of public health ventures, as its focus moves upstream to tackle the broader underlying social and economic determinants of health and inequalities in health.'

There is a belief that traditional approaches to evaluation that emphasise the primacy of experimental approaches are often, although not always, inappropriate for complex, community-based health promotion programmes. This view is reflected in a wide range of publications in the field of health promotion (Speller *et al.* 1997; Green and Tones 1999).

The existing, poorly developed evidence base in relation to health promotion interventions needs to be strengthened. We take the pragmatic view that all research methods have their strengths and weaknesses. Mixed methods and the careful triangulation of evidence offer the best way forward in learning about complex health promotion initiatives. From this perspective theory-driven approaches to evaluation have much to offer.

There are a number of reasons why it is important to consider non-experimental approaches. Health promotion programmes tend to be established in circumstances where evaluation design is a long way down the list of factors considered. At one level it is argued that the very nature of health promotion militates against experimental design (Gillies 1999). In addition, many potentially valuable initiatives are established in ways that simply do not easily lend themselves to evaluation. The aim of this paper is to outline the potential benefits of one particular approach to theory-based evaluation that is being employed to generate learning about Health Action Zones.

Health Action Zones

Health Action Zones (HAZs) were established in 1998 to serve as trail-blazers for a concerted effort to tackle health inequalities as part of an assault on social exclusion. HAZs are complex, partnership-based entities that have set themselves ambitious goals to transform the health and well-being of disadvantaged communities and groups. They have been provided with additional resources, flexibilities and support, but in return they are subject to tough performance management processes. HAZs are expected to set out clear plans that not only indicate how they will achieve social change in the longer term but also demonstrate a capacity to deliver against well specified targets in the form of 'early wins', to satisfy political expectations.

To varying degrees, all of the initial HAZ plans were strong on identifying problems and articulating long-term objectives, and to some extent on specifying routinely available statistical indicators that might be used for monitoring progress. But they were much less good at filling in the gap between problems and goals. Only in very rare cases was it possible at the outset to identify a clear and logical pathway that linked problems, strategies for intervention, milestones or targets with associated timescales and longer-term outcomes or goals. Figure 28.1 illustrates the nature of the problem. Interventions and their associated consequences, or 'targets', are not usually clearly linked to problems and goals.

Many of the HAZs found it difficult to specify precisely how they would intervene to address problems, what consequences they expected to flow from such interventions, and how precisely these related to their strategic goals. As a result, the 'targets' that they included in their plans were not convincing. Many specific 'targets' were not clearly linked with strategic goals or objectives set out elsewhere in the plans. Other 'targets' were not located within a specific timescale. Most importantly, specific 'targets' were highlighted without any accompanying explanation of the mechanisms intended to achieve them. This omission is key. It breaks the critical link between the problems that HAZs are there to address and the ambitious goals that they set themselves.

One of the main reasons why HAZs did not develop clear plans in the early stages is that the timetables that they were expected to work to were hopelessly unrealistic. But haste is not the only issue, and problems of strategic planning are not confined to HAZs. The key difficulty seems to be common to most complex community-based initiatives.

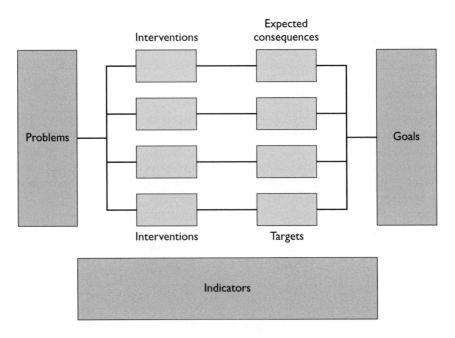

Figure 28.1 Health Action Zones: weak links in the planning process.

Theory-based evaluation

Simply to ignore investments in under-specified programmes, however, would be to seriously reduce the potential for learning about how best to tackle many intractable social problems, including that of social inequalities in health. What is required is an approach that can help to modify or clarify the design and implementation of initiatives in a way that lends itself to evaluation. This is where theory-driven approaches have a crucial role to play.

The concept of theory-based evaluation has evolved over the past 25 years or so in response to the kinds of difficulties outlined above. For example, Wholey (1983) developed the concept of *evaluability assessment* to focus attention on improving the logic that underlies programmes, both to increase their substantive effectiveness and to increase the feasibility of evaluation. The essential aspect 'was that prior to the start of a formal study, the evaluator should analyze the logical reasoning that connected programme inputs to desired outcomes to see whether there was a reasonable likelihood that goals could be achieved' (Weiss 1997a).

Since then a number of contributors (Chen 1990; Weiss 1997b) have made significant advances to thinking about how best to evaluate complex public policy programmes. What has evolved ranges from sophisticated approaches to the evaluation of complex community-based interventions, to more pragmatic and practical uses of 'program logic', 'logical models' and 'logical frameworks' (Funnel 1997). The most comprehensive and persuasive approach to evaluation that follows the logic of theory-based evaluation, and that seems especially applicable to health promotion initiatives, is described as 'theories of change' (Connell *et al.* 1995; Fulbright-Anderson *et al.* 1998).

The theory of change approach to evaluation

This approach to evaluation has been developed over a number of years through the work of the Aspen Institute in the USA (Aspen Institute 1997). It was developed in an effort to find ways of evaluating processes and outcomes in community-based programmes that were not adequately addressed by existing approaches. Comprehensive Community Initiatives (CCIs) aimed to promote positive changes in individual, family and community institutions; develop mechanisms to improve social, economic and physical circumstances, services and conditions in disadvantaged communities; and place a strong emphasis on community building and neighbourhood empowerment.

These characteristics pose a number of challenges for evaluation, because initiatives have multiple, broad goals. They are highly complex learning enterprises with multiple strands of activity operating at many different levels; objectives are defined and strategies chosen to achieve goals that often change over time; many activities and intended outcomes are difficult to measure; and units of action are complex, open systems in which it is virtually impossible to control all the variables that may influence the conduct and outcome of evaluation.

In order to address some of the complexity of CCIs a new conceptual framework for evaluation was developed. This 'theory of change' approach is defined as 'a systematic and cumulative study of the links between activities, outcomes and contexts of the initiative' (Connell and Kubisch 1998). The approach aims to gain clarity around the overall vision of the initiative, meaning the long-term outcomes and the strategies that are intended to produce them.

Connell and Kubisch offer several reasons why this approach is attractive. First, a theory of change can *sharpen the planning and implementation of an initiative*. An emphasis on programme logic or theory during the design phase can increase the probability that stakeholders will clearly specify the intended outcomes of an initiative. Second, *the measurement and data collection elements of the evaluation process will be facilitated*. It requires stakeholders to be clear about not only the final outcomes they hope to achieve but also the means by which they expect to achieve them. Finally, articulating a theory of change early in the life of an initiative and gaining agreement about it by all the stakeholders *helps to reduce problems associated with causal attribution of impact*.

There are difficulties in adopting a theory of change approach to evaluation. The approach requires an analytical stance that is different from the empathetic, responsive and intuitive stance of many practitioners. There is also the challenge, evident from the experience of other evaluators who have employed the approach, of gaining consensus among the many parties involved in implementing community initiatives.

Eliciting theories of change among the diverse groups of individuals involved in planning and implementing an initiative can be a resource-intensive exercise for evaluators. Despite these problems evidence suggests that skilled evaluators can overcome them, and by doing so they enrich both the programme and the lessons to be learnt from it (Jacobs 1999).

Theories of change in HAZs

A theory-based approach informs the national evaluation of HAZs in England (Judge *et al.* 1999; Judge 2000). Figure 28.2 illustrates the approach being adopted. The starting point is the context within which HAZs operate – the resources available in the communities and the challenges that they face. Once this is established, the key challenge is for HAZs to articulate a logical way of achieving social change and to specify

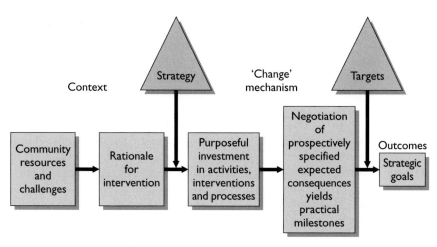

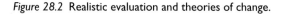

Community health improvement process

Figure 28.2 Realistic evaluation and theories of change.

targets for each of their interventions that satisfy two requirements. First, they should be articulated in advance of the expected consequences of actions. Second, these actions and their associated targets should form part of a logical pathway that leads towards strategic goals or outcomes.

Initial work with HAZs is yielding valuable lessons about the type of information needed if any serious attempt is to be made to learn from their activities. Knowledge is required regarding the ways in which different configurations of contexts, strategies, interventions and their associated consequences contribute to tackling health inequalities and promoting population health. This can be gained only on a continuous basis, through an approach to evaluation that recognises the evolving nature of HAZ plans and activities. Promoting and achieving change in pursuit of ambitious goals will only be possible if HAZs are encouraged to invest in the planning process, to take risks, and to adapt to changing circumstances.

More flexible planning should be matched by adaptive approaches to evaluation if such complex community-based initiatives are to contribute fully to policy learning. The process of monitoring and evaluation has started by trying to persuade HAZ stakeholders to develop and articulate the underlying theories of change that guide their plans.

Practical examples emerging in HAZs

Theories of change need to be developed at a number of different levels. All HAZs start with a vision statement of some kind that embraces their primary goals. A set of strategic goals or 'aspirational' targets are closely related to the vision. These are then pursued through a series of work-streams or programmes that comprise a large number of projects. In their original plans the 26 zones reported that between them they had more than 200 programmes with over 2000 projects (Judge *et al.* 1999). Each is expected to generate a range of outcomes in the short, medium and longer term.

At each stage in this process – the project, the programme and the overall initiative in each HAZ – it is possible and desirable to develop a theory of change. In practice, it has proved easier for the zones to start to develop theories of change for individual projects than it has at the most general level. A key challenge is to develop convincing and acceptable theory of change models for HAZs as whole systems. For the moment we provide a simple illustration of the kind of progress being made.

Smoking cessation services

Smoking cessation services represent one of the most straightforward areas to illustrate how logic models and a theory of change approach are being developed in HAZs. One of the reasons for this is that evidence-based guidelines exist for smoking cessation interventions, which the Department of Health has instructed HAZs to use in developing local services (Raw *et al.* 1998).

Figure 28.3 presents an overview in logic model form of the approach

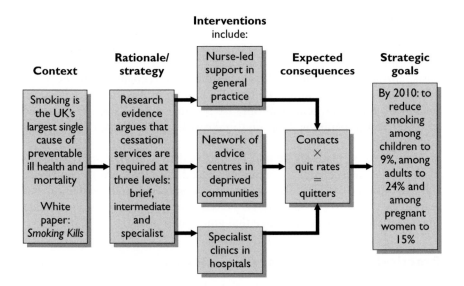

Figure 28.3 Smoking cessation in Health Action Zones.

being adopted by many HAZs. The starting point is the context set out in the White Paper *Smoking Kills* that outlines why smoking is the UK's single biggest cause of avoidable ill health and mortality. The rationale for interventions is evidence-based. The expected consequences of these investments are that contacts will be made with smokers for whom cessation rates can be predicted depending on the package of services that they receive. The number of 'quitters' generated by these interventions will contribute to achieving ambitious reductions in overall smoking prevalence rates in the longer term.

This kind of logical process can then be taken down to a more practical level as shown in Figure 28.4. In this example, from North Staffordshire, the selected intervention is nurse-led support for patients in general practice. The expected consequences of the intervention highlight the critical assumptions that specified numbers of practices will be willing and able to recruit modest numbers of patients on a regular basis for a specified time to receive different levels of service. If these assumptions prove to be valid then the evidence base predicts that a certain number of 'quitters' can be expected.

This relatively simple example draws attention to some critical initial assumptions about the ways in which services will be established and the expected consequences that will result within the context of an overall logical model or theory of change. Moreover the model clearly shows what data are required to test whether or not the assumptions are valid.

Unfortunately, relatively few of the interventions being developed by HAZs are either as straightforward or as clearly linked to evidence-based guidelines as smoking cessation. Many initiatives remain at a relatively

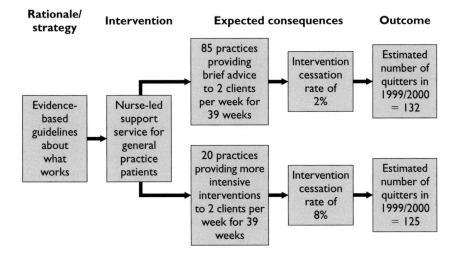

Figure 28.4 Smoking cessation in North Staffordshire HAZ (1).

early stage of development. But these are exactly the kinds of circumstances in which the theory of change approach has much to commend it. Properly applied it helps stakeholders to specify programme properties more clearly and so aids processes of implementation and learning.

Conclusion

Complex community-based initiatives such as HAZs are typically established as demonstration programmes to tackle configurations of long-standing social problems. They are initiatives with very ambitious goals that require sustained investment over time. Their evaluation represents as much of a challenge as does their design and implementation. If they are to achieve their purposes they have to deliver on the promise of substantial social change (impact). It is also essential to understand how any observed benefits were brought about (process). But understanding cause and effect is difficult to establish in complex open systems. It is for these reasons that the more imprecise objective of 'learning' often replaces the more common use of 'evaluation', which often carries with it the unrealistic burden of excessive 'scientific' expectation.

No matter how creative researchers prove to be, the process of learning about and evaluating CCIs will remain a challenging business. Our experience of working with HAZs is that there will be much more scope for productive action and learning if a more theory-based approach to design, implementation and evaluation is adopted at the earliest possible stage (Adams *et al.* 2000).

In following this approach a wide range of methods can be employed to learn about processes and their impact. All those associated with trying to learn about complex community-based initiatives should be encouraged to make a virtue of pragmatism, and to use whatever resources are available to them. But there are some essential requirements associated with the theory of change approach. Policy makers and practitioners must be able to:

- explain their starting assumptions and how they are related to critical aspects of the economic, social and political environments in which they work;
- specify in a plausible and evidence-based way why their chosen investments in interventions and process will take them in the direction of the long-term outcomes they are seeking;
- identify in advance the expected consequences of their actions in ways that lend themselves to being monitored and evaluated;
- commit themselves to a continuous process of learning from feedback;
- be willing to modify their theories of change and the associated investments in the light of what is observed during the life of an initiative.

If these requirements are satisfied, and if politicians and other stake-holders can restrain their impatience, we believe that positive learning can be generated from complex community-based health promotion initi-atives. Practical learning about social problems such as avoidable inequal-ities in health is not only complex in scientific terms but takes time. The pressure of the electoral clock and the demands for instant measures of success may undermine a community's capacity to deliver social change more than any shortage of human and financial resources.

We hope that a wider understanding of theory-based approaches to improving the design, implementation and evaluation of complex community-based initiatives may do something to redress the balance. It is important that they should.

References

Adams, C., Bauld, L. and Judge, K. (2000) 'Baccy to front: smoking cessation in health action zones', *Health Services Journal*, 110: 28–31.

Aspen Institute (1997) *Voices from the Field: Learning from the Early Work of Comprehensive Community Initiatives*, Washington, DC: Aspen Institute.

Chen, H. (1990) *Theory-driven Evaluation*, Thousand Oaks, CA: Sage.

Connell, J.P. and Kubisch, A.C. (1998) 'Applying a theory of change approach to the evaluation of comprehensive community initiatives: progress, prospects, and problems', in K. Fulbright-Anderson, A.C. Kubisch and J.P. Connell (eds) *New Approaches to Evaluating Community Initiatives*, Vol. 2: *Theory, Measurement, and Analysis*, Washington, DC: Aspen Institute.

Connell, J.P., Kubisch, A.C., Schorr, L.B. and Weiss, C.H. (1995) *New Approaches to Evaluating Community Initiatives: Concepts, Methods & Contexts*, Washington, DC: Aspen Institute.

Fulbright-Anderson, K., Kubisch, A.C. and Connell, J.P. (1998) *New Approaches to Evaluating Community Initiatives*, Vol. 2: *Theory, Measurement, and Analysis*, Washington, DC: Aspen Institute.

Funnel, S. (1997) 'Program logic: an adaptable tool for designing and evaluation programs', *Evaluation News and Comment*, July: 5–17.

Gillies, P. (1999) *Evidence Base 2000: Evidence into Practice*, London: Health Edu-cation Authority.

Green, J. and Tones, K. (1999) 'Towards a secure evidence-base for health promo-tion', *Journal of Public Health Medicine*, 21: 133–9.

Jacobs, B. (1999) 'Partnerships in Pittsburgh: the evaluation of complex local initi-atives', in S. Osbourne (ed.) *Managing Public-Private Partnerships for Public Services: An International Perspective*, London: Routledge.

Judge, K. (2000) 'Testing the limits of evaluation: Health Action Zones in England', *Journal of Health Services Research and Policy*, 5: 1.

Judge, K., Barnes, M., Bauld, L., Benzeval, M., Killoran, A., Robinson, R. and Wigglesworth, R. (1999) *Health Action Zones: Learning to Make a Difference*, PSSRU Discussion Paper 1546, Canterbury: University of Kent at Canterbury.

Raw, M., McNeill, A. and West, R. (1998) 'Smoking cessation guidelines for health professionals: a guide to effective smoking cessation interventions for the health care system', *Thorax*, 53 (Suppl. 5): S1–S9.

Speller, V., Learmouth, A. and Harrison, D. (1997) 'The search for evidence of effective health promotion', *British Medical Journal*, 315: 361–3.

Weiss, C. (1997a) 'How can theory-based evaluation make greater headway?', *Evaluation Review*, 21: 501–8.

Weiss, C. (1997b) 'Theory-based evaluation: past, present and future', *New Directions for Evaluation*, 76: 41–55.

Wholey, J.S. (1983) *Evaluation and Effective Public Management*, Boston, MA: Little, Brown.

A complete, unedited version of this article can be found as Judge, K. and Bauld, L., 'Strong theory, flexible methods: evaluating complex community-based initiatives' in *Critical Public Health* (2001) Volume 11, pages 19–38.

Chapter 29

Working together: lessons for collaboration between health and social services

Ray Higgins, Christine Oldman and David J. Hunter

Abstract

The recent community care reforms have placed a high premium on inter-agency collaboration between health and social care agencies to ensure the deliver of high quality services to users. This paper provides a review of the historical record and then illustrates contemporary inter-agency issues through an analysis of a local experiment in joint service delivery. The difficulties encountered by the key actors were a mix of cultural, professional and organisational factors.

Introduction

A principal aim of the recent reform of British community care arrangements as stated in the White Paper, *Caring for People: Community Care in the Next Decade and Beyond* (Department of Health 1989), was the emphasis on inter-agency working. This was identified as a prerequisite for the delivery of responsive and user-led services, particularly with respect to care management.

This paper begins by reviewing the principal issues in collaboration between the health service and local authority social services. These issues are then illustrated by an analysis of a joint venture between the health service and social services in Leeds. This analysis draws on an evaluation carried out over an 18-month period (November 1991–April 1993) of the Rothwell Community Care Project (RCCP) (Higgins *et al.* 1993). The evaluation consisted of: (1) interviews with 46 individuals who were associated with the project, either individually or with professional groups; (2) an analysis of all available documentation; (3) attendance at key project meetings; (4) a validation exercise of interim findings; and (5) a feedback session with health and social services staff working in Rothwell.

Source: *Health and Social Care*, 2, 1994, 269–77.

A review of inter-agency collaboration

A seamless service

Inter-agency collaboration has long been a theme in community care policies (Department of Health and Social Security 1972, 1976, 1977). The need for a seamless service was given fresh impetus at the end of the 1980s (Audit Commission 1986; Griffiths 1988; Department of Health 1989), and subsequent policy guidance reiterated the importance of joint operations.

Numerous research studies, official reports and inquiries have concluded that effective collaboration remains largely an elusive goal (Audit Commission 1986; National Audit Office 1987; Hunter and Wistow 1987, 1991; Griffiths 1988). Hunter and Wistow (1991) have argued that:

> 'A distinction needs to be made between at least three levels of joint activity: (1) joint planning, (2) joint management and (3) joint working or joint service delivery. Concerning the first of these, there is evidence that health and local authority planning was more "joint" by the second half of the 1980s, than a decade earlier.'
>
> (Wistow 1988)

The idea of joint management is less firmly established than joint planning, but appears to be increasing its scope. At this second level of joint activity some degree of integration of structures is implied.

The third level of joint activity, joint working or joint service delivery, is still relatively rare (Dalley 1989). Various studies have found difficulties such as boundary problems between professionals, services and agencies; service overlap and duplication; separatism giving rise to gaps in services; and discontinuities in service (Brown and Wistow 1990; Hunter and Wistow 1991; Higgins and Young 1992; Richardson and Higgins 1992).

Factors facilitating inter-agency collaboration

Improved co-ordination between agencies is often perceived as the cure to the difficulties associated with joint activity. A number of successful inter-agency projects have been undertaken in the last decade. Their success was attributed to developing structures which improved inter-agency co-operation and co-ordination, and which facilitated the provision of services that were flexible and responsive to the needs of users. Hardy *et al.* (1992) have identified the types of organisational structures that will improve inter-agency co-ordination: (1) a single organisational framework (Hunter and Wistow 1991), (2) a dedicated project leader (Friend *et al.* 1984), (3) decentralised resources (Knapp *et al.* 1992), and (4) a common budget (Higgins and Young 1992).

The Rothwell Community Care Project (RCCP): a local experiment in inter-agency collaboration

The project included all client groups (Oldham *et al.* 1989). It was proposed that the totality of secondary health and social care services in Rothwell, including services to children and families, should be delivered by a joint management structure.

The intention was for health and social care services to be brought together under single management, operating from a common base, together with a health and social services joint budget and managed by a specially created joint post, the Rothwell Community Care Manager. The project was established for an initial period of three years (April 1990–March 1993).

Two multi-agency and multi-disciplinary locality teams were to be established and managed by the Community Care Manager. Each team would comprise: a team leader, home care staff, social workers, social welfare officers, district nurses, health visitors and school nurses. One team would be headed by a principal social worker and the other by a clinical nurse team leader.

The overall management of the project was to be undertaken by a Strategic Group. It comprised senior managers from health and social services and representatives from other interested parties, such as the Community Health Council, the Family Health Services Authority and local general practitioners (GPs). A local carer was also a member of the group.

A Local Management Group was established to discuss issues that arose between Strategic Group meetings. Its membership comprised the group manager for neighbourhood teams (social services), the neighbourhood team manager responsible for child care work (social services), the locality manager (health), a local GP, the two team leaders, the Community Care Manager and a carer representative.

Working together in Rothwell

The benefits

As a result of participating in the project it was said that everyone knew each other better; staff understood the scope of each others' roles and how these contributed to a holistic approach to care. It also helped to identify potential overlap between different roles.

The improved level of inter-professional communication had a beneficial impact on service delivery. Home care team leaders, for example, went directly to a district nurse, instead of referring up to their manager.

As a result of this greater understanding about inter-agency working a number of service developments were initiated in Rothwell. These included the following:

1 An **evening home care service**.
2 A **joint duty system** was developed. Its aim was to achieve a holistic approach to an individual's needs.
3 The use of **joint care plans** was established, to provide a more co-ordinated approach to service delivery.
4 A **Case Referral Panel** was initiated to devise alternatives for individuals at risk of entering residential care. The panel was an inter-agency and multi-disciplinary forum in which representatives from residential care and day care services participated.
5 An important aspect of the RCCP vision was the emphasis on **user and community involvement** in its operation. To this end an Open Forum was established and held at regular intervals, a carers' group and a users' group were active, and a local carer joined both the Strategic Group and the Local Management Group.
6 A number of **community development** ventures were initiated. For example, a task group developed a community involvement strategy with residents of a local housing estate.

The difficulties

Despite the benefits of joint activity, health and social services staff did encounter difficulties in working together.

Developing a single organisational framework

The original architects of the RCCP wanted to create a workable organisational framework to facilitate joint working. Cultural and professional differences were the main obstacles to achieving this aim.

There are clear *cultural* differences and different modes of operation between the health service and local authority social services. For instance, a major difference is the presence of elected representatives in local authorities who are periodically held to account at the ballot box. Moreover, there is not one health service culture or one social services culture, but several. In Rothwell, district nurses and health visitors appeared to have different approaches. Within social services there were differences between the roles of social worker, social welfare officer and home carer.

The notion of *professionalism* caused problems for successful joint working between health and social services staff.

Some health service staff perceived social services staff as undisciplined, heavily influenced by union practices and more committed than themselves to a nine-to-five working day. They also believed large numbers of social services staff were untrained and were not, therefore, professionals.

A number of health service staff were also critical of others' approach to assessment. Some community nurses believed that assessment was informed by theory, such as that underpinning the nursing process. Such knowledge was only acquired after years of professional training. There were further differences in the approaches used in service delivery. It was suggested that district nurses were trained to encourage people to be independent. In contrast, home care staff were trained to make people comfortable.

Social services staff had their own views of health service colleagues. They believed that, in some respects, health service colleagues' jobs were easier than their own. They operated within a medical model and their work was more tangible: dealing with peoples' physical illnesses. Social service staff, in contrast, were often looking for underlying social and/or mental health problems, which was perceived as being a more difficult and intangible task. Social services staff argued that they had a more open-ended commitment to people.

A dedicated project leader

The original project architects felt that for joint working to be a success a more formalised and jointly managed approach was required. The core of this joint approach was the Community Care Manager role, together with that of team leader.

For this arrangement to work it required agencies to have confidence to let go of some of their individual powers. This was referred to by some project participants as the *transferability of management* between agencies. This would allow the joint manager to have overall responsibility and accountability for resources, staff management and project development. It would also allow the team leaders to both manage and facilitate joint team working. This clarity was seen as essential to avoid confusion about roles and purposes.

The issue of transferable management skills proved difficult to achieve in practice, particularly in relation to the Community Care Manager. From the health service perspective, it was argued that someone with the background of an occupational therapist could not provide the necessary management for a team leader with a health visiting background. In the event management supervision was provided by a senior manager from the health service.

On the social services side, because the Community Care Manager was not a qualified social worker he could not manage child protection work. Thus, the social services team leader received additional management support from a senior social services manager who had special responsibility for child care work.

A further difficulty encountered by the Community Care Manager was concerned with the *management of change* within an unstable organisational context (Barrett and Fudge 1981; Ham and Hill 1993; Harrison

1994). The detrimental effect of personnel changes on the project's progress was significant. This resulted in a weakening of senior management support and commitment as they were replaced by others who needed time to internalise the project's aims and objectives, and who may not have given it the same priority.

Decentralised resources and a common budget

It was never envisaged that additional resources would be made available to the project, apart from the Community Care Manager's salary for the three-year period. The intention was that health and social services monies should be combined in a common, devolved and localised budget to aid the flexible deployment of services. It was also envisaged that there should be a single base to provide a single point of access for service users.

There was an acceptance, by the project planners, that the creation of a joint budget and a single point of access would not be easy, but was essential to the project's aims. The project architects had also compiled an inventory of local, voluntary, private and statutory resources. There were many resources, but they were not efficiently used. The original planners felt that they required the ability to vire between different agency budgets.

Little progress was made in developing a joint budget or viring between budget heads. The objective of a single operating base proved to be unattainable. It was suggested that the political and organisational obstacles were too great.

Conclusions: lessons for joint working

The Rothwell vision was to develop appropriate structures for effective joint working between health service and social services staff. This was to be achieved by building on the success of earlier experiments in joint working. Thus, health and social care services were to be brought together under single management, operating from a common base and with a joint health and social services budget managed by the Community Care Manager. Much of this original vision remained unrealised, although as discussed above, there were a number of important achievements and benefits.

The RCCP failed to achieve its original vision, the delivery of a seamless service, because it was unable to put into place and/or sustain the necessary conditions for successful joint working.

The paper has indicated the importance of certain structural factors that can help to facilitate successful inter-agency working. The evaluation of the RCCP has also shown that cultural and professional factors are equally important if success in collaborative ventures is to be achieved.

The principal lessons derived from the RCCP experience are outlined below.

1 There is a need for a **balanced** approach between inter-agency **training and education** and **undertaking joint work**, to sustain staff commitment and enthusiasm.

2 There is a need for clarity in **aims and objectives**, which need to be realistic and robust in order to withstand organisational and personnel changes. They also need to be capable of delivering a management of change agenda.

3 There is a need to clarify **joint management arrangements** so that they address the transferability of management issue.

4 There is a need to clarify **resource availability** at the outset.

References

Audit Commission (1986) *Making a Reality of Community Care*, London: HMSO.

Barrett, S. and Fudge, C. (1981) *Policy and Action*, London: Methuen.

Brown, S. and Wistow, C. (1990) *The Roles and Tasks of Community Mental Handicap Teams*, Aldershot: Avebury.

Dalley, C. (1989) *Ideologies of Caring: Rethinking Community and Collectivism*, London: Macmillan.

Department of Health (1989) *Caring for People: Community Care in the Next Decade and Beyond*, Cm 849, London: HMSO.

Department of Health and Social Security (1972) *Management Arrangements for the Re-organised National Health Service*, London: HMSO.

Department of Health and Social Security (1976) *Joint Care Planning: Health and Local Authorities*, Circular HC(76)18/LAC(76)6, London: DHSS.

Department of Health and Social Security (1977) *Joint Care Planning: Health and Local Authorities*, Circular HC(77)17/LAC(77)10, London: DHSS.

Friend, J.K., Power, J.M. and Yewlett, C.J.L. (1974) *Public Planning: The Inter-corporate Dimension*, London: Tavistock.

Griffiths, R. (1988) *Community Care: Agenda for Action*, London: HMSO.

Ham, C. and Hill, M. (1993) *The Policy Process in the Modern Capitalist State*, 2nd edn, Hemel Hempstead: Harvester Wheatsheaf.

Hardy, B., Turrell, A. and Wistow, C. (1992) *Innovations in Community Care Management: Minimising Vulnerability*, Aldershot: Avebury.

Harrison, S. (1994) *National Health Service Management in the 1980s: Policy Making on the Hoof?*, Aldershot: Avebury.

Higgins, R. and Young, E. (1992) *Evaluation of the Development Manager Role within the Derby Elderly People's Integrated Care System (EPICS)*, Project Paper 1, Leeds: Nuffield Institute for Health.

Higgins, R., Oldman, C. and Hunter, D.J. (1993) *'Let's Work Together!': Lessons for Collaboration Between Health and Social Services*, Working Paper 7, Leeds: Nuffield Institute for Health.

Hunter, D.J. and Wistow, C. (1987) *Community Care in Britain: Variations on a Theme*, London: King's Fund Centre.

Hunter, D.J. and Wistow, G. (1991) *Elderly People's Integrated Care System (EPICS): An Organisational, Policy and Practice Review*, Leeds: Nuffield Institute for Health.

Knapp, M., Cambridge, P., Thomason, C., Beecham, J., Allen, C. and Darton, R. (1992) *Care in the Community: Challenge and Demonstration*, Aldershot: Ashgate.

National Audit Office (1987) *Community Care Developments: Report to the Comptroller and Auditor General*, London: HMSO.

Oldham, J., Jordan, D. and Philokyprou, J. (1989) 'Ahead on paper', *Insight* 20 November: 24–5.

Richardson, A. and Higgins, R. (1992) *The Limits of Case Management: Lessons from the Wakefield Case Management Project*, Working Paper 5, Leeds: Nuffield Institute for Health.

Wistow, G. (1988) 'Health and local authority collaboration: lessons and prospects', in G. Wistow and T. Brooks (eds) *Joint Planning and Joint Management*, London: Royal Institute of Public Administration.

A complete, unedited version of this article can be found as Higgins, R., Oldman, C. and Hunter, D.J., 'Working together: lessons for collaboration between health and social services' in *Health and Social Care*, Volume 2, pages 269–77.

Chapter 30

Size, composition and function of hospital boards of directors: a study of organisation environment linkage

Jeffrey Pfeffer

Abstract

In a study of 57 US hospitals in a large mid-western state, the determinants of size, composition and function of boards of directors were examined. The function of boards was partly explained by the organisational context, and particularly the ownership and source of funds. The size of boards was related to the requirements for successful linkage with the environment and with the function of the board. The composition of boards was related to the social context in which the organisation was embedded, and to their function. Board function and composition had an impact on the hospital's ability to obtain community support and on organisational effectiveness.

Introduction

There are two issues raised when hospital boards of directors are considered as linkages between the organisation and its environment. First, there is the issue of the different functions that boards may perform. Second, there are the different forms and methods of linkage between organisations and their environments. Previous studies have emphasised the role of the board as a link between the organisation and its environment. Zald (1969) noted that the board might also have an executive or administrative function. He hypothesised that the conditions of board power in organisational administration were affected by the external detachable resources that board members possessed, by virtue of personal characteristics, and the strategic contingency situations that the organisation confronted. The board of directors, then, may function in a capacity of either linkage or administration.

Source: *Administrative Science Quarterly*, 18.3, 1973, 349–64.

However, there are other mechanisms besides boards of directors that can be utilised to link organisations to their environments. In a study examining hospital–community relations in Mississippi, Saunders (1960) attempted to correlate the characteristics of the hospital administrator with the success of the organisation's linkage with its environment. Litwak and Meyer (1966) developed a model of co-ordination between bureaucratic organisations and primary groups. Their eight mechanisms of co-ordination are also possibly useful between bureaucratic organisations.

It is the purpose of this study to examine the board of directors as a means of obtaining support from the environment, the functions of the board, and the relationships between organisational context and the function, size and composition of the board.

Background

Four main types account for most hospitals in the USA: hospitals funded and operated by governmental units, either city, state, hospital district, federal, or some combination of these; hospitals operated for profit, such as those of the Hospital Corporation of America; hospitals owned and operated by religious denominations; and private, non-profit hospitals without religious affiliation. Hospitals also differ according to the source of their capital and operating funds. Capital expenditures can be funded by bond issues, private donations, foundations, state or federal funds, or through a surplus earned from operations. Operating funds can be derived from private donations, payments made by patients, payment by private insurers and funds from the government, either in the form of direct operating payments, or indirectly through public assistance or Medicare.

The problems of obtaining support and resources, and therefore the function of the board, will differ with both ownership and sources of funding. Members of hospital boards can provide knowledge of hospital administration and engage in directly advising and assisting in the management of the organisation. The board members may be members of the owning or governing organisation, as with government employees serving on the boards of government hospitals, nuns on the boards of Catholic hospitals, and so forth. Board members also may link the organisation to important segments of its environment. They may have contacts in business and financial circles useful for raising money, or political contacts which may be useful to a hospital relying on public funds for either operations or capital expenditures. Finally, they may be selected to represent various consumer, constituent or other interested groups within the community.

This paper tests four main arguments. First, it is argued that the function of the board of directors is related to the context of the organisation. Second, it is argued that the size and composition of the board is related to the environment, as well as to the function that the board is expected to serve. Third, it is hypothesised that the relations of the hospital with the local community will be influenced by the type of hospital, the function of the board, and how well the board links the organisation to its environment. Finally, it is argued that the ability of the hospital to attract resources is a function of its relations with the local community, and of the function, size and composition of its board.

Results

These arguments were tested with data collected from 57 hospitals in a large mid-western state. Data were collected using a questionnaire filled out by the chief administrator of each hospital. Of 100 hospitals initially randomly sampled from the American Hospital Association Directory, 57 co-operated in the study. Only short-term, general care hospitals were initially sampled, so the final sample consisted of no nursing homes, mental illness, or other single illness facilities. Hospitals affiliated with universities were also excluded. The group of co-operating hospitals covered the state geographically.

Data collected included the size of the hospital in terms of profit or loss, the sources of funds for both operations and capital expenditure, the size of the board and organisational and occupational interests of members, attendance at board meetings, and the administrator's opinion of the most important function of the board and the qualifications that should be used in selecting board members. Data on the occupational composition of the counties in which the hospitals were located were obtained from 1970 census data provided by the state department of finance. Data on the size of the hospital and facilities were obtained for both 1970 and 1965, and projections were obtained for five years into the future. Some general characteristics of the hospitals included in the sample are presented in Table 30.1. In terms of characteristics such as size, ownership and facilities, the hospitals co-operating in the study were not different from those in the set originally sampled.

Table 30.1 Characteristics of 57 hospitals in the sample

Type of hospital	(%)	Operating results in 1970	(%)
Government	21.1	Incurred a large deficit	12.30
Religious	28.1	Incurred a small deficit	26.30
Other private, non-profit	47.4	Broke even	7.00
Operated for profit	3.5	Ran a small surplus	47.40
		Ran a large surplus	7.00
Median number of beds		123	
Median annual operating budget		$2.95 million	
Median number of directors on hospital board		9.375	

Functions of the board of directors

The chief administrator of each hospital was asked to rank from 1 to 4 in order of importance, four possible functions of the board of directors, and from 1 to 5, criteria by which board members should be selected. In both cases, the rankings proceed from 1 for the most important.

Table 30.2 indicates that private hospitals, which were larger and relied more heavily on private donations, tended to place more importance on the fundraising function of the board, while the reverse was true for hospitals with religious affiliations and hospitals that received larger proportions of their resources from the federal government. This table also presents the relationships between organisational context and the function of the board in administration. As expected, the less the hospital relied on private donations, the more it relied on the government for its resources, and the more influence the government had on decisions, the more administration was important as a board function, as was knowledge of hospital administration in selecting members of the board.

Predictions concerning the importance of influence in the community as a criterion for selecting board members were also supported (Table 30.3). Influence in the community is more important for larger hospitals and for those in which decisions are more influenced by the local business community, and less important for government hospitals and to the extent that a larger proportion of the operating revenues are received from the government.

The importance of selecting board members for regional or subgroup representation was positively related to the hospital having a religious affiliation and to the proportion of the capital budget obtained from foundations. The importance of regional or subgroup representation was negatively related to the proportion of the capital budget obtained from the federal government and to being a private, non-profit hospital without religious affiliation.

The criterion of selecting board members for their political connections also tended to follow the hypothesised pattern of relationships with variables of the organisation's context. As expected, this was positively related to the reported influence of political organisations on hospital decisions ($r = 0.18$, $P < 0.10$); positively related to the proportion of operating funds obtained from the government ($r = -0.50$, $P < 0.001$); and negatively related to the proportion of funds obtained from insurance payments ($r = 0.47$, $P < 0.001$). Hospitals operating with relatively more government money, and consequently more influenced by governmental organisations, tended to place more importance on selecting board members for their political connections.

Table 30.2 Correlations of importance of board member characteristics and selection with other variables

	Variable	Importance of fundraising as a function of the board	Importance of selecting board members for their ability to raise money
Correlations of the importance of fundraising and recruiting of board members for their ability to raise money and other variables	Size of budget	−0.21*	−0.21*
	Proportion of capital budget from private donations	−0.37**	−0.33**
	Proportion of capital budget from the federal government	0.12	0.06
	Religious classifications	0.29**	0.33**
	Private, non-profit classification	−0.26**	−0.31**

	Variable	Importance of administration as a function of the board	Importance of selecting board members for their knowledge of hospital administration
Correlations of the importance of administration and recruiting of board members for their knowledge of hospital administration and other variables	Proportion of the capital budget from private donations	0.35**	0.17
	Proportion of the capital budget from the federal government	−0.42***	−0.30**
	Influence of the federal government on decisions	0.28**	−0.06
	Size of budget	0.12	0.23*
	Religious hospital classification	−0.21*	−0.12
	Private, non-profit hospital classification	0.27**	0.19*

continued

Table 30.2 continued

	Variable	Correlation	Level of significance
Correlations of the importance of selecting board members for their influence in the community with other variables	Number of beds in hospital	−0.19	0.1
	Proportion of operating budget obtained from the government	0.39	0.005
	Proportion of operating budget obtained from insurance companies	−0.31	0.03
	Influence of local businessmen on decisions	0.21	0.1
	Classification as government hospital	0.21	0.1
	Private, non-profit classification	−0.18	0.1
Correlations of the importance of selecting board members for their regional or subgroup representation with other variables	Classification as religious hospital	0.4	0.01
	Proportion of the capital budget obtained from the federal government	−0.29	0.05
	Proportion of the capital budget obtained from foundations	0.15	Not significant
	Classification as private, non-profit hospital	−0.19	0.1

* $P < 0.10$.
** $P < 0.05$.
*** $P < 0.01$.

Board size and composition

The size of the hospital boards tended to be larger, the larger the hospital budget, the larger the proportion of funds obtained from private donations, and the more important influence in the community and fundraising were as criteria for selecting board members (Table 30.3). Also, the board was smaller, the larger the proportion of funds obtained from the federal government, and the more important hospital administration was as a board function. In general, the data support the argument that the more the hospital requires linkage to the local environment for fundraising and support, the larger the board. The less that linkage is needed, and the more hospital management is emphasised as a board function, the smaller is the board.

The proportion of hospital directors from agricultural organisations was positively related to the proportion of farm owners in the county population ($r = 0.48$, $P<0.001$ and the proportion of persons employed on a farm ($r = 0.56$, $P<0.001$); and negatively related to the proportion of persons employed in manufacturing ($r = -0.28$, $P<0.05$). Although the proportion of board members from manufacturing organisations was not significantly related to the proportion of persons employed in manufacturing, it was negatively related to the proportion of persons employed on farms ($r = -0.36$, $P<0.01$). Furthermore, the proportion of board members from manufacturing organisations was positively, although not significantly, related to the importance of fundraising as a board function ($r = -0.11$, $P<0.25$), and to the importance of selecting board members for their influence in the community ($r = -0.32$, $P<0.05$).

Table 30.3 Correlations of number of directors with other variables

Variable	Correlation	Level of significance
Size of budget	0.59	0.001
Proportion of capital budget obtained from federal government	−0.16	Not significant
Proportion of capital budget obtained from private donations	0.17	Not significant
Importance of the function of fundraising for the board	−0.46	0.001
Importance of administration as a board function	0.36	0.01
Importance of selecting board members for their knowledge of hospital administration	0.36	0.01
Importance of selecting board members for their ability to raise money	−0.28	0.05
Importance of selecting board members for their influence in the community	−0.22	0.1
Classification as government hospital	−0.34	0.01
Classification as private, non-profit hospital	0.39	0.005

The proportion of directors from financial organisations was not correlated with the percentage of persons employed in finance, but was directly correlated with the size of the budget of the hospital ($r = 0.29$, $P < 0.05$), the proportion of the capital budget obtained from private donations ($r = 0.43$, $P < 0.01$), and inversely related to the importance of choosing board members for regional or subgroup representation ($r = 0.30$, $P < 0.05$). These results, plus those for board members from manufacturing organisations, indicate that the selection of the board is only partly based on considerations of relative supply of various types of person. There is evidence that board members are also chosen according to the function they are expected to serve.

Local support

Two measures of local support of the hospital were employed. As expected, the number of volunteers was positively related to private, non-profit classification and to size of hospital: volunteer support was greater for private hospitals and less for government hospitals. This number was positively correlated with total number of board members, the proportion of revenues obtained from private insurance firms, and negatively related to the proportion of operating and capital budgets obtained from government (Table 30.4). Finally, the number of volunteers was negatively related to the extent to which the composition of the board (with respect to financial and agricultural representatives) deviated from the expected proportion.

The second measure of community support was the chief administrator's perception of the quality of the hospital's relationships with various

Table 30.4 Correlations of number of volunteers working at the hospital with other variables

Variable	Correlation	Level of significance
Number of beds	0.45	0.01
Number of directors	0.42	0.01
Proportion of operating funds obtained from the government	−0.4	0.05
Proportion of operating funds obtained from private insurers	0.48	0.005
Proportion of capital budget obtained from the federal government	−0.23	0.1
Private, non-profit classification	0.15	Not significant
Deviation in proportion of finance directors from predicted value	−0.21	0.1
Deviation in proportion of agricultural directors from predicted value	−0.25	0.1

sectors of the environment, such as the business community. The scale for this question ranged from 1 for very good to 5 for very poor. Business relations were better the higher the proportion of finance directors on the board ($r = -0.20$, $P<0.10$) and the more important the criterion of selecting directors for influence in the community ($r = 0.21$, $P<0.10$). Relations with the business community were poorer to the extent that directors were chosen for regional or subgroup representation ($r = -0.18$, $P<0.10$), and for hospitals with religious affiliations ($r = 0.43$, $P<0.01$). They were relatively better for private, non-profit hospitals without religious affiliation ($r = -0.39$, $P<0.01$). Thus, local support is related to characteristics of the organisation's board and the purpose for which it is used, as well as to the ownership characteristics of the hospital.

Organisational effectiveness and the board of directors

Effectiveness was measured by three indices of institutional growth: the number of medical care programmes, pieces of equipment and services the hospital had added in the preceding five years; the percentage increase in the number of beds in the hospital over the preceding five years; and the percentage increase in the budget of the hospital from 1965 to 1970. These measures appear to be reasonable approximations for the ability of the organisation to obtain resources from the environment.

The number of additions in facilities or programmes in the preceding five years was negatively related to the extent to which the function of the board was primarily administrative ($r = 0.27$, $P<0.05$) and was positively related to the extent that board members were chosen for their political connections ($r = -0.24$, $P<0.10$). The number of additions was positively related to the proportion of members who came from financial organisations ($r = 0.29$, $P<0.05$). The correlation of the number of additions with deviations from the expected proportion of members from manufacturing organisations was $r = -0.28$ ($P<0.05$), and with the deviation from the expected proportion of members from agricultural organisations, $r = -0.17$ ($P<0.15$). Of the five variables significantly associated with the addition of new facilities or programmes, all were related to the composition or function of the board of directors.

The percentage increase in the number of beds was positively related to the selection of board members for influence in the community ($r = -0.16$, $P<0.15$), and for their political connections ($r = -0.23$, $P<0.10$), and negatively related to selection of board members for their knowledge of hospital administration ($r = 0.38$, $P<0.01$). It was positively related to the administrator's rating of relations with the local business community ($r = -0.33$, $P<0.05$), and negatively to both the extent to which the board of directors deviated from the predicted size ($r = -0.20$, $P<0.10$) and to the predicted proportion of members from manufacturing organisations (r = −0.18, P < 0.10). Finally, it was positively related to the importance of liaison with the community as a board of director function (r = −0.31, P < 0.05).

A similar pattern was obtained with the percentage increase in size of budget. The budget increase tended to be larger, the more important was linkage as a function of the board (r = −0.30, P < 0.05), and the less important knowledge of hospital administration was as a criterion for selecting board members (r = 0.20, P < 0.10). Budget growth also tended to be larger if the deviations in board size (r = −0.26, P < 0.05) and the proportion of members from financial organisations (r = −0.22, P < 0.10) were smaller, and the budget tended to grow more for government hospitals (r = 0.37, P < 0.01). With the exception of government hospitals, all the significant associations with organisational budget growth were dimensions of board function and composition.

Discussion

Organisations, as open social systems, are inextricably bound up with the conditions of their environments. Organisations must obtain support, both in the form of resources and in social legitimacy, from their social context. In an examination of the organisation's relationships with other organisations and its environment, one potentially useful perspective is to examine the mechanisms through which organisations ensure continued support from their environments. The board of directors is one vehicle for co-opting important segments of the environment. In this study of the boards of 57 hospitals, it was found that the board tended to be utilised relatively more for fundraising in those settings where the local environment provided relatively more of the resource support, while administration and technical expertise were emphasised when the organisation was not as immediately and directly tied to the support of the local environment.

The size and composition of hospital boards of directors can be analysed from an ecological and co-optative perspective. The size of the board was seen to be related to the requirements for co-optation and to the function of the board. The composition of the board was determined partly by the socio-economic characteristics of the environment in which it operated, and again partly by the function it served. If the board is utilised for linkage, then it should be possible to explain variations in support, and in the capacity to acquire resources with dimensions of board structure and purpose. Boards selected for fundraising rather than administration, and boards that more closely fit their environment, tended to be associated with greater organisational effectiveness.

A number of implications can be derived from the data presented in this paper. Firstly, organisational requirements for support are partly determined by the patterns of resource inputs. An organisation is tied to the local environment only to the extent that its resources come from that environment (Levine and White 1961). In the present study, differences between types of hospitals with respect to linkages with their environments are consequences of the different contingencies that the organisations face in obtaining resources. The private, non-profit hospitals were the most closely linked to the local environment because they needed to be, drawing relatively more of their resource support from the local community. This finding has obvious implications for the design of organisations or systems of organisations that are responsive to external demands. Secondly, it is evident that environmental relationships are important to both organisational administrators and to organisation theorists. Variations in support and the ability to obtain resources can be partly explained by organisational attempts at linkage with the environment.

Selznick's (1949) statement that the organisation must come to terms with its environment has been found to furnish an analytical perspective that is useful in examining one form of organisational linkage mechanism, and in assessing the determinants of the organisation's ability to obtain support from its environment. There are, of course, many other organisational behaviours and organisational strategies for dealing with the environment that can also be examined with this perspective.

References

Levine, S. and White, P.E. (1961) 'Exchange as a conceptual framework for the study of interorganizational relationships', *Administrative Science Quarterly*, 5: 583–601.

Litwak, E. and Meyer, H.J. (1966) 'A balance theory of coordination between bureaucratic organizations and community primary groups', *Administrative Science Quarterly*, 11: 31–58.

Saunders, J.V.D. (1960) 'Characteristics of hospitals and of hospital administrators associated with hospital-community relations in Mississippi', *Rural Sociology*, 25: 229–32.

Selznick, P. (1949) *TVA and the Grass Roots*, Berkeley: University of California Press.

Zald, M.N. (1969) 'The power and function of boards of directors: a theoretical synthesis', *American Journal of Sociology*, 75: 97–111.

A complete, unedited version of this article can be found as Pfeffer, J., 'Size, composition, and function of hospital boards of directors: a study of organisation environment linkage' in *Administrative Science Quarterly*, Volume 18, Issue 3, 349–64.

Index

Note: page numbers in *italics* denote references to Figures/Tables.